Cases on Physician Cultural Responsibility, Ethics, and Biases

Christen Johnson
Boonshoft School of Medicine, Wright State University, USA

Michael John Robertson
Wright State University, USA

IGI Global
Scientific Publishing
Publishing Tomorrow's Research Today

Vice President of Editorial Melissa Wagner
Managing Editor of Acquisitions Mikaela Felty
Managing Editor of Book Development Jocelynn Hessler
Production Manager Mike Brehm
Cover Design Phillip Shickler

Published in the United States of America by
IGI Global Scientific Publishing
701 East Chocolate Avenue
Hershey, PA, 17033, USA
Tel: 717-533-8845
Fax: 717-533-8661
Website: https://www.igi-global.com E-mail: cust@igi-global.com

Library of Congress Cataloging-in-Publication Data

Names: Johnson, Christen, 1991- editor | Robertson, Michael, 1989- editor
Title: Cases on physician cultural responsibility, ethics, and biases / edited by Christen Johnson, Michael Robertson.
Description: Hershey, PA : IGI Global, [2025] | Includes bibliographical references and index. | Summary: "This publication will provide material for instructors teaching health equity to medical students and students of other health professions. Rather than focusing on identifying factors that contribute to health inequities, this publication strives to inspire a deeper application and reflection of the practices needed through the utilization of the Physician Cultural Responsibility framework"-- Provided by publisher.
Identifiers: LCCN 2024047669 (print) | LCCN 2024047670 (ebook) | ISBN 9798369336830 h/c | ISBN 9798337300917 s/c | ISBN 9798369336847 eISBN
Subjects: LCSH: Discrimination in medical care | Medical ethics | Social medicine
Classification: LCC RA563.M56 C373 2025 (print) | LCC RA563.M56 (ebook) | DDC 174.2--dc23/eng/20250214
LC record available at https://lccn.loc.gov/2024047669
LC ebook record available at https://lccn.loc.gov/2024047670
British Cataloguing in Publication Data
A Cataloguing in Publication record for this book is available from the British Library.

To following Divine purpose.

To Deedee for allowing your story to teach others.

To all of those whose stories live within us and remind us to aim higher and be better.

To those who will be healers and those who will be healed-

May this book perpetuate a culture of inclusive medical practice and health equity that touches patients for years to come.

Table of Contents

Detailed Table of Contents

Physician cultural responsibility incorporates best practices from cultural humility, anti-oppression, advocacy, intercultural communication, self-awareness, and self-reflection to foster improved experiences for patients of all backgrounds and the healthcare team. This chapter explores best practices to infuse the practice of physician cultural responsibility into clinical training while cultivating safe learning environments that encourage growth, exploration, and the development of both interpersonal and intrapersonal skills. A learning case displays the utility of the physician cultural responsibility framework in the process of caring for a patient.

Biases are untrue assumptions made without evidence. This can happen explicitly or when it is known to the person making the assumptions, as well as implicitly or when it is unknown. Biases impact interactions and relationships, including the physician-patient relationship. Physician biases can impact patients' health outcomes by influencing the options patients are given, the ways in which care is delivered, and interactions with the healthcare team. This chapter explores the social categorization of medicine or biases found within the field of medicine, their impact on patient care, and ways to overcome them.

Intersectionality recognizes how interdependent identities can be linked to multiple sources of oppression. This chapter will explore how health disparities are exacerbated by the broken health infrastructure using the concept of intersectionality as its foundation. Socioeconomic factors including frameworks of past and current discriminatory housing practices, ableism, ageism, and the Black maternal health crisis will be incorporated to highlight the impact of systemic oppression in the context of the community and built environment. Though the four cases presented have different scenarios, they each demonstrate how health disparities and discrimination require solutions in patient-centered care as well as advancements in systems, policy, and law to create more equitable outcomes.

Socioeconomic challenges have multi-faceted causes and implications upon healthcare. These challenges range from purely financial aspects, housing, education, and food availability to negative health outcomes. Socioeconomic status is sometimes falsely portrayed as a byproduct of one's internal work ethic. However, this viewpoint fails to account for historical and institutional factors that limit mobility between socioeconomic levels. In this chapter, two cases will explore the impact of health care expenditure, access to care, and socioeconomic status on patient outcomes through limitations in wealth accessibility, health care payer laws, and resource scarcity.

Race plays a large role in United States history. Because of that history, there has been a large impact of race on healthcare. Race has impacted how we diagnose and treat diseases and there are both overt and hidden ways that race is still ingrained in our healthcare system. Race has also impacted how patients may view the healthcare system and a long history of experimentation on vulnerable populations continues to impact trust in the healthcare system today. Cases include exploration of topics such as diagnosis of psychotic disorders, using race-based correction factors, broader implication of policy change, pain treatment in patients, intersectionality, the importance of informed consent, and the impact of experimentation on current healthcare and research.

Sexism has long been ingrained in medical institutions, impacting patient care, physician representation, and health disparities. This chapter explores the historical significance of barring women from medical education and professional practice, resulting in a male-dominated healthcare system that has impacted representation in medical research and practice, biases in patient care, and health outcomes. The current day ramifications are examined through two case studies highlighting the impacts on representation in medicine and patient health outcomes.

Gender and sexual orientation are significant aspects of personal identity. Likewise, gender-affirming care is a critical and evolving aspect of modern healthcare, centered on supporting transgender and non-binary (TGNB) individuals aligning their physical and emotional well-being with their gender identity. The chapter explores the principles, practices, and challenges associated with issues of sex, gender, and sexual orientation alongside gender-affirming care, highlighting its transformative potential in reducing health disparities and promoting equity. Key topics include shared definitions of sex, gender, and sexual orientation, current medical policies and practices in puberty suppression, hormone therapy, and surgical options, with a focus on ethical considerations, informed consent, and patient-centered care. The chapter also addresses barriers to accessing care, including systemic discrimination, provider bias, financial constraints, and emphasizes the role of multidisciplinary care teams in overcoming these challenges through the nuanced experiences of individuals.

The physician-patient relationship (PPR) is a critical element in medical ethics, built on mutual respect, trust, and knowledge. It ensures that physicians meet patient needs, including providing care and education on diagnoses and treatments while creating a working relationship that allows patients to be centered in their care. Intercultural communication is essential for understanding patient perspectives and building trust. However, physician burnout and biases can negatively affect care. This chapter highlights the importance of utilizing intercultural communication to strengthen the physician-patient relationship allowing for better care and health outcomes.

Oppression surrounding multiple areas of patient identity have been used to stigmatize patient needs and outcomes. This creates barriers to care and impacts health outcomes. This chapter will explore the stigmatization of diverse patients through the lens of pain management. Patients can often have complex pain concerns alongside intersectional stigma which impacts patient-centered care and collaborative decision-making. Equal pain management policies can help stigmatized populations eliminate inequities. Supporting patients with pain from underrepresented groups requires intersectional policy and practice, addressing sociocultural reasons of health disparities among these groups, and integrating an understanding of ethnicity, gender, sexual orientation, ability, age, and socioeconomic status into healthcare practice. By implementing these strategies and promoting patient engagement, individuals with chronic pain can receive the care, support, and validation that is needed to facilitate pain relief regardless of their identity.

Foreword

In the sacred space where medicine and humanity intersect, we find both our greatest challenges and our most profound opportunities for growth. The current increased national and international focus on the feelings of being aggrieved by large segments of our populations, truly underscores the need for cultural awareness to be foundational in eliminating health disparities and improving overall health outcomes for our nation and the world. The work you hold in your hands represents a critical turning point in how we conceptualize and teach cultural awareness in medicine—moving beyond mere competency checklists toward a deeper, more authentic commitment to seeing and honoring the full humanity of every patient.

For too long, medicine has operated under the illusion that clinical excellence alone could overcome health disparities. We've created frameworks and competencies, memorized cultural characteristics, and developed skills to navigate difference. Yet the disparities persist, the trust erodes, and the gap between who we aspire to be as healers and the reality of patient experiences continues to widen.

This text introduces Physician Cultural Responsibility as a revolutionary framework that challenges us to do the harder, deeper work. Rather than positioning physicians as cultural experts who must master knowledge about "others," it calls us to the humbling practice of acknowledging our limitations, examining our biases, and yielding power to our patients as the true experts of their own experiences.

What makes this approach so powerful is its honesty. It acknowledges that medicine has a problem—that bias, stigma, and oppression are woven into the very fabric of our education and practice. It doesn't shy away from uncomfortable truths about how intersecting systems of oppression based on race, class, gender, sexual orientation, and ability impact health outcomes. Instead, it invites us into the difficult but necessary work of untangling these influences from the art of medicine.

As you engage with the chapters ahead, you'll encounter not just theoretical frameworks but practical applications through carefully crafted case studies. You'll be challenged to move beyond surface-level observations to examine root causes. You'll practice the skills of intercultural communication and learn to elevate patient values and needs. Most importantly, you'll be invited to engage in both objective and subjective reflection—pushing yourself to those uncomfortable but fertile learning edges where genuine growth occurs.

The method presented here offers medical educators a structured approach to facilitate these complex discussions in the classroom, providing the scaffolding needed to transform abstract concepts into actionable practice. For practicing clinicians, these pages offer an opportunity to reconnect with the core values that likely drew you to medicine in the first place—the desire to heal, to connect, to serve with compassion and dignity.

Our patients deserve better than what our current systems provide. Health equity remains an aspiration rather than a reality for too many. But within these pages lies a roadmap for change—not through grand gestures or policy reforms alone, but through the daily practice of cultural responsibility embraced by individual physicians and healthcare teams.

The journey ahead is not an easy one. It requires vulnerability, humility, and a willingness to be uncomfortable. It asks us to question assumptions we may not even realize we hold. But it is precisely this journey that offers the greatest hope for transforming medicine into what it has always aspired to be: a healing art practiced with equal skill and compassion for all.

I invite you to approach this text not merely as an academic exercise but as a personal and professional calling—to see in these pages as not just information to be absorbed but an invitation to initiate transformation. Our patients, our profession, and our shared humanity deserve nothing less.

With hope for the journey ahead,

Warren A. Jones
University of Mississippi School of Medicine, USA (Emeritus)

Preface

Physician Cultural Responsibility offers an opportunity to impact health equity as well as benefit the those providing care to patients. But what is it? It's not a solitary fight against an -ism in medicine, whether that be race, sex, class, gender, age, ability or otherwise that must be targeted. It's a systemic battle against intersectional biases that are deeply ingrained within our practice, our teaching, and our plans. We cannot overcome health disparities or change healthcare for the better without facing the ugly truth that medicine has a problem. We have to do the painful work to untangle bias and stigma from the art of medicine in order to care for every patient as they deserve.

Physician Cultural Responsibility is the:

the physician's attitude of responsibility or ethical duty to patients, colleagues, and themselves to transcend personal biases and preconceived notions and uphold the dignity of all through acknowledging one's limitations, biases, knowledge gaps, and power differential, and committing to the ongoing work of improving one's cultural understanding, skillset, and practice to ensure empathetic, professional, and humanistic exchanges in all facets. (Johnson, 2023, p. 2)

It in essence strips away the lists and boxes to check, the need to be competent in any culture other than one's own, and replaces what is assumed with a posture of humility, inquiry and connection. The physician or health care worker yields their power to the patient, to learn about the patient's values and beliefs and to elevate the patient's needs in truly seeing the humanity within them first and the disease process second.

While this sounds like an easy task- it's not. It takes being able to identify the thoughts and assumptions that bridge the gap between who the patient seems to be and who the patient really is. When the health care team acts upon who they think they see, connection is lost to biases and stereotypes within those assumptions. In cultivating trust and relationships with patients, patients can lead those caring for them to the solutions that meet their needs for both their diagnosis and their social determinants of health. When all patient are able to live their healthiest life, regardless of their circumstances, we achieve health equity.

This text aims to assist in doing that work. Within this text, you will find an orientation to Physician Cultural Responsibility. After this orientation is a chapter outlining the basics of bias and oppression, followed by an explanation of the concept of intersectionality. The subsequent chapters cover a selected few of the major areas of oppression including Socioeconomic Status, Race, Sex, Gender, and Sexual Orientation. A discussion of intercultural communication follows this overview. The final chapter in this text discusses stigma and the ways that these topics can impact care for special populations including those with specific diagnoses, of specific ages, and with differing abilities.

The chapter on Physician Cultural Responsibility provides an outline of how to use this innovative framework within the classroom. It yields a better understanding of best practices as well as the implications of using Physician Cultural Responsibility in patient encounters. The cases in this chapter seek to display multiple areas of opportunity in patient care including identifying the impact of stereotypes, biases, and the social categorization of medicine, utilizing intercultural communication skills, and elevating patient values and needs.

From the implications for job opportunities and access to healthy foods to educational opportunities and child care availability, socioeconomic status impacts the social determinants of health, the root cause of health disparities. The chapter on socioeconomic status describes the multifaceted implications on health outcomes and health delivery as associated with socioeconomic status. Through examining the impacts of health care expenditures and complex situations that patients may face, learners will navigate bridging gaps the health gaps that socioeconomic status creates.

The current day implications of racism in medicine are evident in the perpetuation of racial heath disparities. From unethical research to race based pseudoscience, racism has been deeply ingrained in medical education and practice which has impacted patient trust and outcomes. An exploration of patient cases assists learners in identifying racial bias in patient care and its implications, overcoming those biases, and providing equitable care.

The chapter entitled Sex: Enduring Invisibility and Its Impact on Healthcare, focuses on the historical implications of the exclusion of women, both within the medical workforce and in healthcare. This chapter explores the biases and stereotypes that are common when caring for non-male patients. This chapter aims to bridge the gap between diverse representation and medicine and the alleviation of health disparities.

There is much confusion surrounding the concepts of sex, gender, and sexual orientation. The chapter Gender, and Sexual Orientation: Embracing the Intersectionality of Identity offers a dialogue about the nuances of sex, gender, and sexual orientation, providing an in-depth look at the intersectionality of gender and sexual orientation, as well as special topics in gender firming care. The cases assist in showcasing guidelines, best practices, and considerations for providing inclusive medical care for this population.

Supportive physician-patient relationships are built on communication. This chapter provides best practices for intercultural communication that assists in establishing rapport and cultivating relationships between patients and health care team members. The cases provided illustrate the impact of using intercultural communication.

Intersectionality: Where Identities Collide is an overview of the concept of intersectionality. This chapter dives into the multiplicative nature of oppression and the ways in which it complicates patient outcomes, perpetuating health disparities. This chapter considers multiple areas of identity, including race, sex, socioeconomic status, ability, and ageism.

The chapter on stigma considers its impact on patient outcomes in chronic pain management. The author examines the impact of stigma on identity and health disparities. Cases provide an intersectional view of patient needs and barriers.

Bias, whether implicit or explicit, has a destructive impact on physician-patient relationships and patient outcomes. Created by falsehoods, these assumptions involve all areas of identity. This chapter examines common biases noted within the social categorization of medicine and best practices to challenge these notions.

Each of these chapters has its own set of cases that further understanding, reflection, and application through the Physician Cultural Responsibility framework. The Physician Cultural Responsibility framework assists in encouraging both objective and subjective reflection that pushes students to the learning edges and assists in physician development (Johnson, 2023). The cases within this book were created with this framework. They aim to take learners past the surface level observations to examine root causes and identify implicit decision making, and later to integrate this thinking into everyday practice. These cases can be used within the classroom setting, to assist in demonstrating more immediately relevant examples, or even for training instructors.

It is our hope that this text not only provides the background knowledge and guidance to better facilitate this learning within medical education, but that it enriches classroom discussions, inspires questions biases about patients, and cultivates improved patient care and health outcomes.

Our patients deserve better, here is opportunity to inspire lasting change.

Christen D. Johnson
Boonshoft School of Medicine, Wright State University, USA

Michael John Robertson

Wright State University, USA

REFERENCES

Johnson, C. D. (2023). The MONROE Method: A Methodology on Navigating Race, Oppression, and Equity in Medical Education through Physician Cultural Responsibility. https://aura.antioch.edu/etds/979

Chapter 1
Physician Cultural Responsibility:
Teaching a New Way to Practice

Christen D. Johnson
https://orcid.org/0000-0001-8752-0030
Boonshoft School of Medicine, Wright State University, USA

EXECUTIVE SUMMARY

Physician cultural responsibility incorporates best practices from cultural humility, anti-oppression, advocacy, intercultural communication, self-awareness, and self-reflection to foster improved experiences for patients of all backgrounds and the healthcare team. This chapter explores best practices to infuse the practice of physician cultural responsibility into clinical training while cultivating safe learning environments that encourage growth, exploration, and the development of both interpersonal and intrapersonal skills. A learning case displays the utility of the physician cultural responsibility framework in the process of caring for a patient.

INTRODUCTION

Cultural humility is defined by the National Institutes of Health as, "a lifelong process of self-reflection and self-critique [that] does not require mastery of lists of 'different' or peculiar beliefs and behaviors supposedly pertaining to different cultures, rather it encourages [one] to develop a respectful attitude toward diverse points of view" (National Institutes of Health, 2007). The practice of cultural humility can assist in bridging the gap between cultural differences and medical knowledge in creating care plans as well as assisting in one's ability to relate to others with different cultural norms and values (Beavis et. al, 2015; Foronda et.

DOI: 10.4018/979-8-3693-3683-0.ch001

al, 2016; Hunter and Thompson, 2019; Johnson et. al., 2022; Masters et. al., 2019; Nazar et. al., 2015). Not only does this improve the climate of medicine, this is key in ensuring that the care physicians provide is both achievable and relevant to patients' healthcare needs and cultural values.

However, cultural humility alone is not enough to ensure that patients receive the care necessary to achieve their best health status. Curricula associated with social justice, racism, and physician advocacy have also been described as useful in the fight for health equity. Physician Cultural Responsibility incorporates best practices from cultural humility, anti-oppression, Advocacy, intercultural communication, self-awareness, and self-reflection in the classroom.

Defined as,

the physician's attitude of responsibility or ethical duty to patients, colleagues, and themselves to transcend personal biases and preconceived notions and uphold the dignity of all through acknowledging one's limitations, biases, knowledge gaps, and power differential, and committing to the ongoing work of improving one's cultural understanding, skillset, and practice to ensure empathetic, professional, and humanistic exchanges in all facets (Johnson, 2023, p. 2),

Physician Cultural Responsibility offers an opportunity to impact health equity as well as benefit the healthcare team. As patients are intersectional, understanding the many social factors that impact patients and their health outcomes is essential in providing relevant care (Masters et. al., 2019; Corneau and Stergiopoulos, 2012; Sharma et. al., 2018; Staats et. al., 2015). Likewise, understanding they ways in which society impacts patient outcomes and how healthcare workers can be a part of the solution can empower those providing care and lessen burnout rates (Johnson, 2023).

The social categorization of medicine (Blackie et. al., 2019), or biases ingrained within the medical profession, personal biases, and microaggressions, matched with lack of awareness creates a difficult space for learning about these topics. As the current political climate has polarized conversations about identity and disparities, learners and educators are likely to have some trepidation in these discussions. However, deepening one's understanding of the impact of socialization on the development of biases and stereotypes offers space for improved connection with those who are from different backgrounds, and for interactions with both patients and colleagues. Beginning this process within the classroom allows for an in-depth learning experience that can not only build trust and collegiality but improve experiences for patients in the future.

The Practice of Physician Cultural Responsibility

The practice of Physician Cultural Responsibility is a way of thinking and connecting rather than a list of characteristics and specific activities. This makes Physician Cultural Responsibility a multifaceted tool in patient care that can be useful for all interactions. This also assists in dispelling myths and stereotypes regardless of who they're about.

Often when discussing health disparities, the examples used highlight interactions between those who are from a privileged identity like a majority race, culture, or gender and those who are from other oppressed or disenfranchised identities. While this is a concern in many patient experiences, it ignores the stereotypes surrounding those from privileged identities. Just as someone from lower socioeconomic status or a different nationality may encounter biases that impact their health outcomes, so can those who are male or White. Further, medicine also fails if the we don't negate they stereotype that every White male patient who is heterosexual has no health risks, unlimited resources for care, and perfect health literacy. Thus the work of dismantling biases in medicine through Physician Cultural Responsibility serves all patients and should not be politicized or siloed to one area of identity.

Physician Cultural Responsibility demands opening one's mind and seeing every patient as not just an individual, but an intersectional being whose unique beliefs, values, social connections, lived experiences, and future goals will impact health outcomes. While their identity including factors like culture, race, gender, sex, ability, nationality and socioeconomic status will impact those unique traits, understanding how society's categorization of their identity can assist in overcoming the stereotypes and stigma the prevent one's intersectional being from being seen. One must be aware of current beliefs, values, and biases in order to change these patterns of thought. Clinicians must know what they actually know and what they assume, and thus how they see the world. Once there is awareness, one can begin the difficult work of questioning their own assumptions and biases, whether that be through the cognitive dissonance created from exposure to experiences that counter those assumptions and biases, or from classroom experiences that push learners to their learning edges, inspiring growth (King and Castenell, 2001). Reflection is a tool that is easily used to assist in bringing ideas to one's conscious awareness, grappling with alternate ideas and theories, and to identify goals and needs.

Keys to Changing Thought Through Awareness and Reflection

The Physician Cultural Responsibility Framework was created to infuse reflection into activities and discussions with the aim of supporting students in the process of learning and growing in the practice of Physician Cultural Responsibility. In the framework, guided reflection upon the 5 pillars or core values of Physician Cultural Responsibility (Table 1) assists in challenging biases students may have and ask them to dig deeper. Rather that expecting that students will have one answer or one pathway, students are free to examine what they believe to be true and how that may impact interactions with patients in certain scenarios.

Table 1. Physician Cultural Responsibility Framework (Johnson, 2023)

Core Value	Guided Reflection
Cultural Humility	Assessment assumptions of cultural differences and possible labels stemming from biases and stereotypes being utilized
Anti-Oppression	Examination of institutional and societal biases and factor that impact equity in circumstances, environments, and opportunities and thus health outcomes for patients of diverse identities
Advocacy	Analysis of possible interventions and opportunities that improve the access, experiences, and health outcomes that can be impacted by various factors
Intercultural Communication	Analysis of communication styles, word choice, language, and possible assumptions associated with identity, culture, and intersectionality including possible faux pas including microaggressions, tone-policing, gas-lighting, and inherent misinterpretations or misunderstandings
Self-Awareness and Self-Reflection	Awareness of the condition of the self at this time including emotional state, current biases, boundaries, and one's current level of burnout or investment Reflection upon the stimuli, situation, or challenge including areas of strength and opportunity for growth, future needs and interests, and interests in improvement or further development

Best Practices for Cultivating Physician Cultural Responsibility in the Classroom

Teaching this material can be difficult as many instructors do not receive formal training in this area. Considering classroom environment, preparing for content delivery and learner participation, and navigating difficult discussions are a necessity to create a safe learning environment for students to prepare for experiences within the exam room. While these tips are not an exhaustive list, they aim to guide instructors through some suggested best practices.

Classroom Environment

The classroom environment is one of the most important components of teaching Physician Cultural Responsibility. As this material is very sensitive, has been politicized, and can be very difficult for some students to identify with, creating space for a unified learning community is a necessity. Safe learning environments can encourage students to be more open to the uncomfortable, including new experiences and new points of view from classmates which can improve growth and learning (King and Castenell, 2001).

Creating a class code that allows all students to contribute what they need to feel safe within the learning environment can begin to cultivate a positive learning environment (Strasser & Spelocha, 2005). Likewise, encouraging unity through community-building activities and creating diverse, small, and stable groups for classroom discussions increases feelings of support and belonging which can increase classroom learning and participation (Inoue, 2020; Santas, 2000; Strasser & Spelocha, 2005). Leading students through peer evaluations can also assist in opening lines of communication between students. This can allow students to see themselves from another's perspective, contributing to personal growth (Ramani and colleagues, 2017 & Kondrat, 1999).

Preparing for Content Delivery and Learner Participation

Physician Cultural Responsibility spans courses including health equity and disparities, the social determinants of health, advocacy and policy (Boroumand et al., 2020; Coria et al., 2013; Coutinho et al., 2020). Courses teaching this type of material, especially those incorporating community involvement or assessment, should be longitudinal rather than singular sessions (Boroumand et al., 2020; Coria et al., 2013; Coutinho et al., 2020). This can improve the students' ability to reflect and grow with the material as all students will begin with a different foundation of previous learning.

Both learners and educators need the tools to be able to communicate their ideas and experiences effectively within the classroom. This can improve student participation. Being confident in using classroom vocabulary, like naming types of oppression and power structures when recognized can help students to better discuss their beliefs and feelings within the environment (King & Castenell, 2001) while respecting the needs of everyone around them. Introducing goals and objectives for all activities and shared definitions for all vocabulary can help students to conceptualize material that may be completely foreign to their experiences (Hassen and colleagues, 2021).

Likewise, planning classroom activities that incorporates highlighting diversity and inclusion through collaboration while yielding opportunities for individual experiences and intersectionality can improve student growth and the classroom environment. Focusing on intersectionality gives space for seeing each student and later, each patient, as an individual rather than focusing on stereotypical lists for different identities (Betancourt et al., 2003). When choosing activities or assignments, considering the diversity of learning styles and the many levels that learners may already have in foundational learning to ensure that everyone is on the same page.

Activities rooted in narrative medicine are a great example to allow students to hear other's perspectives (American Medical Association and American Association of Medical Colleges Center for Health Justice, 2021; DeVoss et al., 2002) and to identify their own beliefs and biases. Experiences that allow students to question their own beliefs and assumptions can help students process others experiences and focus on their own personal growth (Dobie, 2007; Kondrat, 1999). As such, small group interactions in intentionally diverse groups can assist students in practicing new skills and learning from each other (Briguglio, 2006; Chiper, 2013; DeVoss et al., 2002, Dimitrov et al., 2014; Eisenchlas & Trevaskes, 2007).

Navigating Difficult Discussions

These topics can inherently bring up uncomfortable emotions that learners may try to avoid. For example, those who identify with identities that have privilege can struggle with guilt, fear, or shame that can prevent them from engaging in learning opportunities (Denevi & Paston, 2006; Pieterse et al., 2016) or fight the cognitive dissonance by denying these systems exist at all. Instructors can break through some of the resistance by sharing their own experiences (Brookfield & Hess, 2021). Likewise, learners should be encouraged to work through this discomfort and engage with new ideas (Brookfield & Hess, 2021).

Activities that encourage nonjudgemental communication and inquiry like sharing personal experiences and creating space to identify areas of opportunity within topics (Strasser and Spelocha, 2005) can assist with some of the complex processing with can come with identifying stereotypes and recognizing personal biases (Corneau and Stergiopolos, 2012). Language is key in preventing incidents. Often what offends is not intended to be offensive. Yet the aim is not to teach students tolerance of others and to merely accept that people are different, but inclusion and the practice of forethought to both prevent unintentionally offending others through insensitive language and cultural misunderstandings. Learners should expect to use nonjudgemental active listening skills (Chiper, 2013; DeVoss et al., 2002; Dimitrov et al., 2014) and to avoid using humor, slang, figures of speech, irony, or sarcasm (DeVoss et al., 2002).

Inevitably something will be said, whether in the classroom or otherwise, that impacts the safety of the learning environment. Incorporating opportunities to learn and practice bystander responses can positively impact learners' ability to respond to these experiences (Pieterse et al., 2016; York et al., 2021). These responses include the 5 D's: *Direct* or directly addressing the incident at that time, *Distract* or creating a distraction that prevents continued harm, *Delegate* or encouraging another person to respond, *Delay* or handling the situation at a later time, or to *Display Discomfort* in which one shows discomfort nonverbally to try to discourage the continuation of the situation (York et al., 2021). For those leading sessions, both the Direct and Display Discomfort responses can be very effective to use if concerns arise within the classroom. If choosing to Delegate or Delay individual discussion about the concern, this should be paired with either the Direct or Display Discomfort responses within the classroom to address the harm to the learning environment. Any response that does not directly address the harm to the learning environment can negatively impact both trust in the instructor and trust in other participants, changing the dynamic for all involved.

Impact of Practicing with Physician Cultural Responsibility

Seeking to understand, listening to connect, and responding in compassion are the keys to practicing Physician Cultural Responsibility with all patients. Patients are more able trust their health care team and be open about their needs when they are affirmed and centered in their care plan. Poor experiences with healthcare teams can easily dissuade patients from pursuing the care that they need. Finding real world examples of the impact of care without Physician Cultural Responsibility is not hard to do. The following cases follow a patient through a series of poor interactions where Physician Cultural Responsibility could have positively impacted the patient's experience and ultimately outcomes.

CASES

Case 1-4. Missed Opportunities

Learning Objectives

1. Identify the impact of the core values of Physician Cultural Responsibility in Patient Interactions.
2. Analyze stereotypes and biases through the lens of a patient case.
3. Describe the sources of trauma that patients and their support systems may endure from seeking medical care.
4. Examine the impact of system failures and patient advocacy on health outcomes.
5. Practice skills in self- awareness and reflection through a patient case.

Case Aim: These cases aim to highlight the utility of practicing medicine using Physician Cultural Responsibility.

1. The Impact of an Advocate

An 82 year old African American female with a pertinent past medical history of atrial fibrillation and orthostatic hypotension came to the emergency room in distress. Bought by her family, she was awaiting outpatient pacemaker placement due to atrial fibrillation with slow ventricular response, but with worsening dyspnea on exertion and exhaustion to the point of presyncope, she could no longer wait. Her code status was confirmed as DNR-CCA and admission order was placed. The hospital she went to was unable to place pacemakers so she was sent to another hospital 20 miles away.

Her pacemaker was placed on hospital day 2, seemingly without incident except hypertension during and after the procedure. The patient told the team about a left rotator cuff injury but remembers intense pain with the placement of her left shoulder. The nurse caring for the patient decided that she would hold the patient's medication for orthostatic hypotension because the patient was hypertensive post-op. The family advocated for the patient, describing previous concerns with falls and the need to give the medication. The nurse noted that she would pass the information to the physician and also passed to the oncoming nurse that the medication should be held. When the physician rounded on the patient, intending to discharge her home, she was unable to stand without falling asleep while standing and almost falling. Physical therapy was called and recommended further evaluation as the patient was able to walk to the bathroom prior to the procedure.

2. Questions Without Answers

Over the next 4 weeks, the patient experienced an inability to stand, fatigue, decreased PO intake, acute on chronic absence seizures, and new onset incontinence. This was initially diagnosed as deconditioning, to which the family objected as the patient was previously able to manage her own affairs and move around. Multiple specialists were consulted- Neurovascular, Neuro-Autonomic, Neuro-Stroke, Neurology, Physical Medicine and Rehab, Cardiology, Electrophysiology, who were not able to come up with an etiology for her symptoms.

Neurovascular found intracranial stenosis on CT- angiogram and recommended titrating midodrine and optimizing pacemaker settings with concern for intracranial perfusion. Neuro-Autonomic noted overt dysautonomia possibly acute on chronic versus pacemaker syndrome and recommended IV fluids with ted hose and abdominal binding to assist in maintaining blood pressure. Neuro-Stroke proclaimed that this was not a stroke even though no MRI could be done and signed off while neurology found that the patient's sleeping spells were actually sleep waves on EEG paired with an acute worsening of orthostatic hypotension. They trialed an SSRI for possible narcolepsy, increased Keppra dosing to prevent additional seizures, and agreed with autonomic follow up. Physical Medicine and Rehab agreed with autonomic recommendations and recommended daily physical therapy with a tilt bed to assist the patient in increasing her standing tolerance. Cardiology evaluated and noted no clots or heart damage with the pacemaker placement, deferring to electrophysiology., Electrophysiology refused to evaluate the pacemaker or change settings until a conference was had, describing the inability to stabilize the patient. The settings were initially questioned with the patient remaining at a slow rate. The settings were increased by 10 beats per minute, the patient remained unable to stand. Once the settings were adjusted to pace at 80 beats per minute, the patient started to improve.

3. Stereotypes and Dismay

The patient improved with the changes and multiple follow-ups were recommended. Inpatient rehabilitation was recommended but she was not accepted at the hospital affiliated facility. When asked for more information. The team noted that she was not a good fit but could not note which criteria was used to evaluate her as she still did not have a diagnosis. The patient was ultimately accepted to a skilled nursing facility for rehabilitation. On the morning that she was supposed to transfer, the patient was noted to vagal down while having a bowel movement, had an absence seizure, and was unresponsive. No pulse was lost on telemetry but the nurse present noted not being able to find a radial pulse and began chest compressions. When the patient came to, she was screaming for the staff to stop and get off of her. A review of the incident highlighted that the patient should not have been coded but the damage was done. The patient suffered a back strain and multiple broken ribs. No pain management was offered to the patient who suffered in agony while trying to move for personal care and participate in physical therapy.

The patient's family began to search for another facility for the patient to transition to but was given a very short list of subpar options as the other facilities were worried about the patient's medical stability. When additional options were requested, clinical case managers refused citing hospital policies surrounding length of stay. Arrangements were made without the patient's consent to transfer to a facility without the resources to care for her. All follow up was left for the family to arrange.

4. Heartbreaking Outcomes

One week later, the patient was readmitted to a different hospital for an infection with delirium. The physician teams questioned her initial management and lack of diagnosis. After running many tests, it was discovered that the patient had suffered a stroke during the pacemaker placement secondary to hypotension during the procedure, causing all of her symptoms. The patient was admitted to inpatient rehab however with the delay in diagnosis, continued dysautonomia, and new-onset heart failure caused by the treatment for the dysautonomia, the patient later elected hospice care and passed away.

Case Questions

1. How Do We Address This Patient's Needs?

- When analyzing this case, one may see the glaring lack of appreciation for the patient's needs, values, beliefs, or wishes for her care. Placing the patient at the center of her care is necessary to ensure that her needs are met. If you note there is nowhere within this case that the patient was asked what she wanted or what she needed. The patient's family is often seen advocating for her wishes but are often ignored. When patients are heard and valued in the creation of care plans, physicians have the power to prevent readmissions, additional healthcare costs, and additional trauma for patients.

  In case one the patient presents in distress and is noted to need a pacemaker. While this pacemaker was placed at a hospital outside of the area, it is unknown if the patient has any socioeconomic considerations that would add additional stressors for her or her family in going to that hospital. Evaluation of the patient's needs for support is important in this space, as the patient has no choice but to travel to this hospital for the care that she needs. Later, the patient is noted to have a unrelated medical concern due to a rotator cuff injury but this is not addressed. As the patient is noted to have pain and have elevated blood pressure, it would be appropriate to further discuss this injury and a plan to manage the patients pain prior to assuming the patient has hypertension that needs treated. By centering the patient's needs in her care, we can see that the patient has a history of treated orthostatic hypotension and is planning to return home the next day. It may be harmful to hold the patient's medicine if the hypertension is not urgently concerning.

  Similarly in case 2, the patient is assumed to be deconditioned rather than having had some type of event that has caused her change in mobility. The case notes that the patient has multiple concerns however the family had to advocate for the patient to be evaluated. Again we see that rather than the patient being seen as an individual, the patient has been stereotyped and her needs ignored. There is no discussion in the case of addressing the distress that the patient may be feeling in having had a complication to what is commonly known as a very simple procedure. There is no attention to her emotional health or supporting her support system who continually seems to be advocating while no one else is attending to her needs. We see at the end of case 2 that electrophysiology refused to evaluate the pacemaker or change the settings until external measures were taken, yet the patient improved with increasing the rate. This may have been a very frustrating experience for the patient, especially after having to be bed bound until they were willing to make the change. This also was not addressed and should be to support the patient and her family within this experience.

In case 3, a medical mistake was made. Often, healthcare teams worry about taking responsibility for mistakes in case of litigation. However it is important to ensure that the patient is supported and still cared for within subsequent interactions. Again we see that this patient's pain was not addressed and there was no support given for the psychological distress that this caused. Addressing this is imperative as the patient has now experienced multiple traumatic situations within this admission and is very likely to have less trust in the medical staff caring for her.

Later in the case, it seems as though the patient or her family has been able to voice some needs yet the patient was still discharged to a facility that did not meet her needs. With such a complicated hospital course, this patient's discharge follow-ups should have been arranged to assist in the transition from the hospital to the facility. However they were not, and yet again, the family is left to try to navigate next steps to ensure this patient success. In the event that the patient requested not to have follow up scheduled this would be fine, but the language in the case suggests that this was not the case. Those conversations about additional needs for follow up at discharge are imperative to ensure that each patient's unique home situation is taken into account when transitioning from an acute care setting. In order to address this, it may be helpful to consider current policies surrounding discharge planning as well as improved health care team advocacy for patient needs.

In case #4 we see the consequences of not centering the patient's needs in her care plan. Not only is she readmitted but it is discovered that the patients initial diagnosis was a stroke, a complication of the pacemaker placement, that went undiagnosed. This delay caused the subsequent delay of her rehabilitation plan, additional deconditioning from having to be bed bound during this experience, and a lack of adequate treatment for her condition. Unfortunately this patient lost her life and her family lost a loved one. It's hard to say that the patient's clinical outcome would have changed significantly as the case does not provide details for the appropriate care plan however we do know the patient's experience within the hospital, symptom management, and overall support could have been improved.

2. What Biases May Be at Play Surrounding Areas of This Patient's Identity Consideration? Are There Any Specific Stereotypes That Can Be Identified?

- This case highlights multiple stereotypes and biases associated with multiple areas of this patient's identity. Aligned with intersectionality, each area of her identity that is discussed will be examined. Her socioeconomic standing, nationality, first language, and religion were not discussed here, but may add additional considerations for biases and stereotypes.
- We first learned that this patient is 82 years old. The elderly face many stereotypes about their cognitive and physical abilities within the medical community. Further, the social categorization of medicine often perpetuates the bias that the elderly are unable to manage their own health care decisions, that they are deconditioned at baseline, and that nearing one's life expectancy changes one's zeal to continue living (Allen and Sikora, 2023). This can be seen as the team never asked the patient about her needs but rather made decisions and priorities without patient input. The family had to advocate for her needs. Additionally, assumptions were made about the patient's baseline status, chronic health conditions, and ability to participate in physical therapy. Mistakes were made and this patient endured poor outcomes, both of which were never addressed as if it didn't matter that the patient had life-altering effects from the care she received.

  Likewise, once patients are a certain age, assumptions are made about the types and urgency of interventions they will agree to, their ability to recover, and their interest in additional measures (Allen and Sikora, 2023). If this patient had been a 40 year old woman, is it possible that she may have received a sooner diagnosis with more urgency to identify the cause of her symptoms? It is unlikely that a 40 year old patient would have been assumed to be deconditioned without further evaluation. This patient only received further evaluation because her family advocated for her. Similarly, her discharge was poorly managed and not adequate for her needs, communicating less consideration for long-term management or continuity with follow up.
- Next, we learn that this patient is African American. Specialists made recommendations that were less than the standard of care and likewise, her dis-

charge was known not to be adequate. African American and Hispanic/Latinx patients have reported having to advocate more to just receive the bare minimum of what others receive (Staats, 2015). There is little in the case about how the patient was consented for the procedure or if she felt as though she understood all of the risks as no alternatives were noted. Historically, patients of color were not given opportunities to give full consent for many studies and procedures. Even now, studies show that patients of color are less likely to receive all options for their care (Staats, 2015). Stereotypes include that patients of color are less likely to be able to afford care, follow up, or handle the recovery. Unfortunately, with the power dynamics between patient and physician, many patients do not know that they can ask additional questions, ask for other options, or consent to parts and not all of what is being offered. There may be an intersectional relationship between the impact of her age and the impact of her race on these biases, magnifying the impact of her identity on the biases she is facing.

- We also know that this patient is female. It is well know that the pain and symptoms experienced by women are often brushed aside as a mental health concern (Samulowitz, et. al., 2018). The only complaint that we see that the patient voices herself is shoulder pain which went unaddressed. Again, her family had to advocate for the constellation of symptoms that she experienced to be evaluated. Still, this patient was assumed to be deconditioned until being admitted to another facility who found the culprit- a small stroke that impacted her autonomic system. There may be an intersectional relationship between the impact of her age and race and the impact that her sex on these biases, amplifying the impact of her identity on the biases she is facing.

3. What Cultural Values or Norms Are Being Assumed? Which May Be Missing?

- The cases presented here do not speak directly to this patient's cultural values or norms. One can assume that this patient's cultural values include interconnection with family support and shared decision making as the patient's family is heavily involved in both her care and advocating for her needs. Further, throughout the cases, the patient also aims to improve her condition through health care and trusts that medicine can help her to do that. This is seen first with the pacemaker placement, then through evaluation of her symptoms in search of a modifiable cause, and later through her continued efforts to participate in physical therapy and rehabilitation efforts. We are not privy to any religious ideologies or additional cultural factors. That does not preclude them from being present.

4. How Do Structural Factors Impact This Patient's Care?

- In case 1, this patient is noted to live near a hospital that is not able to give her the care that is necessary. It is unknown whether or not this patient lives in a rural or inner city area however access to care close to home is imperative for maintaining health. Aligned with the social determinants of health, this patient's access to care has been impacted by proximity. Similarly, it is possible that the nurse in case one is following the procedures set forth for patients with hypertension rather than evaluating the patient individually. While these protocols can be very helpful in preventing misdiagnosis or causing iatrogenic harm, further evaluation of each patient is necessary. It is unknown what consequences nursing may face if these protocols are missed which further impacts individualization of care. In both of these examples, patient advocacy is necessary in ensuring appropriate patient care.
- Case 2 highlights structural concerns surrounding the bureaucracy of medicine. Multiple specialists were consulted but few collaborated with her care. It is possible that addressing her symptoms collectively rather than individually may have assisted in sooner diagnosis And better symptom control. This is a common concern for inpatient medicine as managing physicians are given multiple recommendations from different specialists who may not be communicating with all of the teams on board. Again advocating for patient needs is important as the managing physician to ensure both patient safety and the best outcomes possible.
- Case 3 displays multiple system failures. First, this patient had a do not resuscitate order and was unnecessarily resuscitated anyway. Noted as a mistake and the patient did not lose cardiac function, this should have never happened but more so, the patient elected not to be necessitated even if cardiac function was lost. Not only did this oversight cause additional suffering for the patient, it did not align with patient autonomy. Hospital error reporting systems allow for further investigation of events like this. The case does not specify whether any other team members were present however, if mistakes are noticed prior to reaching the patient, it is important to intervene.

    Additionally, many facilities have discharge protocols that heavily relies on metrics like length of stay rather than individually evaluating patients. This is associated with concerns that insurance companies will not pay for additional care that they do not feel was medically necessary. While this is important, safe discharge planning not only prevents poor health outcomes associated with loss to follow up and poor transitional care, it also prevents additional healthcare expenditure associated with readmissions. Patient advocacy can make the difference between patients getting the care and support that they need and them not.

5. Picture Yourself as the Managing Physician in This Case. You've Just Received a Notice That This Patient Has Died With the Cases Outlined Attached. What Emotions Are You Feeling as the Physician in This Case?

- This patient went on to have additional complications associated with delayed care which in just a few months, ended her life. Very strong emotions can surface anytime there are complications in patient care, medical mistakes, unforeseen circumstances, or loss of life. These factors contribute to moral injury, known as the personal impacts that one has after an action or decision has unintended outcomes. This can also happen when one is unable to manage a condition because of poor access to care or provide patients with what they need due to a lack of resources. Moral injury matched with grief, sadness, guilt, frustration, disappointment, or many other uncomfortable emotions contribute to physician burnout (Weisleder, 2023). Being able to identify and discuss the emotions one is feeling can assist in managing moral injury and preventing burnout.
- This is a good opportunity for expanding awareness of one's emotions and practicing identifying emotions. A few questions to consider include: After reading this case what is your immediate reaction? What thoughts are you having that prompt this reaction? How do you feel physically? What emotions would you assign to the feelings and thoughts you are having right now? How do you cope with these emotions? What resources, activities, or supports do you need right now?

6. Are There Any Beliefs That You Have That May Be Stretched Right Now?

- This is a great opportunity for expanding awareness of one's personal beliefs and their alignment with these cases. A few questions to consider include: After reading this case what is your immediate reaction? What thoughts are you having that prompt this reaction? What are your beliefs about patient care, patient autonomy, and communication with families when things don't go as expected? Do the thoughts that you are having align with your beliefs that you've named? What is similar? What is different? What would you have done differently as the physician in this case? What would you have done the same as the physician in this case?

Case Discussion: We cannot know what would have happened without the stroke. We do know that her experience during this very frightening time of her life and the experience of her family supporting her, could have been very different if the medical teams saw her as an individual with value rather than just another medical record number. This is what Physician Cultural Responsibility is all about. When patients are cared for in a way that creates a compassionate space that amplifies their voices, needs, beliefs, and values, medicine becomes the art it was always intended to be, healing the body and the soul. We may not be able to change all health outcomes, but for those that we can, we have a responsibility to set our biases aside and to meet our patients where they are.

CONCLUSION

Physician Cultural Responsibility is a practice that opens doors for physicians to connect more deeply with their patients to improve communication, patient care, and their health outcomes. As noted in the cases above, patients suffer when their needs aren't met, values aren't considered, and their concerns aren't heard. While some complications are inevitable, this patient went without pain control and suffered due to multiple system failures that ultimately delayed her care and cost the patient her life. Often, medical students are taught a standard way to approach patient care which they continue throughout their career. Without consideration of patient intersectionality, health care teams leave themselves open to incorporating biases and stereotypes in their medical practice, and ultimately negatively impacting their patients. However, by encountering each patient as an unique and intersectional individual, centering the patient's needs, beliefs and values in their care, and being aware of the personal biases that they hold, physicians have the power to change medicine and achieve true health equity.

REFERENCES

Allen, J. O., & Sikora, N. (2023). Aging Stigma and the Health of US Adults Over 65: What Do We Know? *Clinical Interventions in Aging, 18*, 2093–2116. DOI: 10.2147/CIA.S396833 PMID: 38116457

Beavis, A. S. W., Hojjati, A., Kassam, A., Choudhury, D., Fraser, M., Masching, R., & Nixon, S. A. (2015). What All Students in Healthcare Training Programs Should Learn to Increase Health Equity: Perspectices on postcolonialsm and the health of Aboriginal peoples in Canada. *BMC Medical Education, 15*(155), 155. DOI: 10.1186/s12909-015-0442-y PMID: 26400722

Betancourt, J. R., Green, A. R., Carrillo, J. E., & Ananeh-Firempong, O.II. (2003). Defining Cultural Competence: A practical framework for addressing racial/ethnic disparities in health and health care. *Public Health Reports, 118*(4), 293–302. DOI: 10.1016/S0033-3549(04)50253-4 PMID: 12815076

Blackie, M., Wear, D., & Zarconi, J. (2019). Narrative Intersectionality in Caring for Marginalized or Disadvantaged Patients. *Academic Medicine, 94*(1), 59–63. PMID: 30134270

Boroumand, S., Stein, M. J., Jay, M., Shen, J. W., Hirsh, M., & Dharamsi, S. (2020). Addressing the health advocate role in medical education. *BMC Medical Education, 20*(28), 1–5. DOI: 10.1186/s12909-020-1938-7 PMID: 32000759

Briguglio, C. (2006). *Empowering students by developing their intercultural communication competence: A two-way process. Educate, advocate, empower.* ISANA International Education Association Inc.

Brookfield, S. D., & Hess, M. E. (2021). *Becoming a White antiracist: A practical guide for educators, leaders, and activists.* Stylus Publishing.

Chiper, S. (2013). Teaching intercultural communication: ICT resources and best practices. *Procedia Social and Behavioral Sciences, 93*(2012), 1641–1645.

Coria, A., McKelvey, T. G., Charlton, P., Woodworth, M., & Lahey, T. (2013). The design of a medical school social justice and curriculum. *Academic Medicine, 88*(10), 1442–1449. DOI: 10.1097/ACM.0b013e3182a325be PMID: 23969356

Corneau, S. & Stergiopoulos, V. (2012) More than being against it: Anti-racism and anti-oppression in mental health services. Academic Press.

Coutinho, A. J., Nguyen, B., Kelly, C., Lin, K., Gits, A., Crichlow, R., & Moreno, G. (2020). Formal advocacy curricula in family medicine residencies: A CERA survey of program directors. *Family Medicine, 52*(4), 255–261. PMID: 32267520

Denevi, E., & Paston, N. (2006, Winter). Helping Whites Develop Anti-Racist Identities: Overcoming their resistance to fighting racism. *Multicultural Education*, 70–71.

DeVoss, D., Jasken, J., & Hayden, D. (2002). Teaching Intracultural and Intercultural Communication: A critique suggested method. *Journal of Business and Technical Communication, 16*(1), 69–94.

Dimitrov, N., Dawson, D., Olsen, K., & Meadows, K. N. (2014). Developing the intercultural competence of graduate students. *Canadian Journal of Higher Education, 44*(3), 86–103.

Dobie, S. (2007). Reflections on a Well-Traveled Path: Self-awareness, mindful practice, and relationship centered care as foundations for medical education. *Academic Medicine, 82*(4). PMID: 17414201

Eisenchlas, S., & Trevaskes, S. (2007). Developing intercultural communication skills through intergroup interaction. *Intercultural Education, 18*(5), 413–425. DOI: 10.1080/14675980701685271

Foronda, C., Baptiste, D., Reinholdt, M. M., & Ousman, K. (2016). Cultural Humility: A Concept Analysis. *Journal of Transcultural Nursing, 27*(3), 210–217. PMID: 26122618

Hassen, N., Lofters, A., Michael, S., Mall, A., Pinto, A. D., & Rackal, J. (2021). Implementing Anti-Racism Interventions in Healthcare Settings: A Scoping Review. *International Journal of Environmental Research and Public Health, 18*(6), 2993. Advance online publication. DOI: 10.3390/ijerph18062993 PMID: 33803942

Hunter, K., & Thompson, B. (2019). A Scoping review of Social Determinants of Health Curricula in Post-Graduate Medical Education. *Canadian Medical Education Journal, 10*(3), e61–e71. PMID: 31388378

Inoue, A. B. (2020). Teaching antiracist writing. *Journal of College Reading and Learning, 50*(1), 1–23.

Johnson, C., Rastetter, M., & Olayiwola, J. N. (2022). Pathways to Equity: Implementing a Health Equity Leadership Curriculum in Residency Education as an Antidote to Systemic Racism. *Journal of the National Medical Association, 114*(2), 141–146. DOI: 10.1016/j.jnma.2021.12.015 PMID: 35078671

Johnson, C. D. (2023). The MONROE Method: A Methodology on Navigating Race, Oppression, and Equity in Medical Education through Physician Cultural Responsibility. https://aura.antioch.edu/etds/979

King, S. H., & Castenell, L. A. (2001). *Racism and racial inequality: Implications for teacher education*. AACTE Publications.

Kondrat, M. E. (1999). Who is the "self" in self-aware: Professional self-awareness from a critical theory perspective. *The Social Service Review*, *73*(4), 451–477. DOI: 10.1086/514441

Masters, C., Robinson, D., Faulkner, S., Patterson, E., McIlraith, T., & Ansari, A. (2019). Addressing Biases in Patient Care with The 5Rs of Cultural Humility, a Clinician Coaching Tool. *Journal of General Internal Medicine*, *34*(4), 627–630. DOI: 10.1007/s11606-018-4814-y PMID: 30623383

National Institutes of Health. (2007). *Cultural Awareness Glossary of Key Terms*. https://www.niehs.nih.gov/news/events/pastmtg/hazmat/assets/2007/wtp_2007ntec_wruc_latino_tips_glossary_508.pdf

Nazar, M., Kendall, K., Day, L., & Nazar, H. (2015). Decolonising medical curricula through diversity education: Lessons from students. *Medical Teacher*, *37*(4), 385–393. DOI: 10.3109/0142159X.2014.947938 PMID: 25156358

Pieterse, A. L., Utsey, S. O., & Miller, M. J. (2016). Development and initial validation of the anti-racism behavioral inventory (ARBI). *Counselling Psychology Quarterly*, *29*(4), 356–381. DOI: 10.1080/09515070.2015.1101534

Ramani, S., Konings, K., Mann, V., & van der Vluten, C. (2017). Uncovering the unknown: A grounded theory study exploring the impact of self-awareness on the culture of feedback in residency education. *Medical Teacher*, *39*(10), 1065–1073. DOI: 10.1080/0142159X.2017.1353071 PMID: 28741446

Samulowitz, A., Gremyr, I., Eriksson, E., & Hensing, G. (2018). "Brave Men" and "Emotional Women": A theory-guided literature review on gender bias in health care and gendered norms towards patients with chronic pain. *Pain Research & Management*, *2018*, 1–14. DOI: 10.1155/2018/6358624 PMID: 29682130

Santas, A. (2000). Teaching antiracism. *Studies in Philosophy and Education*, *19*(4), 349–361. DOI: 10.1023/A:1005298916161

Sharma, M., Pinto, A. D., & Kumagai, A. K. (2018). Teaching the Social Determinants of Health: A path to equity or a road to nowhere? *Academic Medicine*, *2018*(93), 25–30. DOI: 10.1097/ACM.0000000000001689 PMID: 28445214

Staats, C., Capatosto, K., Wright, R. A., & Contractor, D. (2015). State of the Science: Implicit Bias Review 2015. Academic Press.

Strasser, J., & Spelocha, H. (2005). How can university professors help their students to understand issues of diversity through interpersonal and intrapersonal intelligences. *Multicultural Education*, *12*(4), 20.

Weisleder, P. (2023). Moral distress, moral injury, and burnout: Clinicians' resilience and adaptability are not the solution. *Annals of the Child Neurology Society*, *1*(4), 262–266. DOI: 10.1002/cns3.20048

York, M., Davidson, L. M., Hemingway, C., Russell, R., Neeley, M., & Fleming, A. (2021). Becoming Active Bystanders and Advocated: Teaching medical students to respond to bias in the clinical setting. *Academic Medicine*, *2021*(17).

Chapter 2 Bias: Understanding and Addressing Disparities in Patient Care Across Multiple Demographics

S. Srinivasan
https://orcid.org/0009-0002-0179-9849
Department of Humanities and Social Sciences, Graphic Era University, Dehradun, India

R. Vallipriya
https://orcid.org/0009-0008-6692-603X
Department of Physical Science, Institute of Education, India & Tamil Nadu Teacher Education University, Trichy, India

ABSTRACT

Biases are untrue assumptions made without evidence. This can happen explicitly or when it is known to the person making the assumptions, as well as implicitly or when it is unknown. Biases impact interactions and relationships, including the physician-patient relationship. Physician biases can impact patients' health outcomes by influencing the options patients are given, the ways in which care is delivered, and interactions with the healthcare team. This chapter explores the social categorization of medicine or biases found within the field of medicine, their impact on patient care, and ways to overcome them.

DOI: 10.4018/979-8-3693-3683-0.ch002

INTRODUCTION

Biases can be unconscious or conscious, which can lead to disparities in healthcare. Explicit biases are conscious stereotypes while implicit biases involve unconscious attitudes and stereotypes that influence the decision-making of health professionals (Hagihigi, 2023). Bias exists in healthcare services, and are be detrimental to the quality of healthcare a person receives (FitzGerald & Hurst, 2017) even though many physicians and health care team members don't know that they have them (Davis Moore, 2023). Bias and discrimination can happen at several levels, such as policies nationwide or locally, in institutional policy, and individually with healthcare workers. Bias can lead to poor support and services for patients, inaccurate or delays in diagnosis, delays in results, and delays in treatment initiation. In return, patients often face additional stressors, discontinue treatment, and avoid healthcare services all together (Hagihigi, 2023).

Biases are only a part of the problem. Privilege is an unearned right associated with power or influence in society. Thus, when biases intertwine with power dynamics, like within the exam room, they create spaces for oppression which has a much greater impact than the bias alone (Casanova-Perez,2021). This is often described within identities, for example, those without disabilities or special physical needs are in a place of power versus those who have disabilities or need accommodations. Those who are in a position of power don't often have to consider this as the standard set by the societal norm caters to those who do not need any accommodations. This power is more apparent to those who are not in a position of power, or in this example, the people who do need accommodations. We also see this within the physician-patient relationship as physicians hold the position of power within the exam room (Casanova-Perez, 2021). With the knowledge and trust of the patient, patients are relying on physicians to assist them in receiving the care that they need. When biases enter the exam room, patients can be oppressed and have poorer health outcomes (Vela, et. al, 2022).

The Social Categorization of Medicine

Social categorization refers to the way in which judgements or biases are made to group or categorize groups of people (Van Ryn & Burke, 2000). The social categorization of medicine refers to the biases that are circulated throughout the field of medicine. These biases, often learned in training, impact patient care and interactions with the entire health care team (Spencer & Grace, 2016). Unfortunately, while false, many are assumed to be true and have been used in making health care decisions for patients.

Sex and Gender

Biases relating to gender are based upon the idea that women, nonbinary, and transgender individuals are often undervalued in comparison to men (Zhang et al., 2021). This is like the biases seen against sex in the idea that females are in some way less than males. Common stereotypes of women or females include considerations of pain tolerance and hormonal impacts to behavior and mental health. Thus, this leads to symptoms being dismissed as psychological (Chrisler et al., 2016) and health concerns being over-pathologized to reproductive health leading to underdiagnosis and undertreatment. Alternatively, men or males are expected to be inexpressive. This leads to underreporting of symptoms, pain, and mental health concerns and delayed diagnoses from less preventive care or screenings. (Hagihigi, 2023). Those who are nonbinary or transgender often meet biases associated with physicians misunderstanding of medical needs. Misgendering and discrimination may discourage transgender individuals from seeking care (Walkowska et al., 2023).

Sexual Orientation

Medicine operates from a space of heteronormativity or the assumption that all patients are heterosexual. Thus, those who are not heterosexual face risks of the health care team missing relevant care leading to overlooked needs and misdiagnoses. Stereotypes about their health risks and promiscuity as well as the lack of education about providing inclusive sexual health guidance impact health outcomes (Casanova-Perez, 2021). In the worst, physician prejudices may result in substandard care or refusal of treatment which creates a common fear of discrimination, leading individuals who are not heterosexual to avoid seeking care all together (Casanova-Perez, 2021) Additionally, same-sex partnerships may not be recognized in healthcare settings, affecting decision-making rights. Partners may be excluded from care discussions, especially in emergency situations, creating added concerns.

Race

Racial biases focus on assumptions made due to characteristics that would visually assign a patient to one race or another. As race is a social construct, these biases change based upon the culture and society that one is in just like the definitions of the races change based on locations. In America, biases associated with race include Black individuals feel less pain (Vela et.al, 2022), Hispanic and Latinx individuals are less interested in their health (Funk & Lopez, 2022), Native American and American Indian individuals have access to care (ADHS, 2021), and Asian individuals are healthier and have healthier habits (Lee, 2021). These biases lead to disparities in treatment for those from non-White races (Panner et al., 2012, Howe et al., 2022) including poorer pain control for Black patients, lower quality care for Hispanic and Latinx patients (Funk & Lopez, 2022), lesser access to care for Native American and American Indian patients who are not close to Indian Health Service sites (ADHS, 2021), and less preventative care and cancer screenings for Asian individuals (Lee, 2021). For instance, 62% of patients in a minority-predominant cancer center were found to be undertreated for their pain by World Health Organization (WHO) guidelines. This translated to 3-fold increase in undertreatment when compared to non-minority-predominant cancer center setting (Campbell et al, 2012).

Nationality

Biases associated with nationality are complex. While this can incorporate biases about where one is from, it can also include biases about accommodations needed like cultural considerations and interpretation needs. Healthcare teams may assume patients from certain nationalities hold specific cultural beliefs or health behaviors, leading to misunderstandings or misdiagnoses. Some may assume a patient's immigration status, affecting care, especially for undocumented immigrants who fear seeking medical help due to the current politicization of immigration. Further, Xenophobic attitudes towards patients from certain countries can lead to discriminatory behavior, contributing to unequal care. Stereotypes may also include assumptions about a patient's financial resources or access to treatment and assumptions about comprehension, leading to oversimplified explanations, suboptimal care, or fewer referrals to specialists (Lancet, 2022)

Physical Appearance

Common biases surrounding physical appearance include those about weight. Negative stereotypes about overweight patients include having poor lifestyle habits, laziness, and overemphasis on weight as the cause of health problems. This paired with unhelpful comments and the shame associated with inadequate supplies and equipment for those of larger sizes leads to feelings of judgment, erosion of the physician-patient relationship, and a lack of compassionate care. Patients avoid care due to past bias or discrimination, leading to worse outcome (Phelan, 2015). Likewise, judging lifestyle and health behaviors by physical appearance, leading to inaccurate conclusions. The assumption that thin patients are healthy overlooks the prevalence of body dysmorphia, eating disorders, and the development of chronic conditions in those with poor lifestyle habits who also happen to be thin.

Religion

Providers may generalize religious practices or stereotype patients based on their religion, leading to misunderstandings or inappropriate treatment. A lack of knowledge about religious practices can result in offering treatments or foods that conflict with a patient's beliefs, potentially causing non-adherence to treatment plans. Further, religious beliefs may conflict with medical practices (Scheitle, 2023). For example, assumptions about end-of-life decisions based on religion can lead to conflicts or unmet needs, resulting in lower-quality care and reduced trust in healthcare providers.

Ageism

Ageism or age bias refers to stereotypes about older and younger patients. Ageism can lead to improper treatment, especially for older adults, who may not receive proper, regular, or real-time treatment (Wyman et al., 2018). According to the U.S. National Health and Retirement data, about 20% of people over 50 face age-based discrimination in healthcare. Elderly patients' symptoms may be assumed to be related to established health conditions or medications. Maximum recovery of stamina, strength, balance, and fitness is often underestimated. They may be undertreated for their symptoms, which are dismissed as merely a result of normal aging (Pelham, 2023). Although older patients may not prefer advanced treatments or surgeries, they may not be asked or recommended to do the appropriate treatments due to their age (Mannucci et al., 2009). For instance, breast cancer screening guidelines will generally stop at age 75. However, if the patient has a life expectancy greater than 10 years, then ongoing screenings are still recommended. Conversely, young people are generally perceived to be healthy, but that can lead to delays in diagnosis. Hypertension and diabetes are often overlooked in the younger generation (Hagihigi, 2023).

Education Level

Patient education level can impact health disparities especially from a socioeconomic perspective. A clinician may have implicit and/or explicit biases based on the education level (Macias-Konstantopoulos et al., 2023). These predominantly relate to health literacy, financial resources, and communities in which that patient may live. However, health literacy is not directly tied to education. Assumptions made on health literacy may impact the treatment options presented, or the clarity of the health conditions discussed (Hagihigi, 2023; Berkman, 2011). This can affect patients of higher education by overestimating their understanding of complex medical terms, which could lead to confusion or poor adherence. Meanwhile assuming that patients with lower education lack health literacy, could lead to an oversimplification of information (Institute of Medicine, 2011).

Ability

Laws are in place to ensure accessibility, but ableism can extend to vision, hearing, mobility baseline, swallowing ability, bowel / bladder control, reading comprehension, and others. A 2020 showed that 82% of physicians in the United States view patients with disabilities as having a lower quality of life (RTI Health Alliance, 2023). Due to the ingrained nature of this bias in medical practice, this can lead to deeming certain treatments as futile or too extreme despite the patient having been stable with their disability for many years. In addition, healthcare providers have also noted feeling uncomfortable treating patients with disabilities (Janz, 2019), leading to less empathetic care. More exposure to standard life for various disabilities has been noted to curb some of this bias (Janz, 2019).

Socioeconomic Status

Socioeconomic status (SES) is a very prevalent bias especially regarding lower SES patients. Stereotypes including inherently having unhealthy habits and low health engagement with non-adherence leads to stereotyping and stigmatizing low-income patients as "undeserving" of care. Physicians may view higher SES patients as more deserving of care, leading to unequal treatment (Van Ryn & Burke, 2000; Job, 2022)

Chronic Health Conditions

Biases in medicine extend to specific health conditions as well. Clinicians will make assumptions about character, SES, and other lifestyle habits purely based on the health conditions a patient has. Mental health conditions, diabetes, hypertension, substance use disorders, chronic pain, and infectious diseases are common conditions for which clinicians may stereotype patients for having these conditions. Mental health can be overlooked or disregarded due to its intangible nature (Stangl, 2019). Patients with diabetes, hypertension, heart disease, and/or obesity are often stereotyped for the lifestyle habits that exacerbate these conditions issues despite the hereditary predisposition to these conditions. Substance use disorders and infectious diseases (such as tuberculosis, HIV, and sexually transmitted infections) are often stigmatized and marginalized due to a "classic" appearance of having these conditions. This overlooks situations like rape, promiscuous partner, abusive relationships / parents, etc. that can lead into these conditions. It's important for a clinician to be aware of their biases to avoid inequitable care to patients in these situations.

Best Practices to Avoid Perpetuating Biases in Medicine

Stopping the socialization of medicine from impacting patient care is a large task. Combatting biases takes both individual and systemic efforts. Ensuring improved connections with patients means educating healthcare workers, advocating for patients, and diversifying healthcare teams.

Educating Healthcare Workers

Providing training to educate healthcare professionals on cultural diversity and unconscious biases can improve decision-making. Further, ensuring that patients are involved in decision-making, respecting their preferences and backgrounds and avoids assumptions based on demographics. Conducting thorough, non-judgmental assessments allows for physicians to connect with patients and consider all aspects of a patient's health. By learning to use respectful, stigma-free language with patients, teams can foster open, honest communication (Casanova-Perez,2021).

Advocating for Patients

Policy changes have the power to influence workplace culture and expectations (Vela et. al, 2022). Inclusive policies including standardized protocols that rely on evidence-based guidelines to ensure consistent and unbiased diagnosis and treatment and data collection to track health disparities and monitor practices for bias can reveal areas where the healthcare system needs additional training or support to provide inclusive care.

Diversifying Healthcare Teams

Diverse physicians bring varied perspectives, improving communication, and promoting inclusive attitudes. Likewise, studies show diverse providers are more likely to address health disparities and ensure equitable care. By having shared identities with health care team members, patients of disenfranchised identities may feel more comfortable and understood, leading to better adherence and satisfaction (Vela et. Al, 2022).

CASES

Case 1: Physician and Patient Communication Challenges

Learning Objectives

1. Identify biases associated with patient identity.
2. Understand common barriers to care for patients of diverse identities.
3. Discuss the steps to improve communication with patients who need interpretation services.

Case Aim: Biases associated with cultural differences and language barriers within patient encounters can impact health outcomes.

A 45-year-old patient named Maheswari with no past medical history is coming into the office today with her son. She speaks the local language, Telugu, and has a problem with abdominal pain. Her son is also with her; he tries to speak in the local language to accompany her and act as the interpreter. They have a conversation with the physician, but the patient hesitates in speaking with the physician, making it difficult to translate her symptoms and inform the physician.

Her son mentions the pain has been occurring for some time but will fade away on its own for 1-2 weeks every month before recurring. Per her son, she has tried some home remedies and some over-the-counter pain relievers, but the pain persists. Her son notes that she is having difficulty doing routine activities due to this pain. The physician suspects this could be premenstrual symptoms, and that patient is not vocalizing these concerns directly due to not wanting to discuss feminine health concerns in front of her son. The physician orders several diagnostic tests to rule out alternative causes such as infection, gallstones, and ovarian cysts. In the meantime, the clinician recommends starting hormonal treatment to help with the suspected premenstrual symptoms and following up next week to follow up the results and status of the pain.

At the 3 month follow up, Maheswari is accompanied by her son again. The physician's office also has an official Telugu interpreter present for the visit. Maheswari via the official interpreter mentions via the interpreter that the hormonal treatment hasn't helped thus far. It did help her menstrual pains, but that wasn't the reason she came to the office last week. This pain is constant when doing any lifting or physically demanding activities. The pain subsides when doing lighter activities or resting, and thus has stopped doing several household activities and exercising routinely. Her son chimes in and has a conversation with her. The interpreter provides insight into what this conversation was about. Per the interpreter, son was under the impression she wasn't doing activities anymore when the usual menstrual pain got worse instead of the activities causing the pain. She further went on to mention that she was quiet during the first encounter, since she had discussed everything with the son before coming to the doctor's appointment. Her son directly asked her about the menstrual pain previously, so she mentioned to him that menstrual pains have always been uncomfortable. Yet she wanted to keep her menstrual pains discrete.

She's only fluent in Telugu and wasn't sure if her son stated things correctly to the physician, but didn't want to interrupt the discussion. Considering this new information, the physician clarifies a few more things with the patient. She notes that there is also a bulge on her leg when the pain is most intense. The pain first started 4 months ago when she was moving some extra heavy furniture solo. Additional tests were ordered to confirm, and the patient was found to have a femoral hernia. A referral was placed to surgeon for repair.

Case Questions

1. What Biases Can You Identify in This Case?

- This patient's menstrual pain was assumed to be the cause of her abdominal pain. This is noted to be a very common concern as women can have delayed diagnoses due to the expectation that their pain is related to reproductive health concerns when it is not. Likewise, the physician assumed that the patient was not speaking to him due to shame about her reproductive health and that the sone was correctly describing her complaint without directly asking her.

2. How Might Language Barriers Contribute to Inequities in Healthcare Delivery? How Can Healthcare Workers Address Such Barriers to Ensure the Patient Receives Accurate Diagnosis and Care?

- Language barriers present concerns like inaccurate translation, lack of direct translation for words, and patient non-fluency which can lead to miscommunication with the practitioner. In this case, the miscommunication was derived from the son's interpretation of the patient's health concerns, whether that be because she did not want to discuss menstrual concerns with her son or otherwise. These types of miscommunications make it difficult to correctly diagnose the cause of symptoms, which can lead to inaccurate diagnoses and contribute to inequities in healthcare delivery.
- Allowing the family member to describe the exact issues raises ethical concerns, as it can include potential biases, breaches of patient confidentiality,

and inaccurate information. The family members may unintentionally alter or omit some important information, which can affect the quality of communication. Healthcare workers must provide balance and professional experience, which can enhance the confidentiality of information and allow them to provide relevant details to family members to improve their supportive role. This can improve the accuracy of the patient's health information being conveyed, without compromising privacy.

- Professional interpreters should always be used to prevent these types of mistakes. Family members may be able to speak the same language as the health care team but may not be able to adequately discuss the complexities of medical terminology, especially in patient encounters and any consent or treatment discussions.

3. What Cultural Differences Can Be Identified in this Case? How Can the Physician Demonstrate Cultural Humility When Working With Maheswari and Her Son, Particularly Considering the Language Barrier and the Patient's Potential Discomfort With Speaking Openly? How Can They Respect the Patient's Cultural Values While Providing the Best Care Possible?

- The physician should acknowledge Maheswari's cultural values within the encounter, especially since she has never been seen in this setting before. The language in this case suggests that she is uncomfortable. We know that family support is a strong value for her as her son is assisting in her care. We also know that there are some remedies that she has tried for her symptoms, but the physician has not explored what these are or their cultural significance further.
- The physician should use open-ended questions and encourage her to express her health needs. In this case, the physician assumed cultural dynamics with her being more passive and unwilling to speak up. Although some of those cultural dynamics may have been present, when she had a non-family member interpret, she was willing to voice her own concerns.
- The physician should maintain a non-judgmental attitude, offer empathetic and positive body language, and ensure the patient is aware that she has their attention through posture and gestures.

Case Discussion

Healthcare workers must provide a professional approach to create proper communication and a comfortable environment. This can lead to a positive patient experience. By prioritizing cultural sensitivity, using a professional interpreter, and connecting with this patient, the physician could have solved this patient's health at the first visit. Building trust requires respect of the patient's cultural values, personal need, and autonomy which can encourage them to openly share their concerns.

Case 2: To Navigate TB Treatment and Provide Cultural Sensitivity

Learning Objectives

1. To understand the patient's cultural beliefs and provide patient care to improve the decision-making process.
2. To analyze the process of balancing Ethics and Autonomy
3. Consider ethical challenges in diagnosis and treatment when patients have a health care proxy.
4. Develop skills and strategies for patient centered care.

Case Aim: Cultural beliefs and ethical balance for patient autonomy can improve the role of religion in decision-making, address strategies to resolve patient-family conflicts, and ensure ethical assistance for effective TB care and treatment.

The 95-year-old man, named Baashha, went to a private clinic for TB treatment. He was found to be positive, but the medical practitioner did not inform him that he had TB because his family requested that he not be informed. The patient had suffered greatly and already discussed his end-of-life plans with his doctor who shared his Muslim faith including making his family members his health care proxy and requesting not to have any bad news delivered to him. He believed that increasing suffering by medical intervention with hopes of preventing the end of life was wrong and that TB was a bad omen. The patient was treated for TB with the goal to alleviate his suffering but with consideration for preventing side effects and maximizing what quality of life he had left. The health department made an in-home visit and disclosed the patient's diagnosis to him as well as the options for additional treatments. When the patient angrily refused further treatment or additional options, the health department sought a force med order and inpatient hospitalization against his wishes.

Case Questions

1. How Might Cultural Norms and Beliefs Influence the Way Baashha, and His Family View His TB Diagnosis, and How Can Healthcare Providers Navigate These Cultural Concerns While Ensuring the Patient Receives Appropriate Care?

- Awareness of cultural factors allows the healthcare workers to provide the appropriate care for patients. In this case, we see the patient's family request to omit the patient's diagnosis to prevent further harm while ensuring that he was adequately treated to prevent communicable spread. This patient's doctor shared identity with him, leading to additional understanding of the request and greater trust between the physician, the patient, and the patient's family. The healthcare worker from the health department was not aware of the patient's cultural and religious values or their impact on his treatment plan. Ultimately this patient's autonomy was compromised due to cultural differences.

2. What Ethical Considerations Arise When the Healthcare Practitioner Decides Not to Disclose the TB Diagnosis to the Patient Based on Family Requests? How Can Healthcare Workers Navigate the Tension Between Cultural Respect and Their Professional Duty to Inform the Patient?

- Patient ethical considerations can include the patient's right to know, seek a second opinion for their diagnosis, and make an informed decision about their treatment. The diagnosis is based on the family's request, which can provide patient autonomy and improve informed consent. It has the potential to reduce their risk and prevent disclosure of their cultural concerns with empathy.

Case Discussion

Cultural beliefs and patient stigma can cause fear of TB, which may affect patient's adherence to treatment. Communication provided by healthcare workers, like that from the physician in this case, should be free from judgement or bias, and elevate the patient's needs. When assumptions are made, like those by the health-care worker from the health department, patients may feel as though the lack of cultural understanding and demands infringes upon their autonomy. This can erode the physician-patient relationship and deter patients from continuing to seek care.

CONCLUSION

The social categorization of medicine complicates the ways in which care is provided for patients of all identities. Differences in cultural norms, communication, and goals of care can spur health care workers to rely on their biases when providing care for patients whose backgrounds and values they don't understand. When healthcare workers can be aware of their biases, they can provide more equitable care. Policy changes and diversity efforts can assist in overcoming the social categorization of medicine and in turn improving health disparities.

REFERENCES

ADHS. (2021). *Leading Causes of Death and Health Disparities Among The American Indian and Alaska Native Population in Arizona*. Arizona Department of Health Services Interventions.

Berkman, N. D., Sheridan, S. L., Donahue, K. E., Halpern, D. J., & Crotty, K. (2011). Low health literacy and health outcomes: An updated systematic review. *Annals of Internal Medicine, 155*(2), 97–107. DOI: 10.7326/0003-4819-155-2-201107190-00005 PMID: 21768583

Berthold, H. K., Gouni-Berthold, I., Bestehorn, K. P., Böhm, M., & Krone, W. (2008). Physician gender is associated with the quality of type 2 diabetes care. *Journal of Internal Medicine, 264*(4), 340–350. DOI: 10.1111/j.1365-2796.2008.01967.x PMID: 18397244

Campbell, C. M., & Edwards, R. R. (2012). Ethnic differences in pain and pain management. *Pain Management, 2*(3), 219–230. DOI: 10.2217/pmt.12.7 PMID: 23687518

Casanova-Perez, R., Apodaca, C., Bascom, E., Mohanraj, D., Lane, C., Vidyarthi, D., Beneteau, E., Sabin, J., Pratt, W., Weibel, N., & Hartzler, A. L. (2022). Broken down by bias: Healthcare biases experienced by BIPOC and LGBTQ+ patients. *AMIA ... Annual Symposium proceedings.AMIA Symposium,2021*, 275–284.

Chrisler, J. C., Barney, A., & Palatino, B. (2016). Ageism can be hazardous to women's health: Ageism, sexism, and stereotypes of older women in the healthcare system. *The Journal of Social Issues, 72*(1), 86–104. DOI: 10.1111/josi.12157

Davis Moore, T. (2023). Can Provider Bias Impact Patient Treatment Outcomes: A Qualitative Analysis. https://digitalcommons.memphis.edu/etd/3025/

Devereaux, P. J., Choi, P. T., Lacchetti, C., Weaver, B., Schünemann, H. J., Haines, T., Lavis, J. N., Grant, B. J. B., Haslam, D. R. S., Bhandari, M., Sullivan, T., Cook, D. J., Walter, S. D., Meade, M., Khan, H., Bhatnagar, N., & Guyatt, G. H. (2002). A systematic review and meta-analysis of studies comparing mortality rates of private for-profit and private not-for-profit hospitals. *Canadian Medical Association Journal, 166*(11), 1399–1406. https://www.cmaj.ca/content/166/11/1399.short PMID: 12054406

Evans, M. (2019). *Fits and starts: A genealogy of hysteria in modern France*. Cornell University Press.

FitzGerald, C., & Hurst, S. (2017). Implicit bias in healthcare professionals: A systematic review. *BMC Medical Ethics*, *18*(1), 1–18. DOI: 10.1186/s12910-017-0179-8 PMID: 28249596

Funk, C., & Lopez, M. H. (2022). Hispanic Americans' Trust in and Engagement with Science. Pew Research Center. https://www.pewresearch.org/science/2022/06/14/hispanic-americans-trust-in-and-engagement-with-science/

Hagihigi, A. S. (2023). Biases in healthcare: An overview. *Medical News Today*. https://www.medicalnewstoday.com/articles/biases-in-healthcare

Howe, L. C., Hardebeck, E. J., Eberhardt, J. L., Markus, H. R., & Crum, A. J. (2022). White patients' physical responses to healthcare treatments are influenced by provider race and gender. *Proceedings of the National Academy of Sciences of the United States of America*, *119*(27), e2007717119. DOI: 10.1073/pnas.2007717119 PMID: 35749352

Institute of Medicine (US) Roundtable on Health Literacy. (2011). Innovations in Health Literacy Research: Workshop Summary. National Academies Press (US). Available from: https://www.ncbi.nlm.nih.gov/books/NBK209674/

Janz H. L. (2019). Ableism: the undiagnosed malady afflicting medicine. CMAJ: Canadian Medical Association journal = journal de l'Association medicale canadienne, 191(17), E478–E479. DOI: 10.1503/cmaj.180903

Job, C., Adenipekun, B., Cleves, A., & Samuriwo, R. (2022). Health professional's implicit bias of adult patients with low socioeconomic status (SES) and its effects on clinical decision-making: A scoping review protocol. *BMJ Open*, *12*(12), e059837. DOI: 10.1136/bmjopen-2021-059837 PMID: 36523234

Johansson, C., & Chinworth, S. A. (2018). *Mobility in context: Principles of patient care skills*. FA Davis.

Kennedy, M., & Kennedy, M. (2014). Bogan bias: Addressing class-based prejudice in physician-patient interactions. *Journal of Social Inclusion*, *5*(2), 27–43. DOI: 10.36251/josi74

Lee, R. J., Madan, R. A., Kim, J., Posadas, E. M., & Yu, E. Y. (2021). Disparities in Cancer Care and the Asian American Population. *The Oncologist*, *26*(6), 453–460. DOI: 10.1002/onco.13748 PMID: 33683795

Macias-Konstantopoulos, W. L., Collins, K. A., Diaz, R., Duber, H. C., Edwards, C. D., Hsu, A. P., Ranney, M. L., Riviello, R. J., Wettstein, Z. S., & Sachs, C. J. (2023). Race, Healthcare, and Health Disparities: A Critical Review and Recommendations for Advancing Health Equity. *The Western Journal of Emergency Medicine*, *24*(5), 906–918. DOI: 10.5811/WESTJEM.58408 PMID: 37788031

Mannucci, P. M., Schutgens, R. E., Santagostino, E., & Mauser-Bunschoten, E. P. (2009). How I treat age-related morbidities in elderly persons with hemophilia. *Blood*, *114*(26), 5256–5263. DOI: 10.1182/blood-2009-07-215665 PMID: 19837978

Phelan, S. M., Burgess, D. J., Yeazel, M. W., Hellerstedt, W. L., Griffin, J. M., & van Ryn, M. (2015). Impact of weight bias and stigma on quality of care and outcomes for patients with obesity. *Obesity Reviews*, *16*(4), 319–326. DOI: 10.1111/obr.12266 PMID: 25752756

RTI Health Alliance. (2023, June 27). Addressing Healthcare Bias Among People With Disabilities. Retrieved from RTI Health Alliance: https://healthcare.rti.org/insights/health-inequities-of-disabled-persons

Scheitle, C. P., Frost, J., & Ecklund, E. H. (2023). The Association between Religious Discrimination and Health: Disaggregating by Types of Discrimination Experiences, Spencer, K. L., & Grace, M. (2016). Social foundations of health care inequality and treatment bias. *Annual Review of Sociology*, *42*(1), 101–120. DOI: 10.1146/annurev-soc-091715-074226

Stangl, A. L., Earnshaw, V. A., & Logie, C. H. (2019). The Health Stigma and Discrimination Framework: A global, crosscutting framework to inform research, intervention development, and policy on health-related stigmas. *BMC Medicine*, *17*, 31. DOI: 10.1186/s12916-019-1271-3 PMID: 30764826

The Lancet Series on racism, xenophobia, discrimination, and health. (2022). The Lancet. www.thelancet.com/series/racism-xenophobia-discrimination-health

Van Ryn, M., & Burke, J. (2000). The effect of patient race and socio-economic status on physicians' perceptions of patients. *Social Science & Medicine*, *50*(6), 813–828. DOI: 10.1016/S0277-9536(99)00338-X PMID: 10695979

Vela, M. B., Erondu, A. I., Smith, N. A., Peek, M. E., Woodruff, J. N., & Chin, M. H. (2022). Eliminating Explicit and Implicit Biases in Health Care: Evidence and Research Needs. *Annual Review of Public Health*, *43*(1), 477–501. DOI: 10.1146/annurev-publhealth-052620-103528 PMID: 35020445

Walkowska, A., Przymuszała, P., Marciniak-Stępak, P., Nowosadko, M., & Baum, E. (2023). Enhancing cross-cultural competence of medical and healthcare students with the use of simulated patients—A systematic review. *International Journal of Environmental Research and Public Health*, *20*(3), 2505. DOI: 10.3390/ijerph20032505 PMID: 36767872

Wyman, M. F., Shiovitz-Ezra, S., & Bengel, J. (2018). Ageism in the health care system: Providers, patients, and systems. *Contemporary perspectives on ageism*, 193-212. DOI: 10.1007/978-3-319-73820-8

Zhang, L., Losin, E. A. R., Ashar, Y. K., Koban, L., & Wager, T. D. (2021). Gender biases in estimation of others' pain. *The Journal of Pain*, *22*(9), 1048–1059. DOI: 10.1016/j.jpain.2021.03.001 PMID: 33684539

Chapter 3
Intersectionality:
Where Identities Collide

Brittany Iris Hugue
https://orcid.org/0009-0001-6019-2150
Boonshoft School of Medicine, Wright State University, USA

EXECUTIVE SUMMARY

Intersectionality recognizes how interdependent identities can be linked to multiple sources of oppression. This chapter will explore how health disparities are exacerbated by the broken health infrastructure using the concept of intersectionality as its foundation. Socioeconomic factors including frameworks of past and current discriminatory housing practices, ableism, ageism, and the Black maternal health crisis will be incorporated to highlight the impact of systemic oppression in the context of the community and built environment. Though the four cases presented have different scenarios, they each demonstrate how health disparities and discrimination require solutions in patient-centered care as well as advancements in systems, policy, and law to create more equitable outcomes.

INTRODUCTION

Coined by advocate and scholar Kimberlé Crenshaw, intersectionality describes how race, class, gender, sexual orientation and other identities overlap and intersect with one another (Deleven, 2023). For example, if one identifies as a Black woman who is deaf, then each of her three identities overlap with interdependent systems of discrimination. As one may imagine, the more interdependent identities that one has, the more discrimination they may experience. This principle is easily applied

DOI: 10.4018/979-8-3693-3683-0.ch003

in situations involving health and the delivery of healthcare, more specifically, the Black maternal health crisis.

There are innumerable factors that can be explored that many people experience daily. There is extensive research on how health access and outcomes can be dependent on one's zip code. Where one lives can determine how quickly one receives care, where they receive care and the frequency of care. For example, if a patient lives in an affluent neighborhood and owns a car, then they may be more likely to attend their follow-up appointments. If the facility has an abundance of resources, then their quality of care may also be improved. In contrast, if the patient lives in a low-income neighborhood where public transportation is the main mode of transportation such as buses, then they may be less likely to attend follow-up appointments because they may have to take several buses to reach their destination in addition to the extensive time it may take. Also, the health care site may not even be accessible by bus line at all. Additionally, the hospital may have less staff and resources if they are underfunded so the quality of care may suffer. All these factors contribute to health disparities yet only address healthcare access and quality, one of the tenants of Social Determinants of Health (SDOH).

Likewise, even if one lives in an affluent area of an area of low-income yet they are underinsured, then their quality can still be adversely affected as there is a limited selection of physicians, they may be able to choose from, especially if they cannot afford out-of-pocket expenses. Physicians and free clinics who may serve patients within this population oftentimes have limited availability which delays access to care. This becomes more complicated when care needs to be specialized and requires many procedures.

To promote equity, we must focus on SDOH that impacts them. Two categories of SDOH that will be addressed are health care access and quality and neighborhood and built environment. Specifically, regarding health care access, there should be an emphasis on access and approach to care by creating a comprehensive interprofessional team by diversifying roles and cultural backgrounds. When addressing implicit bias and patient outcomes, it is important to encourage a diverse physician workforce, implement health equity training into the education of physicians and health professionals, as well as use data to track health outcomes. Currently, although Black individuals make up 13% of the population, they comprise just about 5% of the active physician workforce. Black female physicians comprise even less, representing only 2% of physicians overall (Bond et al., 2021). Lack of diversity leads to a lack of innovative ideas and lack of cultural understanding among a growing diverse patient population.

While there are efforts to diminish disparities and create equity, there are political interests that are negatively impacting progress made. With the overturning of affirmative action and increasing policies to eliminate education about equity, sociology, and systemic racism in both public and higher education, there will be latent effects that impact undergraduate and graduate medical education. With the Embracing Anti-Discrimination, Unbiased Curriculum, and Advancing Truth in Education (EDUCATE) Act, equity in medicine in still being threatened (AAMC, 2024). It demonstrates a pattern that will have dangerous effects not only on the healthcare of Black people and other minorities, it threatens the advancement of health care for all. Even still, medical schools and health professional programs should incorporate social determinants of health and health disparities education into the curriculum to equip students with an appreciation of cultural humility, to help them identify and address racial bias in themselves and medicine, and to clarify how health disparities can unfavorably affect both patient and healthcare system outcomes (Lacey & Johnston, 2020; Njoku et al., 2023).

For example, authored by Abraham Flexner, a Johns Hopkins trained science administrator and politician, Flexner Report was released in 1910 in commission for the Carnegie Foundation for the Advancement of Teaching. With Johns Hopkins serving as the gold standard, it evaluated medical schools in both America and Canada with the goal of standardizing medicine under the pretense that Complementary and Alternative Medicine (CAM) was "quackery," and should be weeded out of North American medicine (Stanisch & Verhoef, 2012, p.2). His report effectively weeded out 80% of medical schools. Thus, of the many Black medical schools in existence in the 1900's, only two were determined to be "legitimate," by the Flexner Report. including, Howard University in Washington, D.C. and Meharry Medical College in Nashville, Tennessee. (Stanisch & Verhoef, 2012, p.3; Laws, 2021).

With only two Black medical schools, the training of students of color to become physicians was severely diminished impacting the ability to serve underserved populations and populations of color. Moreover, it is significant to note Flexner's thoughts and intentions on why Black physicians should be trained; he suggested that Black students should be well trained to offer a limited scope of medical care to Black patients, (Flexner, 1910). Flexner emphasized Black physicians' duty to keep African Americans healthy enough not to contaminate nearby White people and that training at Howard and Meharry should concentrate on hygiene for Black people rather than surgery (Flexner, 1910). He states, "...ten million of them [negroes] live in close contact with sixty million whites. Not only does the negro himself suffer from hookworm and tuberculosis; he communicates them to his white neighbors," (Flexner, 1910).

The training that Flexner recommended, as modeled by Johns Hopkins, would be even more costly given his recommendation that schools integrate expensive laboratories and hospital-based practice into the structure of medical education (Laws, 2021). Without adequate funding compared to White institutions, both Howard and Meharry had less resources. Currently, there are four Black medical schools with the addition of Morehouse School of Medicine in Atlanta, Georgia and Charles R. Drew University of Medicine and Science in Los Angeles, California that were both established in the late 20th century. There are two more opening, sharing the same mission of serving the underserved.

Data from the 2018-2019 academic years shows that 60.5% of Black medical students plan to practice in a medically underserved area which is more than any other racial group (AAMC, n.d.). This data is consistent with current research in that most minorities are more likely to practice in these areas more than races that are not underrepresented in medicine such as Whites and Asians (AAMC, n.d.). Both Black and Latin physicians continue to be underrepresented in the medical workforce relative to their representation in the US population (Laws, 2021). Of those active in the physician workforce in 2018, 5% identified as Black (AAMC, 2018) although Black people compose 13% of the US general population (US Census Bureau, n.d.; Laws, 2021)

When matriculating to medical school, some students may not have had the opportunity to live, work, or serve in culturally diverse areas and have a lack of understanding of different religions, races or backgrounds. While interacting with patients this could lead to significant cultural bias that could influence patient outcomes. With the incorporation of SDOH and health equity into the curriculum, there is potential to challenge implicit bias and create awareness of health disparities that could be adequately addressed by physicians.

Intersectionality in Action: The Black Maternal Health Crisis

There is a history of systemic racism in our society including in medicine and medical education which has generational effects on minorities, specifically among Black people. Moreover, systemically, there is racial residential segregation because of many factors including historical racist practices such as Jim Crow laws and redlining which contributed to Black Americans being denied access to equitable housing, financial security, and access to care. As a result, there are growing disparities in chronic illness such as heart disease and the current Black maternal health crisis.

Sexism is also compounded in these forms of discrimination. While any gender can be discriminated against, sexism most often affects women and girls which can be a contributor in the Black maternal health crisis. Though not exhaustive, these factors still influence how and where large populations of Black Americans live. For example, recent studies in Chicago showed a relationship between racial residential segregation and its impact on Black maternal and infant health. Segregation was associated with lower odds of hypertensive disorder in pregnancy (HDP) in lower poverty neighborhoods and higher odds of HDP in higher poverty neighborhoods (Mayne et al., 2018).

Additionally, in high segregation areas, the prevalence of overall preterm birth was significantly higher than that in low segregation areas (15.5% vs 10.7%, respectively; $P < .001$) (Salow et al., 2018). This further supports that there is a correlation between health and racial residential segregation. From 2020 to 2021, the increases of maternal mortality for all race and Hispanic origin groups were significant. However, In 2021, the maternal mortality rate for non-Hispanic Black (subsequently, Black) women, like Watkins, was 69.9 deaths per 100,000 live births, 2.6 times the rate for non-Hispanic White (subsequently, White) women (26.6) (Hoyert, 2021). Rates for Black women were significantly higher than rates for White and Hispanic women.

While overall infant death rates have declined since the 19th century, the disparity in death rates between Black and White infants is greater today than it was under prewar slavery (Haines, n.d., CDC n.d.). In short, there is a generation of Black mothers and infants that are dying often preventable deaths at alarming rates. To address these statistics on a patient level, it is vital to focus on the contributing historical and social factors. Contributing factors in this current crisis that will be addressed include biases and lack of training in cultural humility and equity, as well as the systemic racism as it relates to social determinants of health (SDOH). CDC defines implicit bias as a form of prejudice in favor of or against a person or group that occurs unconsciously and unintentionally, but nevertheless affects judgments, decisions, and behaviors (NCCDPHP, 2022). This may seem minor to some; however, if an individual is not aware of their implicit bias, then they may easily act upon them including in their interactions with patients. This could influence diagnosis, management and treatment options which inevitably impacts health outcomes.

Black women are disproportionately more likely to die during and after labor. Even when wealth and education status are accounted for, Black women are more likely to experience adverse outcomes which supports the idea that race is an underlying cause. Contributing factors include but are not limited to access to primary care prior to pregnancy as well as prenatal care, distrust and discrimination among healthcare workers due to bias and systemic racism.

A more diverse inter-professional team positively improves the birthing journey and outcomes. Midwifery and doula care can raise patient satisfaction, reduce medical interventions during childbirth, and improve maternal and neonatal morbidity and mortality, particularly among women at higher risk of these outcomes (CDC n.d.) With this understanding, some women especially if they live in impoverished areas or have inadequate access to care may not be able to afford such services. However, it will cost less as a country to invest in these services than it would to pay for costly interventions that contribute to the Black maternal mortality crisis. Medicaid covers over 40 percent of U.S. births and 65 percent of births to Black mothers; almost 30% of Black women of reproductive age are in the Medicaid coverage gap (Solomon, 2021). A possible solution would be to expand Medicaid to include these services.

Intersectionality has been highlighted regarding not only Black maternal and infant morbidity and mortality but also the criminalization of Black women. Brittany Watts is a 33-year-old, Black woman in Ohio who won her case with a "no bill," or lack of evidence for indictment, from a grand jury for felony abuse of a corpse. Months prior, Watts unfortunately experienced a stillbirth and passed the fetus at home, in most women's cases, in her toilet. She sought medical care prior to the stillbirth and health professionals deemed that her 21-week 5 day old fetus was nonviable. She visited the hospital three times in the four days prior to her miscarriage and left against medical advice twice due to waiting hours to receive medical care including an induction of birth (Jevaid & Bellware, 2023).

When she passed the fetus in her toilet, it was mixed with blood, stool, tissue and other bodily fluid. Watts took out what she thought was clogging the toilet into a bucket that she placed outside near the garage. She again sought medical attention at her local hospital and confided in her nurse what occurred; the nurse asked her where the fetus was in which Watts disclosed to her that it was in the bucket at home. That same nurse was advised by risk management to call the local police without even notifying Watts. Unbeknownst to her, a political storm would ensue around such a deeply personal and tragic event. In Ohio, abortion is legal up to 22 weeks of pregnancy; her pregnancy was 21 weeks, 5 days gestation (Jevaid & Bellware, 2023).

Days later while Watts was still healing and receiving care at the hospital, a local detective interviewed Watts to inquire about the entire incident. Two weeks later, the detective arrested her on charges of felony abuse of a corpse. If she was indicted on the charges and found guilty, she would face up to a year in prison with a fine up to $2,500 (Jevaid & Bellware, 2023).

The law that she was accused of breaking explains that, "No person, except as authorized by law, shall treat a human corpse in a way that would outrage reasonable community sensibilities," (Jevaid & Bellware, 2023). Legal and healthcare professionals alike believe this vague, subjective language can have dangerous legal implications for women in relation to reproductive health when it historically fell under a broader law against grave robbing (Jevaid & Bellware, 2023). Her outcome rested in the decision of the grand jury after first going to her jurisdiction's municipal court. The grand jury returned a "no bill" for the charge stating that there was insufficient evidence for an indictment against Watts (Jevaid & Bellware, 2023).

Watts and her lawyer believe that her criminalization was in part since she was an unwed Black woman. In the climate of the 2022 Dobbs decision, women are faced with more scrutiny regarding their personal health. This case is only one of many that demonstrates the intersectionality of being a Black woman and how they are disproportionately criminalized while pregnant.

Additionally, regarding maternal health, misdiagnosis or delay of diagnosis may result in serious harm or death. This was evident in Watts' cases when she repeatedly sought medical attention and left after hours of not receiving care. When dissecting the events of her arrests, could the professionals who served on the ethics committee have succumbed to their own implicit bias which caused a delay in care? Moreover, could the nurse who originally reassured Watts only to call the police been acting on her own biases in that Watts was a Black woman? Thirty percent of Black and Hispanic women in the United States who delivered in a hospital reported provider mistreatment compared to twenty-one percent of White women (Vedam et al., 2019). In a survey on maternity care among women in California, Black women were ten times more likely to report unfair treatment and discrimination from maternity care providers when compared to White women (California Healthcare Foundation, 2018). On a patient level, if a mother feels unheard or is unfairly treated, she may be more reluctant to disclose important information that could affect diagnosis. Additionally, the patient-physician trust is broken.

Similarly, Regina McKnight who is a 22- year old Black woman in South Carolina, was the first woman in America to arrested, prosecuted, and convicted for experiencing a stillbirth under the notion of "homicide by child abuse." (Goodwin, 2017). The South Carolina jury reached this decision after only fifteen minutes of deliberation (Goodwin, 2017). McKnight had substance use disorder and used crack cocaine during her pregnancy, she also experienced a stillbirth yet the former does not necessitate a causal effect of the latter.

Though stillbirth can be due to a variety of causes, prosecutors assumed that her cocaine use caused the stillbirth and that she was subject to a homicide conviction. McKnight had no prior convictions and had a low-income as a farm worker. She spent seven years in prison but in 2008 her sentence was eventually overturned in a unanimous decision that she had an unfair trial. Critical evidence addressed the question of whether pre-natal exposure to substances causes harm to the fetus (Kasden, 2008). An expert medical testimony stated that, "recent studies showed that cocaine is no more harmful to a fetus than nicotine use, poor nutrition, lack of prenatal care or other conditions commonly associated with the urban poor," (Kasden, 2008). This highlights how the intersectionality of socioeconomic status, race and gender have major roles in the context of crime and its attribution to health disparities.

Social and racial factors are major contributors of the Black maternal mortality epidemic. We must address how systemic racism in medicine and the environment influence this disparity to improve the livelihood of Black mothers and infants. There should be enhanced training and education in maternal–fetal medicine to improve the management and medical care of pregnant women to address racial disparities in maternal mortality and severe morbidity (Njoku et al. 2023, D'Alton et al. 2019). This includes the incorporation of community leaders, social workers, and leaders in health equity into focus groups and continuing education opportunities. To assess baseline data and monitor health outcomes, healthcare providers can use clinical resources and tools to address perinatal safety, establish mindful care, recognize and address unconscious bias and stigma in themselves and in their offices to promote cultural awareness and health equity (Njoku et al., 2023; Hear Her Campaign, 2008).

History of the Wealth Gap and Racial Discriminatory Practices

Classism discriminates against others due to their socioeconomic status and is evident in medicine among patients, healthcare workers and medical students. Dangerous consequences thereof can result in lower quality care for patients, discriminatory treatment of lower paying jobs to for healthcare workers from a lower socioeconomic status, and lack of support and mistreatment to medical students from lower socioeconomic status. These consequences can have implications in communities specifically in the five domains of SDOH: economic stability, education access and quality, healthcare access and quality, neighborhood and built environment, social and community context. While separate domains, they are often interconnected with m magnified effects among many demographics especially marginalized communities.

It is widely accepted that education, especially higher-ed is considered a main avenue to build wealth as it creates opportunities to compete in a variety of fields and industries as well as it teaches valuable skills. When considering higher-education, Black people were often barred from attending existing colleges and universities and if they were permitted, they faced racism and discrimination. For this reason, historically Black colleges and universities (HBCUs) were established with many of them located in the Southeastern region. This afforded many Black students the opportunity to compete with their White counterparts that they otherwise would not have been granted resources to do so.

Black people have historically been denied access to fair housing and opportunities to build wealth through homeownership. Namely, the GI Bill was promised to veterans after World War II however, Southern Democrats ensured that Black veterans were denied access. As a result, the program was administered by states instead of the federal government where they were able to individually regulate access (Blakemore, 2019). The GI Bill also guaranteed low-interest mortgages though they were not administered by the VA; rather, they were given to White-run financial institutions which resulted in Black veterans being refused the same loans that White veterans were granted though they both fought in the same war (Blakemore, 2019). For example, only 2 of the 3,229 VA guaranteed loans made in 13 Mississippi cities in 1947 went to Black veterans (Katznelson & Mettler, 2008, p. 523).

These racist practices were not exclusive to southern states. “In New York and the northern New Jersey suburbs, fewer than 100 of the 67,000 mortgages insured by the GI bill supported home purchases by non-whites,” (Katznelson, 2005, p.140). Another barrier to obtaining fair housing was the implementation of redlining by government and banks. Redlining is the practice of arbitrarily denying or limiting financial services to specific neighborhoods, generally because its residents are people of color or are poor (Hunt, 2019). Redlining was implemented by the New Deal’s Homeowner’s Loan Corporation (HOLC) by instituting a redlining policy by developing color-coded maps of American cities that used racial criteria to categorize lending and insurance risks (Hunt, 2019). These gaps in opportunity initially targeted Black populations but have impacted the health and opportunities of all in the areas affected since.

These new, affluent, racially homogeneous housing areas received green lines while Black and poor White neighborhoods were often circumscribed by red lines denoting their undesirability (Hunt, 2019). Banks and insurers soon adopted the HOLC's maps and practices to guide lending and underwriting decisions. Further, the Federal Housing Administration, created in 1934, also used the HOLC's methods to assess locations for federally insured new housing construction (Hunt, 2019). With the adoption of such policies, Black and poor people were gridlocked into neighborhoods without the funding and accommodations of affluent White neighborhoods. Thus, if homeownership serves as a form of generational wealth, the impacts of redlining are not only confined to one time period, rather its effects are translated into how some communities are still built today.

Most notably, Navy Federal, America’s largest credit union whose membership consists of all branches of the armed forces and eligible family members, is facing a class action lawsuit that alleges they used racial bias in mortgage lending. The lawsuit was filed against the $168 billion-asset institution after a CNN report in December 2023 that the credit union approved about 77% of mortgage applications from White borrowers, but only 56% of applications from Latinos and 48% from Black applicants in 2022. Citing Consumer Financial Protection Bureau data, CNN found that this represented the greatest disparity among the 50 largest residential mortgage lenders in the U.S. The gap remained “even after accounting for variables such as applicants' income, debt-to-income ratio, property value and down payment percentage,” CNN reported (Dobbs, 2023).

Intersectional Ableism

Classism can also result in power dynamics between physicians and other health care professionals alike towards patients. When patients have a disability, these power dynamics can be intensified because disabled patients are easily discriminated against as a minority group whom often requires special accommodations.

An estimated 1 in 4 U.S. adults has a disability (CDC, 2024). Disabilities can include cognition, mobility, independent living, deafness or difficulty hearing, vision and blindness, and self-care with difficulty dressing and bathing (CDC, 2024). Unfortunately, persons with disabilities have historically been mistreated and discriminated against in society including healthcare. They have been denied opportunities for equitable care, housing and employment opportunities. In 1990, the Americans with Disabilities Act (ADA) of 1990 was signed as a federal civil rights law that prohibits discrimination against people with disabilities in everyday activities. The ADA guarantees that people with disabilities have the same opportunities as everyone else to enjoy employment opportunities, purchase goods and services, and participate in state and local government programs.

Though this law has been in effect for over three decades, discrimination against persons with disabilities still occur even among healthcare providers. These discriminatory practices have negative effects the health and well-being for a vulnerable population. Individuals face significant healthcare inequities, including but not limited to inaccessibility and mistreatment (Jean, 2022). For example, health care facilities are commonly do not have proper equipment, resources, or trained staff to provide equitable care to patients with disabilities. Since disabled patients. Lagu et al. found that physicians often felt overwhelmed by the demands of practicing medicine in requirements with the American Disabilities Act of 1990 and felt like they were inadequately reimbursed for accommodations. It was noted that physicians were reluctant to care for people with disabilities and some even attempted discharge people with disabilities from their practice (Lagu, 2022).

The inequities are not just from physicians. There is a history of mistreatment of patients with disabilities including the intentional infection of intellectually disabled children with hepatitis at Willowbrook State School of Staten Island in the 1950s, and the forced sterilization and systematic killing of disabled people by the Nazis during World War II (Jean,2022). This mistreatment of a minority and vulnerable population can be juxtaposed to the mistreatment other minority groups have endured as previously mentioned. When patients have intersection identities, the inequities can be compounded.

The lack of accommodations and increasing bias towards patients with disabilities is both systemic and personal. There is an urgent need to better understand and address clinician- and system-level barriers to care for people with disabilities.

Jean et al outlines a three-step approach to help address inequities faces by patients with disabilities:

1. Medical education should include disability rights education and structured opportunities for medical trainees to work with disabled populations early in and throughout clinical training.
2. Pathways for disabled people to enter medicine needs to be strengthened.
3. Care for disabled patients must be trauma-informed.

Though these recommendations are not exhaustive, they are a start.

Medical education should include people with disabilities in patient and teaching roles to provide direct perspective that is not solely through the medical model lens with the hopes to address the built environment, ableism, and structural barriers that impact patients with disabilities health and wellbeing (Jean, 2022). Moreover, increasing providers with disabilities who will have their own lived experiences and understanding of the trauma that disabled patients may experience and could result in a higher likelihood of thorough care. However, it is not enough to rely solely on disabled physicians to provide this care, and we must produce trained physicians who do not identify as disabled (Jean, 2022). Trauma-informed care (TIC) is an interdisciplinary framework that approaches patient care interactions with the acknowledgement that trauma is pervasive and occurs in all populations (Trauma Informed Care, 2018). This practice can be incorporated into medical education and used as an approach to many patients especially those with disabilities. For example, mandated documentation of disability status and accommodation needs in the electronic health record could help clinicians and practices prepare for the needs of people with disabilities ahead of a planned visit (Morris, 2021). With better preparation, providers may feel less frustrated with time commitments so that they can provide better care and improve work flow.

CASES

Case 1: Birthing While Black

Learning Objectives

1. Recognizing that there is a Black maternal health crisis
2. Analyzing how intersectionality contributes to this crisis
3. Understand how shared cultural background between patients and physicians can impact care

Case Aim: Stress and racist interactions can be indirect contributors in the Black maternal health crisis.

Brianna Watkins is a 33 year-old Black woman in the second trimester of her and her husband's first pregnancy and they are excited to welcome their baby girl. She had a high-level position in economics at a prominent international company; she was only one of two Black people in her department and the only woman in a leadership position. She attended all of her doctors' appointments throughout the pregnancy; since she has been deemed low-risk, she elected to have a birth in the hospital's birth center, Your Birth. Your Birth is a low-intervention option where patients must pass screening and meet a set of requirements that deem them to be acceptable candidates for a low-intervention birth. Other than her mounting stress from work, Brianna was healthy and had an uneventful pregnancy thus far.

Brianna joined a birthing group at Your Birth with moms who had similar due dates. There were no Black instructors, and the only other minority participant was a Hispanic woman. Brianna often felt that the lessons and topics of the group had minimal cultural context. When Brianna expressed to the midwife who led class that she had been experiencing sharp abdominal pain for three days, the midwife only asked two follow-up questions: 1) Was she currently using drugs or other substances during her pregnancy 2) Was there any bleeding. Once she replied no, the midwife shrugged off her concerns and told her that the pain she was feeling was not concerning. Taken aback by the questions, Brianna was enraged and in disbelief.

ED Visit

Brianna went home and a few hours later she had an abrupt leakage of fluid at 32 weeks. She was rushed to the emergency room and was hospitalized. There she was diagnosed with Preterm Premature Rupture of Membranes and preeclampsia. Brianna was induced and received the necessary medication including corticosteroids and antibiotics to ensure the safest delivery possible. Dr. Jennings, the OB/GYN on call was a Black woman who shared a similar cultural background. Brianna disclosed her previous interaction with the midwife and the OB/GYN responded with compassion and cultural humility; she was present during the delivery.

Jayla, was born 4 lbs and 6 oz. She was discharged home after being treated in the NICU for four weeks. Brianna was discharged home after four days. Physiologically, she had greatly improved and her preeclampsia subsided soon after delivery. However, she had postpartum depression because she blamed herself for her diagnosis and her baby's current state. With medication and intense therapy, she gradually began improving prior to Jayla's discharge. Due to her depression, she was not motivated to breastfeed so she did not have this particular bonding experience with Jayla like she previously desired during pregnancy. Dr. Jennings referred her to a diverse mother support group where Brianna navigated being a new mom including her mental health struggles. She strongly connected with two moms in the group and remained friends with them. Because of the group, she learned about relocation and is looking forward to working with a local lactation team to help in this area so that she can get the breastfeeding experience she desires.

Case Questions

1. What Historical Events Have Created a Space for This Current Situation?

- Historically, there Black people commonly have a distrust in medicine due to mistreatment, wrongful, and illegal practices. For example, it was commonly accepted that Black people had a higher pain tolerance and were often experimented on for unethical procedures and practices including the Tuskegee trials and obstetric experimentation by Dr. J. Marion Sims, a white physician who enslaved, abused, and experimented on Black women, specifically Anarcha, Betsey, and Lucy (Zellars, 2018). Historically, these scenarios demonstrate how Black people's dignity, humanity, and concerns are dismissed just like Brianna.

2. What Does the Language in This Scenario Tell Us About the Assumptions Being Made?

- The language tells us that Brianna was already in a situation where she was not understood. She was the only one of two minorities and the only Black person in her maternity circle which can be isolating; this is exacerbated by the lack of cultural connection amongst other mothers or group leaders.

  What was most egregious were one of the two questions asked by the midwife specifically the use of drugs during pregnancy because it implies that since she is Black, her current pain is due to substance use disorder. Th question would have been more appropriate if there were additional questions asked related to her abdominal pain other than just drug use and bleeding especially since she asked about drug use first.

3. What (If Anything) Could Have Prevented This Patient's Diagnosis or a Visit to the ED?

- There is not a clear answer on if anything could have prevented the patient's diagnosis. However, stress can contribute to pregnancy complications. This patient had surmounting stress at work and had an emotionally stressful event during her interaction with the midwife while experiencing ongoing abdominal pain. Had the patient received care sooner, or had not had her concerns dismissed, she may have been less stressed.

4. How Do We Address This Patient's Needs?

- We address this patient's needs by first ensuring the safety of her and her unborn child. She needs immediate care and her desires should be acknowledged and respected by all medical staff. Secondly, we should practice cultural humility and understanding as there may be a level of distrust given her previous interaction with the midwife. She previously expressed her concerns, and she was dismissed with racial implications. Also, we must be aware that she may grieve the fact that she is no longer going to have the low-intervention birth in Your Birth given the severity of her situation. This can be another layer of stress that could be easily overlooked while more pressing matters regarding her delivery are addressed. It's important to practice shared-decision making throughout this process while discussing possible interventions, treatment options and decisions regarding the life of her and her unborn child.

5. What Emotions Are You Feeling as the Physician in This Case?

- Use this time to self-reflect. Here are a few questions to guide you: Are there instances where health care providers should be reprimanded for their behavior? How can we better support Black women in their pregnancy journeys? What biases do we have that may be similar or different than those presented in this case?

6. Are There Any Beliefs That You Have That May Be Stretched Right Now?

- Use this time to self-reflect. There is a current Black maternal health crisis and Black moms and babies have higher mortality rates than other racial groups even when they are more educated or have a higher income. One of the contributing factors to this crisis is discrimination and concerns being dismissed moreso than other racial groups which is evident in Brianna's case. This may stretch one's belief that this may not happen to them because they are an executive at an affluent company or a physician themselves but it can happen to anyone, it just more commonly occurs among Black women.

Case Discussion

Brianna unfortunately had complications during her birth despite being healthy and seeking regular prevention and maintenance. The stress she endured at work related to her race and being a woman as well the discrimination she experienced with the midwife are examples of how intersectionality can influence patient interactions and health outcomes. Would she have experienced the same undue stress if she was a White woman? Feeling unheard and with increased stress are two factors contributing to the current Black maternal health crisis.

Brianna was able to disclose her racist encounter to Dr. Jennings because she felt comfortable to do so. It is widely known that there can be better compliance and health outcomes when the physician and patient share a similar cultural background (Snyder, 2023). Since Dr. Jennings responded to Brianna with compassion, she may have eased some pressure in an acutely high-stressful situation where Brianna had to make important decisions regarding the life and safety of her and Jayla.

Case 2. Dying From Lack

Learning Objectives

1. Understand how health care systems can capitalize from the wealth gap and influence health disparities
2. Explore how hospitals and health systems can take advantage of government and public funding
3. Understand how inability to access equitable health resources can directly impact patient care

Case Aim: Patient has chronic condition that was exacerbated due to preventable social factors.

George Thomas, a 54 year old man living in an under-resourced and underinsured neighborhood, visited the emergency department at his local hospital to receive care for his ongoing chest pain. George had an extensive history of hypertension and was not able to afford his antihypertensive medications for the past four months due to lack of insurance since he was let go from his job. He relied on the bus to take him to work but the city recently changed bus routes to now accommodate the gentrified city center thus displacing some routes in lower socioeconomic areas; he no longer lived on the bus line and had no transportation to work. He had a license but his previous vehicles constantly needed repairs so he decided to take the bus to work until he could save money for a more reliable vehicle. His transportation to work was unreliable and due to repeated tardiness, he lost his job and medical insurance.

He frequented the ER multiple times with similar complaints for the past two weeks and was advised to follow up with his primary care physician whom he could not access due to his lack of insurance. There, it was determined that he had a myocardial infarction and needed advanced care. Instead of being able to receive adequate care from said hospital, the lack of equipment and specialists prohibited necessary treatment. It was not until hours later that he was able to get the care he needed after being transferred to another hospital.

Due to the delay in care, George unfortunately died. However, his case was brought up in leadership meetings at the hospital which motivated important changes. For instance, the ED staff demanded additional support for their patients which led to hiring of more physicians, nurses and techs within a 12-month period. Additionally, there was a policy put in place to have patients without health insurance to follow up at the local free clinic and be given resources for other health insurance options.

It was determined that there was an increase in preventative health-related emergencies following the changed bus route which was costing the local and state-government money. As a result, there have been discussions between governmental and health leaders as local business people on how to rectify this issue.

Case Questions

1. What Socioeconomic Factors Contributed to This Patient's Unfortunate Health Outcome?

- The bus route changed which led to the downward spiral of George losing his job and insurance. The reason for the bus route changed is rooted in prioritizing profit even if it displaces communities with lower incomes such as George. Additionally, since there is not universal healthcare and this patient's insurance was provided by his place of employment, he could no longer afford preventative or maintenance care including medication for his hypertension.

2. How Would a PCP's Role Have Positively Impacted This Patient's Care Plan?

- A PCP could have monitored George's blood pressure more regularly, possibly found solutions for him to receive his blood pressure medication and refer him to the appropriate physician/care if his chest pain still occurred despite interventions.

3. What Resources Could Have Been Offered so That George Could Have Received His Medication?

- Ultimately George needs health insurance to pay for his medication and employment for a source of incomed and reliable transportation so that he can remain employed. Possible resources would be a referral to job readiness sites/agencies that could help with new employment that is more local to him so that he could potentially walk or bike to work, access to carpool or rideshare services, and instructions and/or assistance to sign up for insurance in the healthcare marketplace. In the meantime of finding employment, George may need access to local food bank so that he can still eat regular meals that are align with his health goals.

4. How Do Hospital Funding and Resources Influence Patient Outcomes Such as George's?

- Lack of hospital funding led to the facility being understaffed and under resourced. For acute cases like George's, it caused a delay in care because he had to be transported to another facility. Likewise, in cases of prevention and maintenance such as screenings and imaging, this could also lead to delays in care specifically for local residents thus potentially causing additional barriers to health equity because they have to travel longer distances and have less access to care than residents who live local to a better funded and resourced hospital. With less appropriate staffing, there can also a higher chance of mistakes as available staff may burn out quicker because of being overworked or not adequately supported.

5. What Emotions or Responsibility Are You Feeling as the Physician in This Case?

- Use this time to self-reflect. Here are some questions to guide you: How can the healthcare system be improved for patients without insurance? How can physicians and other healthcare professionals be advocates for their patients who have many social factors contributing to their health? What responsibilities do physicians and other healthcare professionals must advocate for patients in public policy?

6. Are There Any Beliefs That You Have That May Be Stretched Right Now?

- Use this time to self-reflect. Here are some thoughts to guide you. Consider how capitalism impacts healthcare. Think about how where patients live may influence type of care they receive.

Case Discussion

Health systems have a responsibility to serve their patients with integrity while providing equitable care. While many health systems can have challenges related to funding and staffing, it is commonplace for hospitals in low-income neighborhoods to be adversely affected.

Federal money is allocated to health systems to fund underserved communities but there are loopholes that permit organizations to use money for other purposes. Without a lack of transparency, patients in underserved or low-income communities are deprived of access to quality and equitable healthcare which magnifies health disparities and leads to adverse health outcomes such as what George experienced. Oftentimes, due to systemic racism, these communities are comprised of Black people and other minorities.

While this case explores one health system, more than half of the hospitals in the United States are a part of this program. Similar dangerous scenarios could be occurring nationwide thus inflating health disparities that result from the widened wealth gap within this country.

Case 3: Discrimination Against Disabilities

Learning Objectives

1. Understand that patients with disabilities face discrimination in society and healthcare
2. Cultivate skills in prioritizing patient needs
3. Explore how implicit bias impacts patient care

Case Aim: Patient has a disability and seeks medication that is morally conflicting for physician.

32 year old White female, Gina, who is a paraplegic comes in for OCPs and the doctor is a male who is Catholic. Doctor never has never had a patient who is paraplegic and wishes he could send her to another physician in the office. He never

discusses sexual history or pregnancy intention and refuses to prescribe when the patient brings it up.

Gina was in an MVA six months ago which resulted in her paraplegia but the physician never asked about her history. She wanted to get on OCPs because her menstrual cycle has become irregular due to depression following her new lifestyle change. It was more challenging to manage her personal and menstrual hygiene especially with current irregular cycles, so she wanted to try OCPs. She was referred to a family medicine doctor who has a large demographic of patients with disabilities, so she was able to get her OCPs as well as social and mental support through treatment and a support group.

Case Questions

1. How Is This Case Impacted by Intersectionality?

- The patient is a female who is paraplegic. It is important to acknowledge that ableism, or the discrimination against people with disabilities, is common in our society including medicine. One can look down upon persons with disabilities, including physicians who may have implicit bias. Additionally, she is requesting treatment regarding her reproductive health, a vulnerable topic, to a male doctor which can be uncomfortable.

    It is important to understand her sexual history including trauma as well as her needs for OCPs and to respect her autonomy to receive them, if she does not have any contraindications. It is not uncommon for patients with disabilities to be vulnerable to abuse so we must consider this possibility in her story.

2. What Cultural Values or Norms Are Being Assumed? Which May Be Missing?

- It is being assumed that the patient is using OCPs for pregnancy intention which opposes many traditional Catholic beliefs. Some physicians feel a moral obligation to deny patients of OCPs, denying them of their autonomy to be the primary decision maker in their reproductive health. In contrast, the patient may want them to regulate her menstrual cycle or treat painful periods.

3. What Do We Have to Consider in Making a Plan With This Patient?

- We must consider that patients with disabilities are more likely to have medical appointments than the general population and more likely to experience medical trauma (Jean, 2022). Therefore, we must consider a plan that ensures there is no mistreatment. Additionally, many physicians do not properly perform exams on patients with certain disabilities or who are wheelchair bound. Since this patient may require a pap smear, it is vital the physician knows how and feels comfortable performing one on Gina.

    Since prescribing OCPs goes against moral values, then the patient must be directed to another physician who will. Unfortunately, this is a barrier to patient care that presents more challenges to patients with disabilities especially if they require transportation accommodations. However, we must ensure that the physician offices are properly equipped for our patient to have full access.

4. How Do We Address This Patient's Needs?

- We address this patient's needs by acknowledging them and treating her with dignity like we would a patient who didn't have a disability by respecting her decision making. If there are no contraindications, then she should be prescribed OCPs. Patients with disabilities are often victims of abuse of different kinds including sexual abuse (Mailhot, 2022) so it is important to discuss sexual history including trauma.

5. What Areas of This Patient's Identity Have Been Left Out of Our Consideration?

- We have not considered how long this patient has been paraplegic or the cause of her paraplegia. This could be a new condition or preexisting condition. Perhaps this patient has been using OCPs for an extended period and she could simply be requesting this prescription that she is accustomed to taking and he is a new provider. We also have not considered her socioeconomic status which may be severely impacted by an unwanted pregnancy or cultural factors that may impact her support system if she was pregnant.

6. What Next Steps or Resources Are Needed Here?

- If this provider will not prescribe this patient an OCP, then he must refer her to a physician who will and ensure that the facility has accommodations for wheelchair accessibility, with a physician who is comfortable performing necessary examinations on this patient.

7. What Emotions Are You Feeling as the Physician in This Case?

- Use this time to self-reflect. Here are some questions to guide you: How can physicians and other healthcare professionals personal or moral beliefs impact patients goals? When health care professionals personal beliefs directly oppose patient goals, how should this conflict be resolved?

Case Discussion

Patients with disabilities are often discriminated against and often do not have the basic accommodations needed in healthcare and society. Many healthcare facilities may not have wheelchair accessible scales or adjustable height tables in exam rooms. Moreover, medical education rarely includes disability related training among medical students and residents which can result in misinformed or low-quality care.

In this scenario, there was ableism intersected with religious beliefs which resulted in denial of a potentially helpful medication for Gina. Where is the fine line between upholding moral beliefs versus having unethical practices that deny patients the right to autonomy and justice? This ongoing debate often leaves patients without the care they deserve. Even with moral preferences, as a physician, it is important to ensure the best quality care that addresses the patients needs even if it means providing a referral to someone who can provide better care.

Case 4. Golden Age

Learning Objectives

1. Describe how implicit bias against older adults and different cultures impact care
2. Recognize how to prioritize patient care plans that best with patient goals
3. Discuss how professionalism impacts patient care

Case Aim: Patient has specific care goals following injury that caused an unfavorable change in lifestyle

Julio, a 70 y/o Hispanic male visited Riley, a physiatrist for rehabilitation following a surgery for knee replacement. Rehabilitation has lasted longer than expected and Julio cannot ambulate without assistance or walker. His main goal of care is to become fully independent and be able to run 10ks like he did prior to his injury. Julio moved to America from Guatemala when he was a teenager so English is his second language. He is also on the board of directors where Riley works.

Riley often complains that his workplace culture has declined because of DEI efforts in hiring unqualified employees. Riley has not re-assessed Julio after his physical therapy and has rescheduled his appointments at least twice because he says that they are unnecessary even though his care plan states otherwise. Riley often emphasizes that most of his patients are young and healthy and subtly suggests that Julio should consider nursing homes with options for more physical therapy.

Julio requested to work with a different physiatrist that could help him reach his goals. Upon reassessment, it was determined that Julio needed additional physical therapy which Julio was determined to complete. He joined a support group because it was more challenging both mentally and emotionally to adjust to his physical restraints than he originally perceived. He and his patient care team are hopeful that he will still be able to live independently and run again.

Moreover, Julio reported Riley for his discriminatory comments and lack of professionalism when he rescheduled twice without cause. Riley will be required to attend a training on implicit bias and the importance of health equity.

Case Questions

1. How is this case impacted by intersectionality?
    - The patient is a Hispanic immigrant and an older adult. Immigrants can be discriminated against especially from nationalist or other groups if they feel they "do not belong in this country." As an older adult, Julio can also be discriminated against for his age.
2. What cultural values or norms are being assumed? Which may be missing?
    - It is being assumed that DEI is to blame because of Riley's unhappiness with his workplace which could be a direct insult to Julio since he is a part of the board of directors. While one may or may not agree with DEI, his open disdain can be condescending to individuals from multicultural backgrounds because it may imply that equitable and inclusive environments and practices are not valued.
3. What does the language in this scenario tell us about the assumptions being made?

- The language tells us that Riley assumes that Julio should consider a nursing home because of his age although Juilio's goals of care is to live independently and return to running. As a result, Riley does not give him the quality care that he deserves that perhaps he would have given most of his patients who are "young and healthy." It is ageist to discriminate against older adults and assume they are not healthy, can live an active lifestyle, and live independently since they are older.

4. What do we have to consider in planning with this patient?
    - This patient's goals of care must be considered. He clearly states that he wants to live independently and return to running, therefore, his progress needs to be monitored as he completes physical therapy and thereafter, which is a part of Riley's responsibilities.
5. Based upon Riley's actions, how do you think Julio feels?
    - Julio may feel disregarded and undervalued. He seems eager to recover from his injury however, Riley assumes that he should settle for a nursing home instead of living independently. Additionally, he may feel angered that Riley assumes that he is only hired because he is Hispanic and not that he is qualified to serve on the board of directors.
6. What next steps or resources are needed here?
    - Julio needs to be reassessed by a qualified and willing physiatrist to determine his progress. Since he already has goals of care, the reassessment and recommendations thereafter need to align with the goals of care as much as possible. Emotional and social support can be offered because patients who have injuries that alter their lifestyle are at increased risk for depression.
7. What emotions are you feeling as the physician in this case?
    - Use this time to self-reflect. Here are a few questions to guide you: Are there instances where health care providers should be reprimanded for their behavior? How can we hold our colleagues accountable? What biases do we have that may be similar or different than those presented in this case?

Case Discussion

Older adults are often victims of ageism not only in the workplace, but in healthcare as well. It is unjust for healthcare workers to assume younger or older adults are not cognitively astute, or in the case of Julio, able to heal and recover with the goals of independent living.

As physicians and healthcare workers, it is important to evaluate our patients' history and abilities individually and not assume their limitations solely based on what we perceive is age appropriate. Shared-decision making should be incorporated with our patients throughout their wellness journeys.

CONCLUSION

This chapter explored how intersecting identities can impact existing health disparities in the contexts such as race, gender, socioeconomic status, disability, and age. Specifically patients, but healthcare workers, and medical students alike can be discriminated against which adversely affects their quality of care, health outcomes, career decisions, and well-being. With each case, there is overwhelming evidence that disparities are results of years' worth of unjust practices against minority groups even with enforced policies and laws.

Incorporating exposure of how intersectionality contributes to discrimination which negatively influences health outcome is vital to medical education. Strategic plans should be in place to educate students how to provide equitable care to their future patients by addressing implicit and explicit bias. Additionally, it would be impactful for health care professionals to learn how they can influence public policy on a local and national level. Improved understanding of how policies affect care is required to diminish health disparity through patient and political advocacy for the sake of improved heath and health infrastructure in America.

REFERENCES

AAMC. (2024, March 22). *EDUCATE Act Introduced by Rep. Greg Murphy, M.D.* AAMC. https://www.aamc.org/advocacy-policy/washington-highlights/educate-act-introduced-rep-greg-murphy-md

AAMC. (n.d.). *Figure 11. Percentage of U.S. medical school matriculants planning to practice in an underserved area by race/ethnicity, academic year 2018-2019.* AAMC. https://www.aamc.org/data-reports/workforce/data/figure-11-percentage-us-medical-school-matriculants-planning-practice-underserved-area-race

Association of American Medical Colleges. (2018). *Figure 18. Percentage of all active physicians by race/ethnicity, 2018.* AAMC. https://www.aamc.org/data-reports/workforce/interactive-data/figure-18-percentage-all-active-physicians-race/ethnicity-2018

Blakemore, E. (2019, June 27). *How the GI Bill's Promise Was Denied to a Million Black WWII Veterans.* HISTORY. https://www.history.com/news/gi-bill-black-wwii-veterans-benefits

Bond, R. M., Gaither, K., Nasser, S. A., Albert, M. A., Ferdinand, K. C., Njoroge, J. N., Parapid, B., Hayes, S. N., Pegus, C., Sogade, B., Grodzinsky, A., Watson, K. E., McCullough, C. A., & Ofili, E. (2021). Working Agenda for Black Mothers. *Circulation: Cardiovascular Quality and Outcomes*, *14*(2), e007643. Advance online publication. DOI: 10.1161/CIRCOUTCOMES.120.007643 PMID: 33563007

California Healthcare Foundation. (2018). *Listening to Black Mothers in California ISSUE BRIEF.* https://www.nationalpartnership.org/our-work/resources/health-care/maternity/listening-to-black-mothers-in-california.pdf

CDC. (2024, December 10). *Disability Impacts All of Us Infographic.* Disability and Health. https://www.cdc.gov/disability-and-health/articles-documents/disability-impacts-all-of-us-infographic.html?CDC_AAref_Val=https://www.cdc.gov/ncbddd/disabilityandhealth/infographic-disability-impacts-all.html

CDC. (n.d.). *Centers for Disease Control and Prevention User guide to the 2016 Period Linked Birth/Infant Death Public Use File.* https://ftp.cdc.gov/pub/Health_Statistics/NCHS/Dataset_Documentation/DVS/periodlinked/LinkPE16Guide.pdf

D'Alton, M. E., Friedman, A. M., Bernstein, P. S., Brown, H. L., Callaghan, W. M., Clark, S. L., Grobman, W. A., Kilpatrick, S. J., O'Keeffe, D. F., Montgomery, D. M., Srinivas, S. K., Wendel, G. D., Wenstrom, K. D., & Foley, M. R. (2019). Putting the "M" back in maternal-fetal medicine: A 5-year report card on a collaborative effort to address maternal morbidity and mortality in the United States. *American Journal of Obstetrics and Gynecology*, *221*(4), 311–317.e1. DOI: 10.1016/j.ajog.2019.02.055 PMID: 30849353

Delevan, K. (2023, November 4). *Research Guides: FYS 101: Intersectionality*. Researchguides.library.syr.edu. https://researchguides.library.syr.edu/fys101/intersectionality#:~:text=Intersectionality%20(or%20intersectional%20theory)%20is

Dobbs, J. (2023). *Navy Federal faces lawsuit, allegations of racial bias in mortgage lending. American Banker, N.* PAG.

Flexner, A. (1910). Medical education in the United States and Canada. *Science*, *32*(810), 41–50. DOI: 10.1126/science.32.810.41 PMID: 17745880

Goodwin, M. (2017). How the Criminalization of Pregnancy Robs Women of Reproductive Autonomy. *The Hastings Center Report*, *47*(S3), S19–S27. DOI: 10.1002/hast.791 PMID: 29171895

Haines, M. (n.d.). *Fertility and Mortality in the United States*. Eh.net; Economic History Association. https://eh.net/encyclopedia/fertility-and-mortality-in-the-united-states/

Hawkins, B. D. (2023). New Beginnings. *Diverse Issues in Higher Education*, *40*(9), 31–33.

Hear Her Campaign. (2022, September 8). *Clinical Resources and Tools | CDC*. Www.cdc.gov. https://www.cdc.gov/hearher/healthcare-providers/clinical-resources-tools.html

Hoyert, D. (2023, March 16). *Maternal Mortality Rates in the United States, 2021*. Www.cdc.govCenters for Disease Control and Prevention. https://www.cdc.gov/nchs/data/hestat/maternal-mortality/2021/maternal-mortality-rates-2021.htm#:~:text=In%202021%2C%20the%20maternal%20mortality

Hunt, B. (2019). *Redlining*. Chicagohistory.org. http://www.encyclopedia.chicagohistory.org/pages/1050.html

Javaid, M., & Bellware, K. (2024, January 3). She miscarried in her bathroom. Now she's charged with abuse of a corpse. *Washington Post*. https://www.washingtonpost.com/nation/2023/12/15/ohio-woman-miscarriage-abuse-of-corpse-grand-jury/

Jean, C., & Cyr, E. (2022). Accessible Medical Education & TIC: Increasing Equitable Care for Disabled Patients. *Harvard Public Health Review (Cambridge, Mass.), 44*. https://hphr.org/edition-44-su/ and https://pmc.ncbi.nlm.nih.gov/articles/PMC9518008/#R40 PMID: 36176338

Kasden, D. (2008, May 15). *Victory in the Regina McKnight Case | News & Commentary*. American Civil Liberties Union. https://www.aclu.org/news/reproductive-freedom/victory-regina-mcknight-case

Katznelson, I. (2005). *When Affirmative Action was White: An Untold History of Racial Inequality in Twentieth-century America*. W.W. Norton.

Katznelson, I., & Mettler, S. (2008). On Race and Policy History: A Dialogue about the G.I. Bill. *Perspectives on Politics*, *6*(3), 519–537. https://www.jstor.org/stable/20446759. DOI: 10.1017/S1537592708081267

Lagu, T., Haywood, C., Reimold, K., DeJong, C., Walker Sterling, R., & Iezzoni, L. I. (2022). "I Am Not The Doctor For You": Physicians' Attitudes About Caring For People With Disabilities. *Health Affairs*, *41*(10), 1387–1395. DOI: 10.1377/hlthaff.2022.00475 PMID: 36190896

Laws, T. (2021). How Should We Respond to Racist Legacies in Health Professions Education Originating in the Flexner Report? *AMA Journal of Ethics*, *23*(3), 271–275. DOI: 10.1001/amajethics.2021.271 PMID: 33818380

Lucey, C. R., & Johnston, S. C. (2020). The Transformational Effects of COVID-19 on Medical Education. *Journal of the American Medical Association*, *324*(11), 1033. Advance online publication. DOI: 10.1001/jama.2020.14136 PMID: 32857137

Mailhot Amborski, A., Bussières, E.-L., Vaillancourt-Morel, M.-P., & Joyal, C. C. (2021). Sexual Violence Against Persons With Disabilities: A Meta-Analysis. *Trauma, Violence & Abuse*, *23*(4), 152483802199597. DOI: 10.1177/1524838021995975 PMID: 33657931

Mayne, S. L., Yellayi, D., Pool, L. R., Grobman, W. A., & Kershaw, K. N. (2018). Racial Residential Segregation and Hypertensive Disorder of Pregnancy Among Women in Chicago: Analysis of Electronic Health Record Data. *American Journal of Hypertension*, *31*(11), 1221–1227. DOI: 10.1093/ajh/hpy112 PMID: 30010764

Morris, M. A., Hamer, M. K., Eberle, K., Jensen, K. M., & Wong, A. A. (2021). Implementation of Collection of Patients' Disability Status by Centralized Scheduling. *Joint Commission Journal on Quality and Patient Safety*, *47*(10), 627–636. DOI: 10.1016/j.jcjq.2021.05.007 PMID: 34144917

National Center for Chronic Disease Prevention and Health Promotion (NCCD-PHP). (n.d.). https://www.cdc.gov/chronicdisease/healthequity/health-equity-communications/nccdphp-health-equity-glossary.html#:~:text=Implicit%20Bias%3A%20A%20form%20of

Njoku, A., Evans, M., Nimo-Sefah, L., & Bailey, J. (2023). Listen to the Whispers before They Become Screams: Addressing Black Maternal Morbidity and Mortality in the United States. *Health Care*, *11*(3), 438. DOI: 10.3390/healthcare11030438 PMID: 36767014

Quick facts: United States. US Census Bureau. (2018). AAMC. Quick facts: United States. US Census Bureau.

Salow, A. D., Pool, L. R., Grobman, W. A., & Kershaw, K. N. (2018). Associations of neighborhood-level racial residential segregation with adverse pregnancy outcomes. *American Journal of Obstetrics and Gynecology*, *218*(3), 351.e1–351.e7. DOI: 10.1016/j.ajog.2018.01.022 PMID: 29421603

Snyder, J. E., Upton, R. D., Hassett, T. C., Lee, H., Nouri, Z., & Dill, M. (2023). Black Representation in the Primary Care Physician Workforce and Its Association With Population Life Expectancy and Mortality Rates in the US. *JAMA Network Open*, *6*(4), e236687. DOI: 10.1001/jamanetworkopen.2023.6687 PMID: 37058307

Solomon, J. (2021, July 26). *Closing the coverage gap would improve Black maternal health.* Center on Budget and Policy Priorities. https://www.cbpp.org/research/health/closing-the-coverage-gap-would-improve-black-maternal-health

Stahnisch, F. W., & Verhoef, M. (2012). The Flexner Report of 1910 and Its Impact on Complementary and Alternative Medicine and Psychiatry in North America in the 20th Century. *Evidence-Based Complementary and Alternative Medicine : eCAM*, *2012*, 1–10. DOI: 10.1155/2012/647896 PMID: 23346209

Thomas, K., & Silver-Greenberg, J. (2022, September 24). How a Hospital Chain Used a Poor Neighborhood to Turn Huge Profits. *The New York Times*. https://www.nytimes.com/2022/09/24/health/bon-secours-mercy-health-profit-poor-neighborhood.html

Trauma Informed Care. (2018, March 20). *What Is Trauma?* Trauma-Informed Care Implementation Resource Center. https://www.traumainformedcare.chcs.org/what-is-trauma/

U.S. Department of Justice Civil Rights Division. (2024). *Introduction to the Americans with Disabilities Act.* ADA.gov. https://www.ada.gov/topics/intro-to-ada/

Vedam, S., Stoll, K., Taiwo, T. K., Rubashkin, N., Cheyney, M., Strauss, N., McLemore, M., Cadena, M., Nethery, E., Rushton, E., Schummers, L., & Declercq, E. (2019). The Giving Voice to Mothers Study: Inequity and mistreatment during pregnancy and childbirth in the United States. *Reproductive Health, 16*(1), 77. Advance online publication. DOI: 10.1186/s12978-019-0729-2 PMID: 31182118

Zellars, R. (2018, May 31). *Black Subjectivity and the Origins of American Gynecology–AAIHS*. Aaihs.org. https://www.aaihs.org/black-subjectivity-and-the-origins-of-american-gynecology/

Chapter 4
Socioeconomic Status: Challenges From Medicaid Spend-Down to Information Technology Issues

Michael John Robertson
Wright State University, USA

EXECUTIVE SUMMARY

Socioeconomic challenges have multi-faceted causes and implications upon health-care. These challenges range from purely financial aspects, housing, education, and food availability to negative health outcomes. Socioeconomic status is sometimes falsely portrayed as a byproduct of one's internal work ethic. However, this viewpoint fails to account for historical and institutional factors that limit mobility between socioeconomic levels. In this chapter, two cases will explore the impact of health care expenditure, access to care, and socioeconomic status on patient outcomes through limitations in wealth accessibility, health care payer laws, and resource scarcity.

INTRODUCTION

Socioeconomic status is defined as "a way of describing people based on their education, income, and type of job…" (National Cancer Institute, n.d.) The National Cancer Institute describes lower socioeconomic status as a barrier to necessary opportunities in both financial and other areas that increase the likelihood for negative health implications long term. (National Cancer Institute, n.d.) Socioeconomic status is sometimes portrayed as a byproduct of one's internal work ethic. However, this viewpoint fails to account for historical and institutional factors that limit mobility

DOI: 10.4018/979-8-3693-3683-0.ch004

between socioeconomic levels. This chapter will attempt to highlight how some of the areas can lead to health disparities for patients.

Economic Discrepancies

Socioeconomic status is not a static level. Long-term analysis during the 1900s showed that intergenerational mobility has decreased since the baby boomer generation till today. This translates to more people maintaining the same socioeconomic status of their parents. Economic mobility has fallen for the lower 90% of the earnings distribution with the baby boomer generation becoming adults. (Dutko, Ver Ploeg, & Farrigan, 2012) This also has implications on health.

Employment opportunities regardless of wage or salary are less plentiful in lower to moderate income socioeconomic areas. One study placed the ratio of job prospects to residents of the area at 0.73 compared to ratio of 1 job prospect to resident in high income socioeconomic communities. Furthermore, the wages of these jobs are not equivalent in these areas as lower to moderate income socioeconomic areas have lower wages. (Huynh, 2020) Unfortunately, those of lower socioeconomic status often have lower vehicle ownership rates. This requires heavier use of walking, biking, or some form of public transportation to get to work. (Dutko, Ver Ploeg, & Farrigan, 2012) This may limit one to lower paying jobs even if one has the skills to demand higher wages.

ETHICS AND ETHICAL DILEMMAS

In order to discuss various aspects of socioeconomic status in detail, it's important to understand some general versus medical ethical concepts. Ethics are "a system of accepted beliefs that control behavior, especially such a system based on morals." (Cambridge Dictionary, 2025) Philosophers have proposed various systems for ethics.

- ***Supernaturalism***: ethics are inseparable from religion. The only source of moral rules is God.
- ***Intuitionism***: good and bad are real objective properties that can't be broken down into component parts. Something is good because it's good; its goodness doesn't need justifying or proving.
- ***Consequentialism***: bases morality on the consequences of human actions and not on the actions themselves. Morally good actions are actions which produce the greatest number of good consequences.

- ***Non-consequentialism / Deontological ethics:*** concerned with the actions themselves and not with the consequences. Some acts are inherently right or wrong in themselves regardless of the consequences.
- ***Virtue ethics***: based on virtue or moral character, rather than at ethical duties / rules, or consequences of actions. In order for it to be a good action, then it would be the same action that that a virtuous person would do in the same circumstances, and that a virtuous person is someone who has a particularly good character.
- ***Situation ethics***: rejects prescriptive rules and argues that individual ethical decisions should be made according to the unique situation. The decision in that specific situation should follow a desire to seek the best for the people involved. There are no moral rules or rights - each case is unique and deserves a unique solution. (BBC, 2014)

Medical ethics utilizes a virtue ethics approach. (Lyon, 2021) Four main pillars define medical ethics:

- ***Beneficence***: the obligation of physician to act for the benefit of the patient and supports a number of moral rules to protect and defend the right of others, prevent harm, remove conditions that will cause harm, help persons with disabilities, and rescue persons in danger.
- ***Non-maleficence***: the obligation of a physician not to harm the patient (i.e. do no harm). This simply stated principle supports several moral rules – do not kill, do not cause pain or suffering, do not incapacitate, do not cause offense, and do not deprive others of the goods of life.
- ***Autonomy***: all persons have intrinsic and unconditional worth, and therefore, should have the power to make rational decisions and moral choices, and each should be allowed to exercise their capacity for self-determination.
- ***Justice***: fair, equitable, and appropriate treatment of persons. (Varkey, 2020)

These pillars overlap and can sometimes conflict with each other. Additionally, some pillars are superseded by other pillars. For instance, patients may lack the capacity to make medical decisions depending on the situation. At these times patient autonomy is superseded by the pillars of beneficence and non-maleficence. A surrogate decision maker has autonomy to make decisions on the patient's behalf at those times. Furthermore, there are many situations where the pillars of non-maleficence and beneficence collide (e.g. medication benefits vs side effects, discomfort of mechanical ventilation vs sustaining life, etc.). There are also many situations where autonomy and beneficence collide (e.g. patient refusing life sustaining treatment, parent / guardian refusing care for their children, etc.). In these circumstances, it is important for the clinician to weigh these pillars to determine the appropriate course of action. (Varkey, 2020)

In contrast, other organizations and groups have different ethical foundations. The United Nations's fundamental ethical values include independence, loyalty, impartiality, integrity, accountability, and respect for human rights. (United Nations, 2025) Meanwhile the National Association of Colleges and Employers (NACE) uses a different foundation: practicing reasonable / responsible / transparent behavior, acting without bias, ensuring equitable access, complying with laws, and protecting confidentiality. (NACE, 2025) These are simply different systems and approaches. However, these can translate to various ethical dilemmas between a physician's medical ethics and corporate interests despite both parties acting in an "ethical" manner.

Likewise, the approach an individual can take to moral questions can vary and generally fall into one of these types:

- ***Moral realism***: based on the idea that there are real objective moral facts or truths in the universe.
- ***Subjectivism***: moral judgments are nothing more than statements of a person's feelings or attitudes, and that ethical statements do not contain factual truths about goodness or badness.
- ***Emotivism***: moral claims are no more than expressions of approval or disapproval. In contrast to subjectivism, emotivism's moral statements don't provide information about the speaker's feelings about the topic but expresses those feelings.
- ***Prescriptivism***: ethical statements are instructions or recommendations. If something is good, then it's a recommendation to do it; conversely if something is bad, then it's a recommendation not to do it. (BBC, 2014)

Medical ethics relies on a moral realism approach to determine the best course of action. However, each individual will have differing viewpoints for their approach to ethics before considering the system of ethics that ethical dilemmas are based.

The Socioeconomics of Medical Ethics

Socioeconomic status is an area of identity with many ethical implications. Aside from questioning the morality of cost impacting health care accessibility, multiple parts of socioeconomic status impact health outcomes. Because of this, when considering direct patient care, the 4 pillars of medical ethics can get very complicated. For example, autonomy's importance is undeniable as one of those four pillars. However, two separate pillars of beneficence and non-maleficence can be more complex. Doing a total knee replacement surgery on someone with knee arthritis who desires it would follow beneficence and the patient's autonomy. However, if going into the surgery, the physician knew that the patient had no means of doing the necessary physical therapy after the knee surgery would this still be following beneficence? The artificial knee will fail if appropriate therapy is not done. One could even argue this is maleficence since the patient will have added surgical complications and costs associated with getting this procedure.

HOUSING

Social aspects of socioeconomic status can be location specific, however overarching similarities exist between regions, since socioeconomic status limits the locations one can live. Exclusionary zoning laws limit what types and how many housing projects can be constructed for certain regions. In the early 1900s, exclusionary zoning laws were done mainly on racial lines. The 1917 Supreme Court decision of Buchanan v Warley was the first to forbid city zoning ordinances from discriminating along racial lines. A series of legal cases and government intervention in the mid-1900s lead up to the 1968 Fair Housing Act which prohibited discrimination along "race, color, national origin, religion, sex, ability, and familial status." This however still allows for discrimination along economic lines.

Tactics such as minimum lot size requirements, single versus multi-family dwellings, building height limits, and landscaping requirements are just some of the legal means causing the income level discrimination. (Rigsby, 2016) Therefore, lower economic classes are unable to have the same level of housing mobility as higher economic classes. This is one of the reasons that the 2008 housing crises caused stronger and longer housing insecurity for those of lower socioeconomic status than their higher socioeconomic counterparts. (Wang, 2022) High poverty areas have become increasingly more concentrated due to exclusionary zoning, nearly doubling 7.2 million to 13.8 million citizens living in high poverty areas. Concentrated levels of poverty contribute to underperforming schools and fewer recreational spaces. This often perpetuates a cycle of high poverty in these areas.

Food Deserts

A USDA study of census data noted family income, unemployment rates, poverty rates, and the proportion of households receiving public assistance were all indicators of food deserts. Most of these gaps were exacerbated in rural areas. Poverty rates were the leading indicator with almost 90% higher poverty rates for urban food deserts than non-food deserts. Median family income was 18% lower in food deserts regions. Unemployment rates were 60% higher in urban food deserts compared to non-food desert regions. (Dutko, Ver Ploeg, & Farrigan, 2012)

Transportation

Vehicle ownership is 15-25% lower in food desert regions. This aligns with access to job opportunities, ability to go outside of food desert region for food, and housing infrastructure. When transportation is more complex and potentially unreliable, it becomes challenging to seek better opportunities and resources. (Dutko, Ver Ploeg, & Farrigan, 2012)

EDUCATION

Education is a foundation for increasing opportunities and thus income levels. In the current community-based school system, educational opportunities can be determined by location of residence. As noted previously, boundaries exist for those of lower socioeconomic to mitigate this by living in a different school district. Gaps in academic achievement between levels of socioeconomic status for grade school students have been noted. Studies have even shown the toxic stress of growing up in poverty had direct impacts on cognitive, memory, and motor function through decreased quantities of gray matter and delayed brain development. This is separate from the impacts on emotional development which can lead to a survival mindset and more difficulty focusing on class. (Bradley, 2022)

Resource Allocation in Schools

There are stark differences in the resources allocated to poorer community schools versus wealthier community schools. In 2018, the United States spent $1,000 less per student in impoverished areas compared to wealthier counterparts. The majority of funding is based on the state and local levels (school levies, etc.). For those states that provide more consistent funding to all students, there are decreased achievement gaps between students of poorer versus wealthier socioeconomic backgrounds. This can be noted in teacher turnover rates, inadequate teacher training programs and resources, library resources, college preparatory programs, and amount of Advanced Prep and International Baccalaureate classes. (Bradley, 2022)

The concept of school choice and school vouchers have been used in several states in an attempt to combat these issues. This is often met with arguments including the philosophical questions of public money for religious and/or private schools, school vouchers introduce the possibility of discriminatory entrance requirements for private / charter schools, potential for talent drain from the area's public school, and potential for discriminatory curriculum. However, these school choice and voucher programs are not getting the academic benefits intended over public schools alone. Recent in-depth analysis on lower income students in 4 states showed that math scores actually fell with the transition to a private school in 3 of the 4 states. The last school saw initial drops, but recovery to baseline test scores by year 3 at the private school without further increases in scores. Likewise, 2 of the 4 states saw similar drops in English test scores with the transition while the others were neutral. (Barnum, 2017) Graduation rates paint a more positive picture of these programs with a neutral to upwards of 21% increase in high school graduation rates, and neutral to 10% increase in bachelor's degree obtainment. (Barnum, 2017)

School Achievement Rates

Dropout rates are five times higher for lower socioeconomic students to higher socioeconomic peers. Similarly, college degree obtainment is 8 times less likely for a student from the bottom 25% than top 25%. (Bradley, 2022) This adds additional barriers to socioeconomic mobility. Since college / trade schools can provide a person with additional expertise to increase their income level and thus socioeconomic status, but the feasibility is not shared across the socioeconomic spectrum. One, often cited, factor is the rising costs of college tuition. College tuition alone has risen 180% from 1980 to 2020 when adjusted for inflation over the same period. (McGurran, 9) Sadly, there has not been a commiserate increase in income from obtaining a high school diploma versus college degree; instead, the bump in income has fallen over time. Student loan debt is at an all-time high with 1.77 trillion dollars split across over 45 million people as of March 2022. (Schulz, 2023) The opportunity cost of college becomes much different for a student paying for their own college, than someone who has the privilege of a higher socioeconomic background. The lack of that socioeconomic privilege at birth may translate to less schooling, higher individualized costs to education, and/or an inability to afford other life expenses in the future.

Child Care

The cost of childcare has risen 36% over the past decade in the United States outpacing inflation. Families spent more than a quarter of their income on childcare in 2023 equating to $15,000-40,000 per year for one child depending on the type of care used. (Schonberger, 2024) Naturally at a time when median household income is around $75,000 per year in the United States, this is not sustainable for those of low and even those of moderate socioeconomic status. (Guzman & Kollar,

2023) Some two parent households had one parent leave the workforce to defray the increased costs of childcare.

In addition to cost, access to childcare can be affected by socioeconomic status. This was illustrated in a recent study on early childcare up to age 6. This study used mother's educational obtainment as a proxy for the socioeconomic status of the family. Yet there was a discrepancy between mothers who never went to college versus mothers who obtained a college degree. Mothers who never went to college had to spend an average of 12.5% more time (equivalent to 8 hours more weekly) on childcare duties compared to mothers who obtained a college degree. This may suggest decreased access to childcare options (family members, daycares, early childhood education programs, etc.) with lower socioeconomic status. (Flood, McMurry, Sojourner, & Wiswall, 2022) This additional time spent on childcare diminishes a person's ability to increase their earnings potential and socioeconomic status.

Another study evaluated the utilization of early childhood education programs which have shown improvements in academic performance down the lin. Yet again, children of lower socioeconomic status are less likely to be enrolled in early childhood education programs. (Wiederhold, Lergetporer, Peter, & Hermes, 2021) These discrepancies contribute to health disparities for the child in the future.

Education and Healthcare

Educational achievement and income level have direct correlations for several child health factors. When tracking childhood healthy eating behaviors, childhood activity limitations due to health conditions, and infant mortality, all of these factors have more favorable outcomes at higher parental income levels and educational attainment levels than when compared to the lower parental income and educational attainment counterparts. Additionally, educational attainment impacted how a person would rate their health status. The higher the educational achievement a person obtained made them more likely to rate their health as very good or excellent on a Likert scale. Each of these studies was controlled for race and ethnicity, but unfortunately these socioeconomic status inequities can be compound along other areas of identity.

HEALTHCARE COSTS

In the United States, health care costs continue to rise. On a macro level, healthcare spending grew 4% in 2022 to $13,493 per person per year. Although a mean average can be misleading, since 5% of the US population is responsible for over 50% of healthcare expenditures with each person paying over $71,000 annually in

2021. Likewise, the top 1% paid nearly $167,000 in health expenditures per year. The bottom 50% of healthcare utilizers spent only $385 out-of-pocket not including premiums each year. (Peterson-KFF, 2024)

These figures don't capture the under-utilization of the healthcare system due to these costs. 28% of adults went without or delayed care due to concerns about cost in 2022. This is more pronounced from those at 200% of the federal poverty limit or below. (Peterson-KFF, 2024) In order to further discuss patient facing costs, it is important to define some terminology for USA healthcare. First, there are three main classifications of insurance: private, Medicare, and Medicaid.

- Private insurance is often through an employer but can also be purchased through state-run insurance marketplaces.
- Medicare is for elderly (those aged 65 and older) and people with disabilities.
- Medicaid is for low-income individuals / families.

The Medicaid expansion was a component of the Patient Protection and Affordable Care Act of 2010. This expanded Medicaid coverage to anyone up to 138% of the federal poverty level. Since Medicaid is run by each state but partially financed by the federal government, this expansion was left to each individual state. As of 2024, 10 states have not adopted the Medicaid expansion. This means those within the 100-138% of the federal poverty limit are not eligible for federal government subsidies on the health care marketplace like those citizens would be if they were slightly above the 138% mark. This roughly equates to 1.5 million people who are uninsured. (Drake, Tolbert, Rudowitz, & Damico, 2024)

Every health plan is required to cover ten categories: outpatient services, emergency services, hospitalization, pregnancy / maternity / newborn care, mental health services, prescription drugs, rehabilitative services and devices, laboratory services, dental / vision care for children (for adults this is not an essential category), and preventative / wellness services. (HealthCare.gov, n.d.) Different insurances will cover these and other categories to varying degrees. In practice, varying levels of coverage is accomplished by having different premiums, deductibles, copayments (generally referred to as copays), out-of-pocket maximums, coverage limits, and in-network versus out-of-network coverage. (Nall, 2020) (Bauer, 2023)

- Premiums: the amount paid per month for insurance coverage.
- Deductible: the amount the patient has to pay throughout the year before the insurance covers a portion of the bill. This amount resets every year. As a general rule, the higher the premium is the lower the deductible will be.
- Health Savings Accounts (also known as HSAs): a mechanism for a patient to save money for these costs prior to meeting one's deductible.

- Copayments ("Copays"): the amount a patient has to pay for the respective appointment or service while the insurance is billed the rest. Generally, co-payments are paid at time of service.
- Out-of-pocket maximums: the total amount a patient will have to pay before the insurance will cover 100% of services.

These can be category specific or more commonly have different levels for in-network versus out-of-network providers and facilities. In-network and out-of-network providers / facilities are defined by the insurance and are not always intuitive. For instance, a doctor may be in-network but the only hospital that they work at is out-of-network, this causes patient's payments to fall into both categories increasing costs before meeting the out-of-pocket maximum.

- Coverage limits: a maximum amount the insurance will cover for a certain type of service over the year until the patient has paid the out-of-pocket maximum.

Since 2014, coverage limits only apply to Medicare due to the Patient Protection and Affordable Care Act of 2010. This leads to a concept called the "Medicare Donut Hole" where patients have to pay large portions of their prescription drug costs until reaching the out-of-pocket maximum. This was lessened by the Patient Protection and Affordable Care Act of 2010, but not eliminated for Medicare. (Medicare.gov, n.d.)

HEALTH DISPARITIES

These various socioeconomic factors intertwine to contribute to the health disparities that are currently noted in the United States. Before looking at the individual patient considerations, let's analyze some of the macro data. For those people that lived to 25years old, income level showed a linear contribution to life expectancy from then onward as income levels increased. This equated to a 10-year difference in live expectancy among the lowest income classification (someone making less than the federal poverty level) and the highest income classification (someone making more than 400% of the federal poverty level). Starting at 25years eliminates outliers from congenital conditions and infant mortality from impacting the data. Income level also correlated with prevalence of diabetes in those aged 20-64 years old. The higher the income translated to lower rates of diabetes.

Tackling Health Disparities as a Healthcare Worker

Socioeconomic status will impact healthcare outcomes for individual patients. Institutional level changes are undoubtedly needed on the local, state, and federal levels to improve these inequities. In the meantime, it becomes imperative to be mindful of the healthcare system limitations that could impact adherence to treatment regimens and diagnostic work ups. Far too often patients are labeled as "non-compliant", but factors outside of their control made them unable to follow through on healthcare provider recommendations. A more apt term is "non-adherent", and it becomes part of the healthcare provider's responsibility to determine why that non-adherence occurred. (Kleinsinger, 2010)

Working through non-adherence, first and foremost, requires knowing each individual patient. This improves trust in the provider-patient relationship and allows patients to be more open about adherence challenges. For medications alone, non-adherence rates of 43-78% have been documented in studies. (Braveman, Cubbin, Egerter, Williams, & Pamuk, 2010) Even outside of medications, treatment plans can stall with gaps in provider knowledge of the patient's situation. For example, telling a patient to stop eating a granola bar with every meal and eat more protein to control their diabetes is definitely a way to decrease their carbohydrate intake. However, if that person has no access to a grocery store selling perishable foods and can only consume what's at the local gas station, then perhaps that simple statement is not a realistic treatment plan to control the diabetes. One must be open to creative ways to work through these solutions that work for patients, but it is also important not to stereotype solutions by demographic factors. For instance, every lower socioeconomic patient won't be in a food desert.

Shared-Decision Making

Shared-decision making creates a treatment and diagnostic plan that is agreed upon between the patient and their healthcare team. (Braveman, Cubbin, Egerter, Williams, & Pamuk, 2010) This is in contrast to a pure directive which was the paradigm for provider-patient relations. During a shared-decision making process, open conversation allows space for patients to disclose socioeconomic factors or other concerns judgement-free to craft treatment plan that fits their needs.

CASES

Case 1: Taking Care of Aging Parents

Learning Objectives

1. Recognizing high-cost health care system burdens.
2. Recognize patient's priorities.
3. Recognize situations where support networks can be improved.
4. Practice strategies that align patient's priorities with patient's most urgent health conditions.

Case Aim: This case highlights the impact of socioeconomic status on health outcomes when managing chronic conditions.

48yo cisgendered female recently moved to the area to be closer to parents. Patient is somewhat of a poor historian who is establishing care. Patient has morbid obesity, prediabetes, hypertension, and a history of breast cancer but unsure of the status of treatment. Patient was also in the process of being worked up for some type of arthritis but was unsure if anything was determined. Patient currently takes no medications.

Follow-up Visit #1: 4-week follow-up visit (consider pausing to run through questions 1-10 before reading next section of the scenario)

After completing some blood work, patient returns to your office for a 4-week follow up. You learn that patient has a Hemoglobin A1c of 6.7% placing her slightly in the diabetes range now instead of prediabetes. Blood pressure is slightly high, and you also note an increase in patient's weight. Your office also received some of the records from her prior primary care provider (PCP). It's noted that patient is only 2 years out from breast cancer treatment and is still supposed to be on a selective estrogen receptor modulator (SERM) for an additional 3 years. Additionally, patient has rheumatoid arthritis for which the prior rheumatologist was adjusting the disease-modifying anti-rheumatic drugs (DMARD) treatment before patient left the state. You recommended the appropriate lifestyle changes to improve her diabetes / obesity / hypertension, started patient on the appropriate medications, and referred patient to a rheumatologist for further management of the rheumatoid arthritis.

Follow-up Visit #2: 6 weeks after initial follow-up visit (consider pausing to run through questions 1-10 to see if there are any additions before reading next section of the scenario)

The patient returns 6 weeks later. You find that patient has not heard from the Rheumatologist but has been awaiting a call. Her A1c increased further to 7.8%. Meanwhile blood pressure and weight have also increased. Patient has not started any of the lifestyle changes that were discussed at her previous visit. Upon additional discussion, patient's parents are in their late 70s. Parents are struggling with worsening memory and mobility issues, respectively. Patient was considering moving in with parents, since her father will wander off due to his poor memory and her mother has difficulty walking even with the walker, having multiple falls each month. Patient is concerned about the cost of getting elderly services started and is considering increasing the amount of shifts at work but has been actually doing fewer shifts due to her responsibilities for her parents.

After the visit, you reach out to the Rheumatologist's office to see what issue there may be with scheduling. You learn that this Rheumatology office only schedules via text or their online portal. After relaying this information to the patient, the patient notes that she dropped her text and internet packages from her phone bill to save on costs.

Case Questions

1. What Historical Events Have Created a Space for This Current Situation?

- Lawmaking and privatization of elder care has made it expensive for most people to take care of aging parents. (AARP, 2020) For instance, social security and salaries have not been increasing at the same rate as inflation / cost of living needs. (Bremen, 2023) Patient / parents' heritage may be impacting generational wealth as well due to lack of knowledge or what government programs past generations were able to obtain (housing loans, G.I. Bill benefits, etc.). One could question the ethical implications of the patient having to either sacrifice their health or their financial security to care for aging parents.

2. Whose Story Is Needed to Understand the Patient's Needs in This Situation?

- The parents' story would be beneficial, since patient moved here for them. Other family members (spouse, children, siblings, etc.) who could assist in parents' care would be beneficial. Potentially neighbors and friends who are willing to assist in parent's care could also be beneficial.

3. What Cultural Values or Norms Are Being Assumed? Which May Be Missing?

- There is an assumption that family ties are a strong part of this patient's culture. Furthermore, that patient can do any caretaking duties for parents if needed. We are missing insight into religious beliefs and the expression of those beliefs for patient and patient's parents. This could perhaps be another area of support for this patient.

4. How Do Structural Factors Impact This Patient's Care?

- The complex nature of being on Medicare and transitioning to Medicaid are impacting this patient. This patient needs the additional assistance for her parents however they have too many assets. Only the immediate 100-day stay in a nursing home after a hospitalization is covered by Medicare. Long-term nursing home stays beyond 100 days are covered by Medicaid. This means someone would have to spend down assets or pay for their care until they run out of money to qualify for Medicaid before being able to have Medicaid pay for the remainder of a nursing home stay. The intricacies of the Medicaid spend-down are beyond the scope of this discussion, but pointing the patient to a resource to further explore this option is necessary. (Iversen, 2024) (American Council on Aging, 2024)

5. How Do We Address This Patient's Needs?

- Ascertain additional support avenues and elevate priorities. For instance, if patient wants to be able to take care of parents long-term, then her health conditions must be a priority. Many caregivers sacrifice their health to care for others which impacts their own health outcomes. Creating a list that assists in prioritizing her health conditions and necessary follow ups may help her to decide which appointments are most important to do no and what can wait to prevent overwhelm.

6. What Next Steps or Resources Are Needed Here?

- Determine if any barriers exist for completing additional diagnostic workup, taking medications, doing lifestyle interventions. If so, it would be ideal to work through those barriers by connecting with resources. For instance, local libraries, community centers, and YMCAs are often overlooked resources for support and opportunities to exercise. Religious entities may also be able to setup a similar support. Depending on financial need, resources like food pantries, Supplemental Nutrition Assistance Program (SNAP) benefits, housing assistance programs, transportation assistance programs, etc. could be utilized to help.

Getting records from prior out-of-state healthcare providers to limit repeat testing locally can decrease cost for patient. Although the parents are not the patient, connecting the patient with local aging resource groups and Alzheimer's association resources would help patient's health as well. Discussing long-term strategies on managing patient's parents' situation and support for the patient is key (rotation with other caregivers, patient applies to be the parents' paid caretaker through insurance, planning for long-term nursing home care).

7. What Emotions Are You Feeling as the Physician or Health Care Provider in This Case?

- Use personal self-reflection to determine these emotions. However, you can use these questions to help work through this self-reflection. Did this case seem challenging to you? Did you already desire to obtain some of the additional information before it was revealed? If so, why do you think that was? If not, why do you think that was? If you didn't think to ask for some of this information, then how do you think you could go about getting this info from a patient to improve your treatment plan?

8. Are There Any Beliefs That You Have That May Be Stretched Right Now?

- Use personal self-reflection to determine these beliefs. However, you can use these questions to help work through this self-reflection. Would any of these beliefs be considered a stereotype? If so, what's the basis for that stereotype? Regardless, does this belief or these beliefs have a basis in fact? Does it have a basis in experience? Should this belief be adjusted or changed after reviewing additional data?

***Case Outcome*:** Due to your interventions, patient was able to get one of her two siblings and both neighbors more involved with assisting parents' care. Patient and her sibling trade off days. Meanwhile the neighbors will give patient or her sibling a call if they don't see a light turned on in the morning or if her father tried to go for a walk again. This allowed patient to exercise more which has been helping the weight, blood pressure, and glucose levels. Patient has also been to the Rheumatologist, since you reached out to them and worked out a solution. Patient scheduled online at a local library initially. Afterward patient would check on the online portal for responses twice a week at the library. This also helped to get additional walking in, since the YMCA was near the library. Patient has been able to get her parents into some senior activities at the YMCA while she completes activities at the library and then comes back to the YMCA for a walk.

The additional support has also helped patient pick up more / longer trucking shifts which has improved her finances considerably. Patient no longer has concerns about affording her cancer surveillance imaging and blood work. Additionally, patient started looking into nursing home options for eventual transition to nursing home care in the future.

Case Discussion

A patient establishing care with unknown status to several conditions is a common patient encounter. This patient has recently treated breast cancer, known rheumatoid arthritis, diabetes, and hypertension. Sometimes patients can be labeled as non-compliant or non-adherent to a treatment regimen very quickly. However, this does a dis-service to the patient who has legitimate barriers to care. Sifting through those issues and assisting a patient through these can be the difference between conditions being controlled and uncontrolled. As technology improves some medical offices are moving to online portals to eliminate the need for as much phone staff. This highlights the importance of knowing specialist workflows to be able to prepare patients. If someone doesn't have a cell phone to receive text, then you can advise them prior to referral that they need to schedule online.

Case 2: Pitfalls of Employer-Based Health Care Insurance

Learning Objectives

1. Recognizing high-cost health care system burdens.
2. Recognize patient's priorities.
3. Recognize situations where support networks can be improved.
4. Practice strategies that align patient's priorities with patient's most urgent health conditions.

Case Aim: This case aims to highlight the mental health implications of additional stressors caused by socioeconomic status.

Case 2 Scenario

35yo cisgendered male has a history of depression with past suicide attempt and notes doing well now. He is married with 2 children, aged 7 and 9. The patient hasn't been in to see you in some time. Patient did complete a wellness screen for work that noted that patient had high blood pressure, cholesterol, and may be a diabetic. Thus, patient was recommended to come back in to see his healthcare provider for further evaluation. You perform a hemoglobin A1c in the office to find his A1c is 5.8% placing him slightly into the prediabetes range. Fortunately, his blood pressure was in the normal range, but he does have a family history of hypertension.

Patient gave up his gym membership since his children's school started requiring fees for the children's athletic programs this past year. Patient doesn't feel safe walking in his neighborhood, and thus has stopped any regular exercise routine, but notes he will start exercising at work more instead. He has been trying to make more of his kid's soccer games and practices after work as well.

Follow-up Visit #1: 6-month follow-up visit (consider pausing to run through questions 1-10 before reading next section of the scenario)

Patient is in poor spirits upon coming back in. Patient has lost his job. He has health insurance for this month but will be losing his health insurance at the end of the month for him and his kids. His spouse has their own insurance. He's not sleeping as well. He also stopped exercising and has started to gain weight. You note that his blood pressure has also increased to hypertensive ranges.

After further discussion you learn that patient is also moderately depressed based on a PHQ-9 scoring. Patient has become estranged from his family, since they did not approve of his marriage or subsequent adoption of children. His husband's insurance cannot cover the children, which is another point of stress for patient. Patient is further worried that he may have to pull his kids out of their sport programs, because he and his spouse have depleted most of their savings, but he notes that he will become even more depressed if he has to go that route.

Case Questions With Answers

1. What Historical Events Have Created a Space for This Current Situation?

- The decision to make health insurance tied to employment has made several people and families go through similar situations. (Scott, 2023) Chronic underfunding / decreased funding to public schools have caused some schools to turn to fees for athletics to help finance school operations. (Wermiel, 2023)

2. Whose Story Is Needed to Understand the Patient's Needs in This Situation?

- Spouse and children's story would be beneficial.

3. What Cultural Values or Norms Are Being Assumed? Which May Be Missing?

- We are assuming caring and providing for children is part of patient's culture. We are missing insight into religious beliefs and the expression of those beliefs for patient and patient's parents. This could perhaps be another area of support for this patient.

4. What Does the Language in This Scenario Tell Us About the Assumptions Being Made?

- The language implies a that this job loss is assumed to be a surprise based on the timing of the office visit with this news. Patient is also assumed to be the main breadwinner for the family considering the loss of patient's job has sent the family into this situation. There is the assumption that patient's depression is spiraling downward perhaps even toward a potential suicide attempt, since patient has attempted suicide before.

5. How Do Structural Factors Impact This Patient's Care?

- The employer-based healthcare system has created situations where job loss potentiates loss of access to care. This can compound both the stresses of unemployment and the financial impacts of needing medical care which can cause financial ruin if a health need arises. This can also cause the worsening of chronic health conditions as seen in this case. Additionally, this raises the ethical question of the cost of care precluding access to necessary but nonemergent care.

6. How Do We Address This Patient's Needs?

- Ascertain additional support avenues and resources, elevate the patient's priorities. Ensuring this patient is psychologically and physically safe are key in beginning to address his needs. Creating a safety plan and evaluating if the patient is in need of mental health resources or care (referrals, medications, etc.) can address the pressing mental health concerns. This patient may qualify for Medicaid. Even if he doesn't, his children will qualify for the Children's Health Insurance Program (CHIP). For physical health concerns, considering options that lower costs such as using medication coupon sites, manufacturer coupons, or office medication samples can assist in his treatment. Likewise virtual messaging or phone calls can be used to evaluate progress rather than in person visits to save money as he will have to pay for visits. If mental health services are too expensive, volunteer therapy services or various therapy programs that are low cost may provide an avenue to additional mental health services until patient can get back on insurance.

Providing the patient with options to discuss additional needs or concerns can allow for connection to pertinent resources. For instance, the patient may have concerns about losing housing or transportation. Resources for unemployment and job services may be needed if the patient hasn't already looked into these. This can help provide income during the immediate future. Patient may also be able to utilize food pantries, Supplemental Nutrition Assistance Program (SNAP) benefits, school lunch programs, housing assistance programs, transportation assistance programs, etc. that could be utilized to help as well.

7. What Emotions Are You Feeling as the Physician or Health Care Provider in This Case?

- Use personal self-reflection to determine these emotions. However, you can use these questions to help work through this self-reflection. Did this case seem challenging to you? Did you already desire to obtain some of the additional information before it was revealed? If so, why do you think that was? If not, why do you think that was? If you didn't think to ask for some of this information, then how do you think you could go about getting this info from a patient to improve your treatment plan?

8. Are There Any Beliefs That You Have That May Be Stretched Right Now?

- Use personal self-reflection to determine these beliefs. However, you can use these questions to help work through this self-reflection. Would any of these beliefs be considered a stereotype? If so, what's the basis for that stereotype? Regardless, does this belief or these beliefs have a basis in fact? Does it have a basis in experience? Should this belief be adjusted or changed after reviewing additional data?

Case 2 Outcome

Due to your interventions, patient was able to start on a low-cost antidepressant medication that was on $4 list at a local pharmacy. Furthermore, patient applied and received unemployment until a new job could be obtained. This along with getting the children into the school lunches program allowed patient to keep the children in their athletics. Patient has also used this opportunity to go to more of the children's practices and walk around the field while waiting for them to finish which has really helped patient's mood. The patient and children are eligible for Medicaid.

The following month, the patient's blood pressure and weight started to decrease. His mood and sleep are much better. Patient wants to continue on this current antidepressant to prevent another exacerbation of his depression. He even has some job interviews coming up, so he's really excited.

Case 2 Discussion

Socioeconomic factors have the ability to create stressors that initiate or exacerbate mental health conditions like anxiety or depression. As noted in this case, major life changes impacted this patient's depression. Patients may not follow up specifically for mental health disorders, but left untreated then these can impact other health conditions as well. In this case, the patient had an increase in body weight and blood pressure. It's important to recognize the signs of mental health concerns, screen, and work to find solutions that are applicable to the patient's needs and resources.

CONCLUSION

Socioeconomic status has far reaching implications to patient outcomes associated with social determinants of health. Unfortunately, these situations are a byproduct of several macro-factors outside of patient's control. Patient actions are only one aspect driving these situations, but they will be impacted by these forces on a regular basis. Patient's socioeconomic status is a topic that is often omitted from clinician to patient discussions. However, the omission can lead to non-adherence to a diagnostic workups or treatment regimens and unethical medical practices. It becomes imperative to be aware of and incorporate these aspects into determining next steps for patients.

REFERENCES

AARP. (2020, May). *Caregiving in the U.S.* Retrieved from AARP: https://www.aarp.org/content/dam/aarp/ppi/2020/05/executive-summary-caregiving-in-the-united-states.doi.10.26419-2Fppi.00103.003.pdf

American Council on Aging. (2024, January 26). *Spending Down Assets to Become Medicaid Eligible for Nursing Home / Long Term Care.* Retrieved from American Council on Aging: https://www.medicaidplanningassistance.org/medicaid-spend-down/

Barnum, M. (2017, July 12). *Do school vouchers 'work'? As the debate heats up, here's what research really says.* Retrieved May 31, 2023, from Charlkbeat: https://www.chalkbeat.org/2017/7/12/21108235/school-choice-vouchers-system-pros-and-cons-research/

Bauer, B. (2023, October 19). *How to Avoid the Medicare Part D Donut Hole.* Retrieved from National Council on Aging: https://www.ncoa.org/article/how-to-avoid-the-medicare-part-d-donut-hole

BBC. (2014). *Ethics: a general introduction.* Retrieved from What is ethics?: https://www.bbc.co.uk/ethics/introduction/intro_1.shtml

Bradley, K. (2022). *The Socioeconomic Achievement Gap in the US Public Schools.* Retrieved from Ballard Brief: https://ballardbrief.byu.edu/issue-briefs/the-socioeconomic-achievement-gap-in-the-us-public-schools

Braveman, P. A., Cubbin, C., Egerter, S., Williams, D. R., & Pamuk, E. (2010). Socioeconomic disparities in health in the United States: What the patterns tell us. *American Journal of Public Health, 100*(S1), 186–196. DOI: 10.2105/AJPH.2009.166082 PMID: 20147693

Bremen, J. M. (2023, December 14). *Will Pay Increases Exceed Inflation In2024?* Retrieved from Forbes: https://www.forbes.com/sites/johnbremen/2023/12/14/will-pay-increases-exceed-inflation-in-2024/?sh=233bb2c72266

Cambridge Dictionary. (2025). *Meaning of ethic in English.* Retrieved from Cambridge Dictionary: https://dictionary.cambridge.org/us/dictionary/english/ethic

CDC. (2021, July 22). *Sexually Transmitted Infections Treatment Guidelines,2021.* Retrieved from Adolescents: https://www.cdc.gov/std/treatment-guidelines/adolescents.htm#:~:text=All%2050%20states%20and%20the,the%20allowable%20deductible%20is%20reached

CDC. (2023). *National Overview of STIs in 2023*. Retrieved from STI Statistics: https://www.cdc.gov/sti-statistics/annual/summary.html

Drake, P., Tolbert, J., Rudowitz, R., & Damico, A. (2024, February 26). *How Many Uninsured Are in the Coverage Gap and How Many Could be Eligible if All States Adopted the Medicaid Expansion?* Retrieved from KFF: https://www.kff.org/medicaid/issue-brief/how-many-uninsured-are-in-the-coverage-gap-and-how-many-could-be-eligible-if-all-states-adopted-the-medicaid-expansion/

Dutko, P., Ver Ploeg, M., & Farrigan, T. (2012). *Characteristics and Influential Factors of Food Deserts*. United States Department of Agriculture: Economic Research Service.

Flood, S., McMurry, J., Sojourner, A., & Wiswall, M. (2022). Inequality in Early Care Experienced by US Children. *The Journal of Economic Perspectives: a Journal of the American Economic Association*, 199–222.

Guzman, G., & Kollar, M. (2023, September 23). *Income in the United States:2022*. Retrieved from United States Census Bureau: https://www.census.gov/library/publications/2023/demo/p60-279.html

HealthCare.gov. (n.d.). *What Marketplace health insurance plans cover*. Retrieved May 2023, from Health benefits & coverage: https://www.healthcare.gov/coverage/what-marketplace-plans-cover/

Hopkins, C. S.-B., & Kennedy, E. B.-A.-P. (2024). Caring for survivors of sexual violence in primary care. *Women's Health Care*, *11*(1), 25–30. DOI: 10.51256/WHC022425

Huynh, L. N. (2020, March). *Employment barriers within low- and moderate-income communities*. Retrieved from U.S. Bureau of Labor Statistics: https://www.bls.gov/opub/mlr/2020/beyond-bls/employment-barriers-within-low-and-moderate-income-communities.htm

Iversen, J. (2024, February 27). *Medicaid's Look-Back Period Explained: Exceptions & Penalties*. Retrieved from Paying for Senior Care: https://www.payingforseniorcare.com/medicaid/look-back-period

Karas, K. (2005). Must Doctors Report Underage Sex as Abuse? *The Virtual Mentor*, •••, 234–238. PMID: 23249492

Kleinsinger, F. (2010). Working with the noncompliant patient. *The Permanente Journal*, *14*(1), 54–60. DOI: 10.7812/TPP/09-064 PMID: 20740133

Lyon, W. (2021). Virtue and medical ethics education. *Philosophy, Ethics, and Humanities in Medicine; PEHM*, *16*(1), 2. DOI: 10.1186/s13010-021-00100-2 PMID: 34039382

McGurran, B. (9, May 2023). *College Tuition Inflation: Compare The Cost Of College Over Time*. Retrieved from Forbes Advisor: https://www.forbes.com/advisor/student-loans/college-tuition-inflation/

Medicare.gov. (n.d.). *Costs in the coverage gap*. Retrieved from Medicare.gov: https://www.medicare.gov/drug-coverage-part-d/costs-for-medicare-drug-coverage/costs-in-the-coverage-gap

NACE. (2025). *Principles for Ethical Professional Practice*. Retrieved from NACE: https://naceweb.org/career-development/organizational-structure/principles-for-ethical-professional-practice/

Nall, M. C. (2020, March 4). *What is the Medicare donut hole?* Retrieved from Medical News Today: https://www.medicalnewstoday.com/articles/what-is-the-medicare-donut-hole#donut-hole-in-2020

National Cancer Institute. (n.d.). *Socioeconomic Status*. Retrieved May 2024, from National Cancer Institute: https://www.cancer.gov/publications/dictionaries/cancer-terms/def/socioeconomic-status

Nelson, K. M., Skinner, A., & Underhill, K. (2022). Minor Consent Laws for Sexually Transmitted Infection and HIV Services. *Journal of the American Medical Association*, *328*(7), 674–676. DOI: 10.1001/jama.2022.10777 PMID: 35972493

Peterson-KFF. (2024, January 4). *How do health expenditures vary across the population?* Retrieved from Health System Tracker: https://www.healthsystemtracker.org/chart-collection/health-expenditures-vary-across-population/#Average%20total%20health%20spending,%20by%20age%20and%20sex,%202021%C2%A0

Peterson-KFF. (2024, January 12). *How does cost affect access to healthcare?* Retrieved from Health System Tracker: https://www.healthsystemtracker.org/chart-collection/cost-affect-access-care/#Percent%20of%20adults%20reporting%20delaying%20or%20going%20without%20medical%20care%20due%20to%20cost,%20by%20selected%20characteristics,%202000-2022

Rigsby, E. A. (2016, June 23). *Understanding Exclusionary Zoning and Its Impact on Concentrated Poverty*. Retrieved from The Century Foundation: https://tcf.org/content/facts/understanding-exclusionary-zoning-impact-concentrated-poverty/

Schonberger, J. (2024, January 28). *The threat that high childcare costs pose to the US economy*. Retrieved from Yahoo Finance: https://finance.yahoo.com/news/the-threat-that-high-childcare-costs-pose-to-the-us-economy-124248273.html

Schulz, M. (2023, August 10). *Student Loan Debt Statistics*. Retrieved from LendingTree: https://www.lendingtree.com/student/student-loan-debt-statistics/

Scott, D. (2023, October 16). *Why the US is the only country that ties your health insurance to your job*. Retrieved from Vox: https://www.vox.com/23890764/healthcare-insurance-marketplace-open-enrollment-employer-sponsored-united-blue-cross-shield-aetna

United Nations. (2025). *What Is The UN Ethics Office?* Retrieved from UN Ethics Office: Listen - Advise - Respect: https://www.un.org/en/ethics/#:~:text=The%20UN%20Ethics%20Office%20promotes,and%20respect%20for%20human%20rights

Varkey, B. (2020). Principles of Clinical Ethics and Their Application to Practice. *Medical Principles and Practice : International Journal of the Kuwait University, Health Science Centre*, •••, 17–28. https://pmc.ncbi.nlm.nih.gov/articles/PMC7923912/ PMID: 32498071

Wang, K. (2022). Housing Instability and Socioeconomic Disparities in Health: Evidence from the U.S. Economic Recession. *Journal of Racial and Ethnic Health Disparities*, *9*(6), 2451–2467. DOI: 10.1007/s40615-021-01181-7 PMID: 34837164

Wermiel, S. J. (2023, January 6). *Inequitable and Inadequate School Funding*. Retrieved from American Bar Association: Human Rights: https://www.americanbar.org/groups/crsj/publications/human_rights_magazine_home/wealth-disparities-in-civil-rights/inequitable-and-inadequate-school-funding/

Wiederhold, S., Lergetporer, P., Peter, F., & Hermes, H. (2021, December 7). https://cepr.org/voxeu/columns/socioeconomic-gap-childcare-enrolment-role-behavioural-barriers. Retrieved from CEPR: https://cepr.org/voxeu/columns/socioeconomic-gap-childcare-enrolment-role-behavioural-barriers

World Population Review. (2024). *Age of Consent by State 2024*. Retrieved from World Population Review: https://worldpopulationreview.com/state-rankings/age-of-consent-by-state

Chapter 5
Race:
The Implications of Historical Oppression on Healthcare

Katherine Art
Wright State University, USA

EXECUTIVE SUMMARY

Race plays a large role in United States history. Because of that history, there has been a large impact of race on healthcare. Race has impacted how we diagnose and treat diseases and there are both overt and hidden ways that race is still ingrained in our healthcare system. Race has also impacted how patients may view the healthcare system and a long history of experimentation on vulnerable populations continues to impact trust in the healthcare system today. Cases include exploration of topics such as diagnosis of psychotic disorders, using race-based correction factors, broader implication of policy change, pain treatment in patients, intersectionality, the importance of informed consent, and the impact of experimentation on current healthcare and research.

INTRODUCTION

The history of how race has impacted treatment by physicians is complicated. This history has shaped, and continues to shape, how patients perceive the medical field. History also impacts biases that healthcare providers may have before entering the medical field or are taught during training. The chapter will also explore current disparities that people of color experience in the United States today and will challenge implicit bias healthcare learners may have through educational cases.

DOI: 10.4018/979-8-3693-3683-0.ch005

History of Race in Medicine

Historically, medicine and science have been used to justify different political positions by taking different stances on the question: is there an inherent biologic or medical difference in people of different races? Scientific racism was created of false scientific and medical theories positing that there was an inherent difference between races, which were used to justify slavery as a practice and mistreatment of slaves. In the mid-1800s, an American physician Samuel Morton used his large collection of human skulls, which he measured as a proxy for brain size, to invent an intellectual hierarchy that placed White people at the top and Black people at the bottom. He also used these measurements as justification that different races were different species. (Fabian, 2010)

In the antebellum south, the health of slaves was important to plantation owners as they attempted to protect their investment in purchasing the slaves. Physicians often treated slaves on plantations, with the objective of preventing time off of work. This importance of slave health for productivity caused interest in which diseases could be prevented and the quickest treatment of diseases that could prevent slaves from working. In DeBow's Review, a journal on management of slaves, an American physician coined the name *drapetomania*, a disease that caused slaves to desire freedom and run away. He also described *dysaethesia aethiopis*, which was a disease causing "rascality" in Black people and could be cured by stimulating the skin, liver and kidneys. (Cartwright, 1851) Although there were many calls for books or medical school classes on caring specifically for slaves, there were no books published or classes taught on the topic. (Savitt, 1978)

The belief that Black people did not feel pain or anxiety was used to justify surgery or painful experiments without the use of anesthetic. In one example, Dr. Marion Sims performed experimental gynecologic surgeries to close vesicovaginal fistulas on enslaved Black women. When performing the surgeries, he did not use analgesia on the Black women because he claimed the procedures were not painful enough, but several years later when doing the same procedures on White women several years later he did use analgesia. (Washington, 2006) This false belief of differences in pain tolerance has been noted in writings throughout the nineteenth and twentieth centuries.

This bias that Black patients feel less pain is still persistent today and studies have found that in the emergency room, Black and Hispanic patients are less likely to receive equivalent levels of analgesia than White patients for similar injuries or diseases. (Lee et al., 2019; Mills et al., 2011) This may lead to a host of negative consequences from letting patients suffer in pain to worsening minority patients' distrust in the medical system. In a study of 418 medical students and residents, half of the medical trainees endorsed false biological beliefs about the differences between Black and White patients and were more likely to rate a Black patient's pain as lower than the White patients, and make less accurate treatment recommendations. (Hoffman et al., 2016) Although this is a small sample size, this study is jarring for how important it is to incorporate anti-bias teachings into medical training and how these beliefs still persist today. The historical myths of innate differences of sensation of pain between races and history of denying Black patients adequate pain treatment continues to impact patients today.

The Human Genome Project demonstrated that race had no genetic basis and that there is more genetic variation between people within a race than between different races. (Collins et al., 2003) Despite the scientific acceptance that there is no biologic difference between races, there continue to be many who posit that differences in disease prevalence or treatment are due to biologic or genetic differences in disease because of race. Alan Goodman, a biological anthropology professor, explained it well, "Geographic ancestry is not the same thing as race… geographic ancestry, which does indeed matter to genetics, can be conflated with race, which does not." (Goodman, 2020)

Experimentation Throughout History:

People in minority races have been taken advantage of in medical experimentation, especially when they were unable to consent or were coerced into participating. Of particular concern is the large number of examples of experimentation on minority peoples in trials with no conceivable benefit to the patient.

There are many examples of experimentation on slaves. Slaves were often used, or even exclusively purchased, for medical experimentation and were forced into painful and dangerous experiments. In one example, a slave was put in a hole with a fire until he fainted to determine which medicine would best prevent heat stroke. (Savitt, 1982) Another notable example is that many pioneering gynecologic surgeries were developed on enslaved women including treatment for vesico-vaginal fistula, cesarian sections, and early ovariectomies. (Cooper Owens, 2017) Also, slaves' deceased bodies were used without consent for medical training to perform autopsies and anatomy dissections all around the country. (Savitt, 1982)

After slavery ended, unethical experimentation on people of color did not end. The most commonly known example is the Tuskegee syphilis studies that were conducted from 1932-1972 in which syphilis was observed in Black men. The study prevented the men from seeking treatment and did not inform them of their condition, allowing them to pass the disease on to sexual partners and their children. 276 of the 600 participants died as a direct result of untreated syphilis and additional 154 participants died of heart disease which cannot be confirmed to be related or unrelated to the untreated syphilis. (Heller, 2022) These terrible outcomes in a now very well-known historical example highlights the extent of unethical medical experimentation on Black individuals. In another example, the U.S. Atomic Energy Commission conducted more than two thousand experiments between 1944 and 1994, disproportionately on Black Americans, without their knowledge or consent, to determine the effect of radiation on human subjects. These experiments were not to treat any medical conditions, but conducted to study how radiation affects the human body. (Washington, 2006)

Forced sterilization is another area where a lack of consent led to detrimental effects for patients of many minority races and people of lower classes. Many Black, Native American, and Latina women were sterilized without their consent from the early 1900s to the 1970s. Women of color were disproportionately victims of involuntary sterilization when eugenics was popularized in the early 1900s and the procedures of sterilizing Black women while they were unconscious, without their knowledge or informed consent, became so common it began to be known as the "Mississippi Appendectomy". (Washington, 2006) In the early 1970s, a physician Dr. Pinkerton-Uri and other Native Americans accused the Indian Health Services (IHS) of sterilizing one in four Native American women between the ages of 15 and 45 and accused them of not receiving true informed consent, as many of the women thought the surgeries were reversible or were coerced into signing the documents. (Lawrence, 2000) Dr. Pinkerton-Uri brought this information to a US Senator, James Abourezk of South Dakota, who requested a federal investigation. (Lawrence, 2000) The federal investigation found between the years 1973-1976, three thousand and one sterilizations occurred on women ages fifteen to forty-five, and of the sterilizations reviewed in depth, most of the consent forms did not fulfill the requirements the IHS had for informed consent. (Staats EB, 1976) Latina women were also victim to forced sterilization. By the mid- 1960s, an estimated one third of mothers between the ages 20-65 in Puerto Rico had been sterilized. (Presser, 1969) Also, California had a sterilization program in the early 1900s that disproportionately targeted Latino patients. (Novak et al., 2018)

Many have pointed to Tuskegee as a large reason for mistrust from Black patients, although some research has suggested that mistrust of the medical system results from a broader history of inequality. (Brandon et al., 2005; Scharff et al., 2010) Medical mistrust is associated with lower participation in biomedical research. (George et al., 2014; Scharff et al., 2010) Medical mistrust is also associated with lower healthcare utilization, (LaVeist et al., 2009) and lower rates of preventative screening. (Powell et al., 2019) Understanding sources of mistrust in patients can help healthcare professionals when obtaining informed consent today and when explaining treatment options, including experimental treatments and clinical trials. Overall, the historical context of mistreatment and experimentation influences mistrust and is an important factor in the disparities seen today between minority patients and their White counterparts.

Current Disparities

There continues to be significant disparities in the United States between the health of different racial groups. Black American and Hispanic Americans continue to suffer from chronic disease at a higher rate than White Non-Hispanic Americans. (Odlum et al., 2020) There is a complex set of likely reasons for these disparities including systemic and institutional racism, the intersection of socioeconomic differences, and bias from healthcare professionals. Access to a primary care provider and having health insurance are important for obtaining preventative healthcare services, managing chronic conditions, and getting diagnosis and treatment for new conditions. A smaller percentage of minority patients in the United States have a primary care provider or healthcare insurance than White patients. (*Adults Who Report Not Having a Personal Doctor/Health Care Provider by Race/Ethnicity*, 2022) A study of Medicare patients found that Black patients had less specialist referrals than their White counterparts (Landon et al., 2021), so even for Black patients that have a primary care provider, they may not receive the same level of care. In the electronic medical record, some studies have found that stigmatizing language appeared most frequently about non-Hispanic Black patients. (Himmelstein et al., 2022) The institutions of healthcare have also been predominantly designed for White patients. One example of this is that skin color affects the accuracy of pulse-oximetry sensors, (Sjoding et al., 2020) which could prolong therapy that could be urgently needed for people of color.

Healthcare providers' bias, both implicit or overt, plays an important role in current disparities today. A 2003 US Institute of Medicine study reviewed how a large portion of observed disease prevalence differences between races can be attributed to unequal healthcare treatment, specifically assessing how race impacts the clinical encounter. (Institute of Medicine (US) Committee on Understanding and Eliminating Racial and Ethnic Disparities in Health Care, 2003) Increased implicit bias may cause healthcare providers to take use a condescending tone with patients, use less effective communication methods, or recommend treatment options based on the biases or assumptions about adherence. This poor communication can cause patients to feel less satisfied and/or less likely to understand or follow recommendations, which can perpetuate the biases held by the healthcare provider. (Saluja & Bryant, 2021) Healthcare provider bias and poor communication can also lead to patient mistrust of the healthcare system.

Use of Correction Factors

Another large area of discussion where race continues to impact medical decision-making today is the use of correction factors for race in many different diagnostic/prognostic parameters. Some examples include the correction values in estimated glomerular filtration rate (eGFR), in pulmonary function testing (PFTs), vaginal birth after cesarian section (VBAC) success estimates, and in a fracture risk assessment tool (FRAX). Estimated glomerular filtration rate (eGFR) is an estimated value for how effectively the kidneys are working, so lower eGFRs are used to classify worsening chronic kidney disease. The equations used to calculate eGFR includes adjustments for age, sex, and race. Due to some small studies in the late 1900s, researchers concluded that being from the Black race was an independent predictor for GFR. The correction factors increase Black patients' eGFR compared to patients from other races. (Uppal et al., 2022; Vyas et al., 2020) In pulmonary function tests, spirometry is used to estimate the function of the lungs. These function results can help with diagnosis of lung disease such as COPD or interstitial lung disease. There are correction factors for patients that are identified as Black or Asian, that increase lung function compared to other patients' spirometry. (Bhakta et al., 2023; Vyas et al., 2020) These correction factors can cause disease to be under-estimated leading to decreased or delayed treatment. The correction factor makes it harder for patients to get kidney transplants for chronic kidney disease or lung transplants for interstitial lung disease. (Schluger et al., 2022; Vyas et al., 2020)

Another example of the use of correction factors is in a calculation for successful vaginal birth after caesarian section (VBAC). The calculation uses a correction factor that causes the equation to predict a higher chance of failing VBAC for African American or Hispanic patients. This increased calculated risk may decrease shared decision making with providers and push African American or Hispanic women away from attempting a trial of labor after a cesarean section. (Faulkner et al., 2021; Vyas et al., 2020) There are already disparities in the United States leading to increased maternal and infant mortality for minority patients (Holdt Somer et al., 2017; Jang & Lee, 2022), and this adjusted calculation could be worsening these disparities.

Another commonly applied assumption is in osteoporosis. In the FRAX algorithm, Asian, Hispanic, and Black women will be adjusted to have lower risk of fracture. (Vyas et al., 2020) A 2016 article was published that demonstrated wide variation of osteoporosis risk in African patients based on the country within Africa (80-fold risk difference between the widest varying countries) and the risk includes not only genetic risk factors but differences in lifestyle and cultural factors that vary by country. (Hilliard, 2016) If osteoporosis rates vary so widely within African countries, it would be unwise to apply this assumption about genetic predisposition to all Black people in the United States. These correction factors are an example of systemic racism that has been built in to clinical decision making.

Schizophrenia

Physicians diagnose Black and Hispanic patients with schizophrenia at a rate 3-4 times higher than White patients, even when a diagnosis of schizophrenia are not justified. (Schwartz & Blankenship, 2014) Several possible theories for why have been suggested such as clinician racial bias or clinician misinterpretation of symptoms, but little research has been conducted into why there is such a large difference in rates of schizophrenia diagnosis. Misdiagnosis with schizophrenia has significant impacts a patient's medical treatment and their ability to advocate for themselves. Patients with schizophrenia often end up in the legal system, which makes it more difficult to get housing or a job. Further, how the schizophrenia is treated varies by race, as Black patients are more likely to be labeled as "dangerous" and overtreated with higher potency anti-psychotics at higher doses (Segal et al., 1996) Black patients are less likely than White patients to be given second generation anti-psychotics, which have a more favorable side effect profile than the first-generation anti-psychotics. (Herbeck et al., 2004)

While there are many large topics covered here, this is in no way comprehensive for the vast and multifactorial historical relationship between race and medicine. Beginning with beliefs of biologic inferiority, historically medicine and biology have been crafted to appear to justify racism. Experimentation on minority races has impacted all disciplines of medicine and is an important part of history that continues to impact trust of medical professionals. Today, race is still a factor in diagnosis of diseases, such as schizophrenia and impacts treatment including eligibility for surgeries based on correction factors.

CASES

Case 1. Acute Psychosis: An Example of Diagnosis Influenced by Race

Learning Objectives

1. Assess the history leading to disparities in schizophrenia diagnosis by race.
2. Distinguish biases that occur in treating psychiatric patients.
3. Create a differential diagnosis for psychosis including other medical causes of psychosis.

Case Aim: The case details a Black woman who presents with acute psychosis with other medical complaints including gastrointestinal distress. The case challenges assumptions and asks students to think about the consequences of bias. The case emphasizes the ethical importance of creating a broad differential for all patients.

The patient is a 21-year-old Black female. The patient is transferred to the inpatient psychiatric unit you are working on after being admitted from the Emergency Room (ER). The patient reports she took "mushrooms" four weeks ago and since that time has been having abdominal pain, diarrhea and vomiting. Her parents joined her in the ER and reported she has been acting strange lately. They report she has been missing her classes and friends had not seen her in days, has been suspicious of people at the university saying they are "poisoning her" and described her diarrhea as "cleansing the devil from her". The patient's parents report she has never had an episode like this before and report she has continued having 5-6 episodes of painful, non-bloody diarrhea daily. Mental status exam is significant for a patient oriented to person, place, and time. The patient endorses delusions and reports she has been having some auditory hallucinations of voices.

The patient is a senior at a local college. She has had several successful internships and has signed on for a job at a major company after graduation. She is active on campus in several groups. She endorses drinking on the weekends (4-5 standard drinks on Fridays and Saturdays), no tobacco use past or present, she has tried marijuana two times over a year ago, and endorses a month ago she took "a handful" of mushrooms that a friend gave to her. You talk to the family and they have no past medical history of psychiatric illness. Her mother has diabetes. Maternal grandparents both have diabetes and are otherwise healthy. Her father has had several episodes of abdominal pain and diarrhea, but has had two negative diagnostic work-ups. His family history is unknown as he was adopted. On physical exam the patient has some diffuse tenderness to abdominal palpation, without guarding or rebound tenderness.

You talk to the attending physician and they suggest the patient's parents may be denying true psychiatric history because it can be "cultural to downplay psychiatric issues". They would like to put schizophrenia at the top of differential and begin treatment with an anti-psychotic.

Case Questions

1. Are There Assumptions About This Patient That Are Impacting Her Care? Would Your Assumptions Change if the Patient Was Homeless and Did Not Have Supportive Parents?

- There are assumptions being made by the attending physician. The physician is assuming the parents are not being truthful, which may be due to bias from past cases or may be a racially led bias. There is likely an assumption that the mushroom consumption triggered a psychotic disorder to present. Because Black patients are diagnosed with schizophrenia at a higher rate than White patients, there may be some implicit bias that the patient has schizophrenia also. The case does not give us what the team's next steps will be, but ruling out medical causes of psychosis would be an important next step. Assumptions of what the patient's diagnosis may be influenced away from schizophrenia based on the patient's history of success academically and professionally. This may be due to stigma and bias towards people with psychotic disorders, assuming they cannot be successful members of society.

2. What Are the Implications of Hospitalization and Documenting That This Patient Has Schizophrenia or a Psychotic Disorder?

- Often when patients have an undifferentiated psychotic disorder, it can get put into the chart as schizophrenia under medical history. This can cause this diagnosis to be linked with them in the medical chart. When patients come into the emergency room, some providers may use anchoring bias to attribute many complaints or issues to a psychiatric disorder, impacting their care in the future. Also, patients who have psychosis can become involved in the legal system or may be placed on an involuntary hold through a probate court, which can impact future jobs and housing opportunities.

  If schizophrenia, or another psychotic disorder, is incorrectly identified as the etiology for the episode, anti-psychotics may be administered. There are many side effects to anti-psychotics, which are worse with first generation anti-psychotics than the second-generation anti-psychotics. Black patients are more likely to get first generation anti-psychotics or to be labeled as "dangerous". (Herbeck et al., 2004; Segal et al., 1996) Also, this hospitalization may cause distrust from the patient or the patient's family, if they feel that the patient has been mistreated.

3. Are There Aspects to This Case That Suggest There Could Be Another Cause to the Patient's Psychosis?

- This patient is having other symptoms besides psychosis. This episode of psychosis was sudden onset and from the history given, it appears to be unusual for the patient and she was without a prodrome. Although the mushroom use may have triggered the psychosis, the effects appear to be longer lasting than a normal reaction to the hallucinogenic compounds. The patient also is having abdominal pain and diarrhea and has a family history of a father with episodes of gastrointestinal issues. These medical manifestations may also suggest that there could be a medical cause to her psychosis. It is important that all patients with features suspicious for underlying medical causes get an appropriate diagnostic work-up, regardless of their race.

4. What Are the Next Steps When Caring for This Patient?

- Some other potential causes of acute psychosis include acute intermittent porphyria, autoimmune disease, ovarian teratoma, brain tumor, and thyroid dysfunction. These could be ruled out with appropriate laboratory testing or imaging. A drug screen could also be useful, although many hallucinogens are not commonly tested for on standard drug screens. If the patient has continued to use hallucinogens during this episode, being in the hospital may offer time away from active use of the hallucinogens.

  People with psychotic diseases may be triggered by substance use, such as mushrooms, so it is possible that the mushrooms unmasked an underlying pre-disposition to have a psychotic disorder such as schizophrenia. There is little research done about long-term effects of mushrooms, but as more research is done on psilocybin, studies may be conducted on whether effects can last longer term or alter brain chemistry.

Case Discussion: A diagnosis of schizophrenia is life-changing and Black patients have been inappropriately diagnosed. It is important to get background information to ensure patients meet the definition of schizophrenia before a diagnosis is made. Alternate causes should be explored for the cause of psychosis in all patients as other medical causes can lead to acute psychosis, but have a different pathophysiology and treatment. There may be bias in patients with mental health disorders and a diagnosis may change future treatment and can impact legal and social factors for patients. Having background knowledge about bias may impact diagnosis and treatment could change a patient's life.

Case 2: Race Related Correction Factors in Diagnostic and Prognostic Tools

Learning Objectives

1. Explain race as a social construct.
2. Distinguish institutional/systemic racism practices in medicine.
3. Analyze the implications of broader policy changes.

Case Aim: This case is an example of institutional racism that has continued in diagnostic and prognostic tools. This case will spark discussion about implications both medically and socially for patients with broader diagnostic tool change.

Patient is a 25 year old Asian man. He wants to join the military. He got pulmonary function tests during his eligibility assessment because of a history of exercise induced asthma when he was younger. The patient doesn't remember needing an inhaler and is currently having no symptoms. With the correction factors it shows that he has no lung disease and without the correction factors it is showing that he has mild obstructive lung disease. For family history, his parents were born in the Philippines. There is no known lung disease in either parent or either set of grandparents.

Case Questions

1. Are There Inherent Biologic Differences With Different Races?

- Race is a social construct. There is no biologic difference between races. Geographic ancestry can influence genetics. In the case of the patient, it is clearer where his family originated, but many patients will not have clear geographic lineage and race reduces people into a small number of arbitrary categories.

2. What Assumptions Are Made Using Correction Factors?

- Overall, using correction factors assumes that there is a biologic difference in lung function based on a patient's race. One assumption that can come with adding correction factors is assuming race based on appearance. This judgement by providers can significantly impact a patient's care based on an assumption. A problem that comes with using correction factors is if a person is mixed race or has multiple races. If the patient in the case did not have clear geographic heritage, it may not be as easy to select a correction factor for Southeast Asians or to find a geographic correct factor.

3. What Implications Could Happen From Using the Race-Based Correction Factors?

- Implications from using a correction factor could include a patient not getting a diagnosis or appropriate treatment if they do have disease. For pulmonary function tests this can impact patient's quality of life if they are having trouble breathing and can impact eligibility for certain treatments based on insurance. For other correction factors, this may include having another major abdominal surgery in the case of a low VBAC score or not receiving treatments that could prevent further kidney damage in the case of a higher than true GFR. Another implication of these correction factors is impacting the patient's eligibility for transplant. This is specifically true for PFTs and GFR. Patients with pulmonary fibrosis or chronic kidney failure have a cut-off to be considered for transplant eligibility, so having a higher lung or kidney function may limit minority patients' ability to be on the transplant list.

4. Are There Implications From Removing the Correction Factors?

- Removing the correction factors will cause lower lung function values for African American and Asian patients. In kidney function, removing the correction factors will show lower kidney functions for African American patients. In the case of some lung cancer treatment, PFTs determine whether the patient has enough residual lung function to support a lobectomy. If the patient's lung function is determined to be lower than certain thresholds, it may limit minority patients' treatment options or patients may be deemed to not have enough lung function to get elective surgeries. Economically, it may make it harder to get some job, such as in this case for the military, but some other jobs like firefighters, pilots, and commercial diving, also require normal lung function. It also, may make insurance more costly or deductibles higher for patients if they are diagnosed with more severe disease, which can further exacerbate race related health disparities.

Case Discussion: Correction factors used in diagnostic algorithms are an example of institutional racism that continues to perpetuate the belief that there are genetic differences by race. In some correction factors, race may be included as a proxy instead of the true factors that underlie biologic differences. For example, lung function based on geographic origin, or because patients in minority races suffer at higher rates of type 2 diabetes, using their race instead of type 2 diabetes in a diagnostic calculation. These calculations misconstrue correlation and causality and further the idea that there is a biologic difference between races.

Case 3: Informed Consent in Experimental Treatment

Learning Objectives

1. Identify key components of informed consent.
2. Describe the historical context for importance of informed consent, research on vulnerable populations, and reasons for mistrust.
3. Illustrate discussions about informed consent.

Case Aim: This case highlights patient hesitancy associated with experimental treatments due to the history of harmful experimentation without consent on minority patients. This case can help students understand informed consent, practice how they would obtain informed consent from a patient, and build trust with patients.

A Black 85-year-old man is in the ICU with sepsis and respiratory failure. A new virus has been severely impacting older adults. He tested positive for this virus. There is a treatment that is being used off-label without FDA approved, but has shown promising research results. When asked to give consent for the experimental treatment, the patient's daughter tells you they know about people being victims of poorly conducted research that takes advantage of Black people. The report they don't want their dad to "be a guinea pig" and they would like to decline the treatment.

Case Questions

1. What Are the Components of Informed Consent?

- There are four components to informed consent: disclosure, understanding, voluntariness, and authorization. Disclosure includes reporting all important information including what the intervention is and risks and benefits of accepting or declining the intervention. Understanding is confirming that the patient or their surrogate decision maker have capacity and understand the information that was given. Voluntariness is the principle that informed consent is conducted without coercion and authorization is documentation of the decision to accept or decline the intervention after ensuring the patient or their decision maker are informed.

2. What Emotions Are You Bringing as a Physician to This Discussion With the Family? Are There Things You Could Discuss With the Family to Help Reduce Some of the Mistrust?

- This family discussion may feel overwhelming or like the patient's family is accusing the physician personally of continuing oppressive tactics as they are a part of the medical system. Mistrust of the medical system from minorities is still common, and is understandable because of the historical context. Identifying if you feel defensive or upset that the patient's family does not trust you as an extension of the medical system can help separate an emotional response from doing the best thing for the patient and respecting patient autonomy. Some things you could talk about with the patient's family include asking about what concerns they have with the treatment, asking about concerns they have for their father's health, and answering questions they have honestly. You could also ask what the family has heard about experimentation so that you can address specific apprehensions about ensuring that the patient is treated fairly and is not undergoing unnecessary treatment for experimentation. Making sure the patient's family understands the risks and benefits of both accepting and declining the treatment is an important step to ensure they have equitable care. Even if a discussion does not result in the patient getting the treatment, it may be an important step in beginning to build trust with the family. Honesty and respect for their autonomy are key principles to keep in mind during the family discussion.

3. What Is the Historical Context for Mistrust From This Family?

- There is a long history of lack of informed consent from vulnerable populations, specifically a long history in the United States of experimentation on Black patients. There is a larger history of mistreatment of Black Americans that impacts mistrust today, including interpersonal, institutional, and structural racism. It is important to understand examples from history such as experimentation on slaves or the Tuskegee Syphilis experiment, and medical procedures performed without consent such as forced sterilization. If the patient's family gives a specific example from history they have heard about, researching it may help the physician understand some of their mistrust.

4. Because This Therapy Could Help With the Patients' Treatment, What Are the Lasting Implications of Historical Experimentation?

- Because this could be a beneficial therapy, it may be that patients are being harmed indirectly due to the mistrust that experimentation caused. The actions of historical providers may be harming patients secondarily as research on this treatment may be performed on a less diverse population and the patients who could benefit from the experimental treatment may decline treatment.

Case Discussion: In order to obtain informed consent, healthcare professionals need to understand the essential parts of obtaining consent: disclosure, understanding, voluntariness, and authorization. Informed consent is an important part of providing ethical medical care and conducting ethical research. Having knowledge about the historical context for exploitation of vulnerable people that lacked informed consent is essential for building trust with patients and their families. This case offers an opportunity for students to practice having these discussions, which is a key skill in being a culturally sensitive physician.

Case 4: Intersectionality and Bias in Pain Treatment

Learning Objectives

1. Identify bias in pain management
2. Assess objective signs of substance use/drug seeking behavior
3. Design methods to advocate for patients

Case Aim: This case is an example of intersectionality and how bias can impact patient care. This case will assist students in identifying bias and finding ways to equitably assess and advocate for this patient.

You are a student working in the emergency room your patient is a 52-year-old Black Hispanic man. He reports he does not have insurance and has not seen a doctor for at least ten years. The patient smokes a pack of cigarettes a day, smokes marijuana several days a week, and has a history of substance use with cocaine, but reports he has not used cocaine in a few years. He came to the emergency department for foot pain. On physical exam there is a large open wound that has some purulent discharge on the plantar side of his first metatarsal joint. The patient has been reporting 10/10 severe pain in the foot. You notice that the resident saw the patient and only added as needed ibuprofen for pain management.

Case Questions

1. What Biases Are Present in This Case?

- This patient has many identities intersecting that cause him to be at risk for being denied pain medications. Race, ethnicity, history of substance use, lack of insurance, and potential lack of health literacy. The case does not address whether the patient speaks English, but this may be another barrier for the patient to receive treatment and pain management. There may be an implicit bias that the patient does not feel pain as strongly because of his race or that he is seeking pain medication because he has a history of substance use.

2. What Are Some Objective Signs Providers Can Use to Assess for Substance Use or Drug Seeking Behaviors?

- One objective data point to assess whether a patient is seeking inappropriate pain medication is to check government-led databases of prescriptions for other monitored substances from other providers and look through the electronic medical record for whether the patient has a history of coming in recurrently for pain medication. Other objective "red flags" include the patient being unwilling to try any treatment except the medication they are seeking, asking for drugs by name or amount, or being more interested in getting a prescription for pain medication than being assessed to move towards a diagnosis. Also, the setting of where the patient is asking for pain medication matters. In outpatient settings, patients who frequently ask for increased dosage of opioid medications, run out of pills before the prescription should be up, or drive long distances to seek new providers to prescribe them pain medication can also cause suspicion. The clinical decision is also different based on suspected pathology. In this case, the patient may have a diabetic foot ulcer and with the physical exam finding of purulent material, it could suggest osteomyelitis. Further clinical work-up will need to be conducted, but osteomyelitis is very painful and may require treatment with opioid medications.

3. In What Ways Can You Advocate for the Patient?

- Talking with the attending physician or resident and seeing what pathologies are on their differential diagnoses would be a good first step. If they also think this patient has osteomyelitis, a student could politely ask about treatment and at what point opioid pain management would be recommended. Students will be better able to advocate for patients by understanding the patient's history well, already having screened for "red flags" for drug seeking behavior, and being up to date on guidelines for management of the most likely causes of the patient's pain.

Case Discussion: The patient has many identities that could put him at risk for not receiving adequate pain medication. Race plays an integral role in this and his different identities may compound on each other to worsen bias against him. There is significant bias in pain management and this can impact patient quality of life. Students can improve their ability to identify their own bias, use objective tools to ensure patients are treated equitably, and advocate for patients that may be victims of bias from the healthcare system.

CONCLUSION

Historically, medicine and biology has been used illegitimately to support biases and discrimination against minority races. Medical research was often performed without informed consent, sometimes without explicit benefits to patients. The history of which has led to mistrust of medical professionals by vulnerable populations. There are still ways these biases impact medicine today including the way diseases are diagnosed and treatment is prescribed. The assumptions and biases on race must be challenged to restore patient trust, such as in the correction factors for race for calculated diagnostic and prognostic values, how pain is assessed, certain diagnoses, and even the practice of receiving informed consent. History gives both background to the viewpoint with which patients approach the medical field and can help physicians reflect on their own biases and the basis for some of the bias that is taught in their training.

REFERENCES

Adults Who Report Not Having a Personal Doctor/Health Care Provider by Race/ Ethnicity. (2022). KFF.

Bhakta, N. R., Bime, C., Kaminsky, D. A., McCormack, M. C., Thakur, N., Stanojevic, S., Baugh, A. D., Braun, L., Lovinsky-Desir, S., Adamson, R., Witonsky, J., Wise, R. A., Levy, S. D., Brown, R., Forno, E., Cohen, R. T., Johnson, M., Balmes, J., Mageto, Y., & Burney, P. (2023). Race and Ethnicity in Pulmonary Function Test Interpretation: An Official American Thoracic Society Statement. *American Journal of Respiratory and Critical Care Medicine, 207*(8), 978–995. DOI: 10.1164/ rccm.202302-0310ST PMID: 36973004

Brandon, D. T., Isaac, L. A., & LaVeist, T. A. (2005). The legacy of Tuskegee and trust in medical care: Is Tuskegee responsible for race differences in mistrust of medical care? *Journal of the National Medical Association, 97*(7), 951–956. PMID: 16080664

Cartwright, S. (1851). Diseases and Peculiarities of the Negro Race. *De Bow's Review, 1*(2).

Collins, F. S., Morgan, M., & Patrinos, A. (2003). The Human Genome Project: Lessons from Large-Scale Biology. *Science, 300*(5617), 286–290. DOI: 10.1126/ science.1084564 PMID: 12690187

Cooper Owens, D. (2017). *Medical Bondage: Race, Gender, and the Origins of American Gynecology*. University of Georgia Press., DOI: 10.2307/j.ctt1pwt69x

Fabian, A. (2010). *The Skull Collectors: Race, Science and America's Unburied Dead*. University of Chicago Press. DOI: 10.7208/chicago/9780226233499.001.0001

Faulkner, S., Haas, M., Wang, D., Walker, C., Lee-Parritz, A., Perkins, R., & Chinkam, S. (2021). The effects of removing race from the VBAC calculator: Implications for counseling. *American Journal of Obstetrics and Gynecology, 224*(2), S467–S468. DOI: 10.1016/j.ajog.2020.12.769

George, S., Duran, N., & Norris, K. (2014). A Systematic Review of Barriers and Facilitators to Minority Research Participation Among African Americans, Latinos, Asian Americans, and Pacific Islanders. *American Journal of Public Health, 104*(2), e16–e31. DOI: 10.2105/AJPH.2013.301706 PMID: 24328648

Goodman, A. (2020, June 25). *Race Is Real, But It's Not Genetic*. Discover Magazine.

Heller, J. (2022, July 25). *AP exposes the Tuskegee Syphilis Study: The 50th Anniversary*. Associated Press.

Herbeck, D. M., West, J. C., Ruditis, I., Duffy, F. F., Fitek, D. J., Bell, C. C., & Snowden, L. R. (2004). Variations in use of second-generation antipsychotic medication by race among adult psychiatric patients. *Psychiatric Services (Washington, D.C.)*, *55*(6), 677–684. DOI: 10.1176/appi.ps.55.6.677 PMID: 15175466

Hilliard, C. B. (2016). High osteoporosis risk among East Africans linked to lactase persistence genotype. *BoneKEy Reports*, *5*. Advance online publication. DOI: 10.1038/bonekey.2016.30 PMID: 27408710

Himmelstein, G., Bates, D., & Zhou, L. (2022). Examination of Stigmatizing Language in the Electronic Health Record. *JAMA Network Open*, *5*(1), e2144967. Advance online publication. DOI: 10.1001/jamanetworkopen.2021.44967 PMID: 35084481

Hoffman, K. M., Trawalter, S., Axt, J. R., & Oliver, M. N. (2016). Racial bias in pain assessment and treatment recommendations, and false beliefs about biological differences between blacks and whites. *Proceedings of the National Academy of Sciences of the United States of America*, *113*(16), 4296–4301. DOI: 10.1073/pnas.1516047113 PMID: 27044069

Holdt Somer, S. J., Sinkey, R. G., & Bryant, A. S. (2017). Epidemiology of racial/ethnic disparities in severe maternal morbidity and mortality. *Seminars in Perinatology*, *41*(5), 258–265. DOI: 10.1053/j.semperi.2017.04.001 PMID: 28888263

Institute of Medicine (US) Committee on Understanding and Eliminating Racial and Ethnic Disparities in Health Care. (2003). *Unequal Treatment: Confronting Racial and Ethnic Disparities in Health Care* (Smedley, B. D., Stith, A. Y., & Nelson, A. R., Eds.). National Academies Press. DOI: 10.17226/12875

Jang, C., & Lee, H. (2022). A Review of Racial Disparities in Infant Mortality in the US. *Children (Basel, Switzerland)*, *9*(2), 257. DOI: 10.3390/children9020257 PMID: 35204976

Landon, B. E., Onnela, J.-P., Meneades, L., & James O'malley, M. (2021). Assessment of Racial Disparities in Primary Care Physician Specialty Referrals. *JAMA Network Open*, *4*(1), 2029238. DOI: 10.1001/jamanetworkopen.2020.29238 PMID: 33492373

LaVeist, T. A., Isaac, L. A., & Williams, K. P. (2009). Mistrust of Health Care Organizations Is Associated with Underutilization of Health Services. *Health Services Research*, *44*(6), 2093–2105. DOI: 10.1111/j.1475-6773.2009.01017.x PMID: 19732170

Lawrence, J. (2000). The Indian Health Service and the Sterilization of Native American Women. *American Indian Quarterly*, *24*(3), 400–419. DOI: 10.1353/aiq.2000.0008 PMID: 17089462

Lee, P., Le Saux, M., Siegel, R., Goyal, M., Chen, C., Ma, Y., & Meltzer, A. C. (2019). Racial and ethnic disparities in the management of acute pain in US emergency departments: Meta-analysis and systematic review. *The American Journal of Emergency Medicine*, *37*(9), 1770–1777. DOI: 10.1016/j.ajem.2019.06.014 PMID: 31186154

Mills, A. M., Shofer, F. S., Boulis, A. K., Holena, D. N., & Abbuhl, S. B. (2011). Racial disparity in analgesic treatment for ED patients with abdominal or back pain. *The American Journal of Emergency Medicine*, *29*(7), 752–756. DOI: 10.1016/j.ajem.2010.02.023 PMID: 20825892

Novak, N. L., Lira, N., O'Connor, K. E., Harlow, S. D., Kardia, S. L. R., & Stern, A. M. (2018). Disproportionate Sterilization of Latinos Under California's Eugenic Sterilization Program, 1920–1945. *American Journal of Public Health*, *108*(5), 611–613. DOI: 10.2105/AJPH.2018.304369 PMID: 29565671

Odlum, M., Moise, N., Kronish, I. M., Broadwell, P., Alcántara, C., Davis, N. J., Cheung, Y. K. K., Perotte, A., & Yoon, S. (2020). Trends in Poor Health Indicators Among Black and Hispanic Middle-aged and Older Adults in the United States, 1999-2018. *JAMA Network Open*, *3*(11), e2025134. DOI: 10.1001/jamanetworkopen.2020.25134 PMID: 33175177

Powell, W., Richmond, J., Mohottige, D., Yen, I., Joslyn, A., & Corbie-Smith, G. (2019). Medical Mistrust, Racism, and Delays in Preventive Health Screening Among African-American Men. *Behavioral Medicine (Washington, D.C.)*, *45*(2), 102–117. DOI: 10.1080/08964289.2019.1585327 PMID: 31343960

Presser, H. B. (1969). The Role of Sterilization in Controlling Puerto Rican Fertility. *Population Studies*, *23*(3), 343–361. DOI: 10.1080/00324728.1969.10405290 PMID: 22073953

Saluja, B., & Bryant, Z. (2021). How Implicit Bias Contributes to Racial Disparities in Maternal Morbidity and Mortality in the United States. *Journal of Women's Health*, *30*(2), 270–273. DOI: 10.1089/jwh.2020.8874 PMID: 33237843

Savitt, T. L. (1978). *Medicine and Slavery: The Diseases and Health Care of Blacks in Antebellum Virginia*. University of Illinois Press.

Savitt, T. L. (1982). The Use of Blacks for Medical Experimentation and Demonstration in the Old South. *The Journal of Southern History, 48*(3), 331–348. DOI: 10.2307/2207450 PMID: 11645888

Scharff, D. P., Mathews, K. J., Jackson, P., Hoffsuemmer, J., Martin, E., & Edwards, D. (2010). More than Tuskegee: Understanding Mistrust about Research Participation. *Journal of Health Care for the Poor and Underserved, 21*(3), 879–897. DOI: 10.1353/hpu.0.0323 PMID: 20693733

Schluger, N. W., Dozor, A. J., & Jung, Y. E. G. (2022). Rethinking the Race Adjustment in Pulmonary Function Testing. *Annals of the American Thoracic Society, 19*(3), 353–356. DOI: 10.1513/AnnalsATS.202107-890PS PMID: 34784493

Schwartz, R. C., & Blankenship, D. M. (2014). Racial disparities in psychotic disorder diagnosis: A review of empirical literature. *World Journal of Psychiatry, 4*(4), 133–140. DOI: 10.5498/wjp.v4.i4.133 PMID: 25540728

Segal, S. P., Bola, J. R., & Watson, M. A. (1996). Race, Quality of Care, and Antipsychotic Prescribing Practices in Psychiatric Emergency Services. *Psychiatric Services (Washington, D.C.), 47*(3), 282–286. DOI: 10.1176/ps.47.3.282 PMID: 8820552

Sjoding, M. W., Dickson, R. P., Iwashyna, T. J., Gay, S. E., & Valley, T. S. (2020). Racial Bias in Pulse Oximetry Measurement. *The New England Journal of Medicine, 383*(25), 2477–2478. DOI: 10.1056/NEJMc2029240 PMID: 33326721

Staats EB. (1976). *Letter report (HRD-77-3) investigation of allegations concerning Indian Health Service. Comptroller General of the United States.* Author.

Uppal, P., Golden, B. L., Panicker, A., Khan, O. A., & Burday, M. J. (2022). The Case Against Race-Based GFR. *Delaware Journal of Public Health, 8*(3), 86–89. DOI: 10.32481/djph.2022.014 PMID: 36177174

Vyas, D. A., Eisenstein, L. G., & Jones, D. S. (2020). Hidden in Plain Sight — Reconsidering the Use of Race Correction in Clinical Algorithms. *The New England Journal of Medicine, 383*(9), 874–882. DOI: 10.1056/NEJMms2004740 PMID: 32853499

Washington, H. A. (2006). *Medical Apartheid.* Doubleday.

Chapter 6
Sex:
Enduring Invisibility and Its Impact on Healthcare

Jasmine N. Bauknight
Shore Physicians Group, USA

Tamika M. Reese
https://orcid.org/0009-0009-1312-0638
Antioch University, USA

EXECUTIVE SUMMARY

Sexism has long been ingrained in medical institutions, impacting patient care, physician representation, and health disparities. This chapter explores the historical significance of barring women from medical education and professional practice, resulting in a male-dominated healthcare system that has impacted representation in medical research and practice, biases in patient care, and health outcomes. The current day ramifications are examined through two case studies highlighting the impacts on representation in medicine and patient health outcomes.

INTRODUCTION

The word sex pertains to one's reproductive structures being either male or female (Merriam Webster). Those born with sex characteristics that do not fit typical binary definitions of male or female are described as intersex. Not to be confused with gender which pertains to one's identity, sex is solely distinguished on physical attributes. Common language refers to non-male individuals as women, a gendered term, further isolating those who do not fit into binary definitions. Non-male individuals have held multiple roles within their cultural settings, however in western society,

DOI: 10.4018/979-8-3693-3683-0.ch006

they have had to endure historical oppression that barred them from advancement and inclusion in regular society. This power dynamic that deemed non-male individuals as lesser than males, also known as sexism, has impacted all facets of life (Lewis and Tabacco Mar, 2022).

Structural sexism creates a social climate that disenfranchises non-male individuals both within individual institutions through institutional sexism and within society as a whole. The pay gap between males and non-male individuals, the politicization of female health needs, and biases surrounding non-male individuals' educational and professional attainment create oppressive forces for their lived experiences (Lewis and Tabacco Mar, 2022). For example, a someone who aspires to work in a male dominated field will have to overcome sexist microaggressions, negative stigma, and mistreatment through-out her education and professional life to find the same title of success yet earning less than their male colleagues. This occurs while also navigating the impact that possible marriage, pregnancy, or future caretaking responsibilities will have on their career as laws like the Family Medical Leave Act will protect their job but not their upward trajectory. Still, they may endure less health coverage, poorer interactions with the medical community, and increased risks of chronic diseases as compared to their male counterparts (Lewis and Tabacco Mar, 2022). These disparities magnify when matched with other oppressed areas of identity through intersectionality, like race, socioeconomic status, or sexual orientation (Lewis and Tabacco Mar, 2022).

SEXISM IN MEDICINE

Sexism has long been ingrained in medical institutions, impacting patient care, physician representation, and health disparities. Historically, non-male individuals were systematically barred from medical education and professional practice, resulting in a male-dominated healthcare system that persists today. The consequences of this systemic exclusion extend beyond the workforce, affecting medical research, patient treatment, and health outcomes. Given that female physicians often achieve better results for female and non-male patients (Tsugawa et al., 2017), their ongoing underrepresentation exacerbates existing inequities care.

Historical Perspectives

Ancient and Medieval Medicine

Non-male individuals have historically played essential roles as healers, midwives providing care to other non-male individuals, and herbalists, yet they faced increasing exclusion as medicine became professionalized. In ancient Greece, non-male individuals like Agnodice practiced medicine in secrecy, while in medieval Europe, female healers were often accused of witchcraft and persecuted (Ehrenreich & English, 1973). During the Middle Ages, the Church and medical guilds formalized restrictions on non-male individuals' participation in medicine, barring them from universities and regulating midwifery to undermine their autonomy (Schiebinger 1987).

The 19th and Early 20th Century

The rise of formal medical education in the 19th century further institutionalized gender-based exclusion. When Elizabeth Blackwell became the first female physician in the United States in 1849, she was admitted to Geneva Medical College only because her male classmates thought her application was a joke (Morantz-Sanchez, 1985). Even after graduation, female doctors were funneled into lower-paying specialties such as pediatrics and obstetrics, which reinforced gender hierarchies in medicine and widened pay gaps for female physicians.

Intersectionality didn't help. Black non-male individuals physicians faced even greater challenges. Rebecca Lee Crumpler, the first Black female to earn a medical degree in the U.S. in 1864, encountered limited career opportunities due to both sexism and racism (Beckford & Johnson, 2018). Historically Black medical schools like Meharry Medical College and Howard University provided crucial entry points; however, Black non-male individuals in medicine remained severely underrepresented. By 1940, non-male individuals made up only 4.4% of all U.S. physicians, while Black non-male individuals represented an even smaller fraction (U.S. Census Bureau 1940).

Sexism and Patient Care

Sexism in medicine has not only influenced the profession but also impacted patient outcomes. Historically, medical research and treatment have been centered around male bodies, resulting in significant disparities in non-male individuals' healthcare.

- **Pain Management**: Studies indicate that non-male individuals are 25% less likely than males to receive opioid pain relief in emergency rooms (Hoffman et al., 2016).
- **Cardiac Care**: Non-male individuals experiencing heart attacks are significantly less likely to receive appropriate diagnostic tests and treatments compared to males, contributing to higher mortality rates (Mehta et al., 2016).
- **Autoimmune Diseases**: Non-male individuals are disproportionately affected by autoimmune disorders, yet they frequently experience delayed diagnoses due to medical bias (Ngo et al., 2014).

These disparities are even more pronounced for Black and Brown non-male individuals. Structural racism and sexism contribute to alarming maternal mortality rates: in the U.S., Black non-male individuals are 2.6 times more likely to die from pregnancy-related complications than white non-male individuals (Creanga et al., 2017). Research also indicates that Black non-male individuals' pain is systematically undertreated due to racist myths surrounding pain tolerance (Hoffman et al 2016).

Sexism and the Medical Workforce

The underrepresentation of non-male individuals in medicine—particularly in leadership roles and specialized fields—aggravates these disparities.

- **Workplace Discrimination**: Non-male individuals physicians report higher rates of gender-based discrimination, which adversely affects career advancement (Jena et al., 2016).
- **Pay Disparities**: Non-male individuals doctors earn approximately 25% less than their male counterparts, even when accounting for specialty and experience (Sege et al., 2015).
- **Leadership Gaps**: Non-male individuals continue to be underrepresented in crucial decision-making roles. As of 2022, only 18% of U.S. medical school deans were non-male individuals (AAMC, 2022).

For physicians who are Black and non-male individuals, the obstacles are even greater. They encounter both racial and gender discrimination, resulting in lower hiring rates, fewer mentorship opportunities, and limited access to professional networks (Nunez-Smith et al 2010).

SEXISM AND THE PERPETUATION OF HEALTH DISPARITIES

Health disparities are a direct consequence of the social determinants of health (Office of Disease Prevention and Health Promotion, n.d.). The social determinants of health are the supplementary factors that impact health including where people live, their access to food and health care, and their access to opportunities including education and employment (Office of Disease Prevention and Health Promotion, n.d.). For example, jobs associated with caregiving like teaching remain underpaid and what is historically non-male individuals' work may not have overtime or minimum wage protections (Lewis and Tabacco Mar, 2022). This not only impacts health through socioeconomic means but impacts access to healthy neighborhoods and food, educational attainment, social supports, and workplace exposures. Thus, as sexism impacts these factors, sexism directly influences the creation of health disparities.

Sexism in Direct Patient Care

Aside from the impact that sexism has on health overall, studies have shown that non-male individuals are more likely to have their medical concerns overlooked (Lewis and Tabacco Mar, 2022; Samulowitz et al., 2018) or attributed to emotional factors (Staats, 2015). In the current climate, the polarization of non-male individuals' health concerns surrounding pregnancy and contraception has directly impacted access to care and maternal health outcomes (Lewis and Tabacco Mar, 2022). The differences in outcomes are amplified for non-male individuals of color, lower socioeconomic status, and those from rural areas.

Additionally, intersex individuals face significant disparities in healthcare, many of which are rooted in sexism and rigid gender norms. Many intersex infants and children undergo medically unnecessary surgeries to "normalize" their genitalia, often without their consent (Human Rights Watch, 2017). These interventions are based on sexist assumptions that bodies must conform to binary standards of male or female.

Furthermore, intersex people are often excluded from both males' and non-male individuals' health research, leading to gaps in medical knowledge and inadequate healthcare access (Richards et al., 2016). Because medical studies are typically designed around binary sex models, intersex individuals may not receive appropriate screenings or treatments tailored to their needs. This exclusion strengthens the sexist belief that only binary bodies merit comprehensive medical care.

Beyond the exclusion of intersex individuals, gender disparities in healthcare also manifest in the representation of medical professionals. The underrepresentation of female physicians directly impacts patient health. Research indicates that patients treated by female doctors have 4% lower mortality rates and 5% lower hospital readmission rates compared to those treated by male doctors (Tsugawa et al., 2017). For Black non-male individuals, this underrepresentation is particularly detrimental. Research demonstrates that when patients see doctors of the same race, health outcomes improve. Black infant mortality rates decrease by 50% when Black newborns are treated by Black physicians (Greenwood et al., 2020). Yet, Black non-male individuals comprise only 2% of all U.S. physicians (AAMC, 2021), significantly limiting access to culturally competent care.

Medical Research

Historically, female hormonal physiology was assumed to have large implications on the validity of study data based on cyclic changes in hormonal levels during studies. While this easily could have been standardized to look at differences between males and females or to address hypothesis during different parts of the menstrual cycle, non-male individuals were omitted from studies. Much of the data that is currently available on chronic disease, commonly used medications, and many treatments were standardized by male physiology and extrapolated to work on female populations. For example, this is seen in heart attack, or myocardial infarction symptoms as non-male individuals display different symptoms than males (Bibbins-Domingo & Helman, 2022). These discrepancies leave large research gaps for non-male individuals' health and wellness, not just in reproductive health but for chronic disease management.

The following cases highlight the impact of sexism on medical practice from both the medical team and within patient care.

CASES

Case 1. Sexism in Medical Training

Learning Objectives

1. Understand the barriers non-male individuals face entering majority male specialties
2. Discuss the difference in vocabulary used to describe female versus male leaders
3. Discuss ways in which the institution of medicine can be more female friendly

Case Aim: This case aims to examine the difficulties female medical students and residents face in medical training

A 3rd year female medical student is interested in becoming an Orthopedic Surgeon. She notices that there is only one female in the department at her institution. She meets with the male faculty advisor who tells her that surgical subspecialities are very difficult for women, and hard to maintain a work-life balance, and that women don't have the physical strength required to do orthopedic surgery, and if she is set on sports medicine, to apply to Family Medicine.

Discouraged, the student continues with her rotations. During her residency interviews, she notices that some of the programs only have one or two female residents. The faculty strongly discourages her from getting pregnant during residency, which would cause them to have coverage issues.

Still, she matches into an Orthopedic Surgery program and finds that she is consistently assigned to smaller surgeries than the men. She has a hard time asserting herself during rounds and often is being spoken over. She finds that the male residents are referred to as "Doctor" while she is often called by her first name by staff and is mistaken to be a nurse by patients. She gets called into the program director's office, who tells her they have gotten complaints from the nursing staff that she is "angry, abrasive, rude, dismissive and condescending," although she has routinely witnessed the men be much ruder, with no complaints.

She continues to work hard in residency but is becoming increasingly frustrated. She talks to one of the female faculty who tells her that "to be a woman in surgery you have to be tough".

Case Questions

1. How Does the Faculty Advisor's Advice Reflect Societal Biases About Non-Male Individuals in Surgical Specialties?

- The faculty advisor's comments are rooted in traditional gender stereotypes, suggesting that non-male individuals are not suited for the physical demands of orthopedic surgery or that they would struggle with work-life balance. Such advice dismisses the capabilities of female students and reinforces the outdated belief that certain specialties are inherently male. It also implies that non-male individuals should prioritize family medicine over more physically demanding fields, placing an undue limitation on their career options based on gender rather than individual capability or interest.

2. How Does the Situation Reflect the Double Standards Non-Male Individuals Face When They Express Assertiveness in the Workplace?

- In this case, the female resident is labeled as "angry, abrasive, rude, dismissive, and condescending" for behaviors that are likely similar to the assertive, confident behavior exhibited by her male counterparts. This double standard—where non-male individuals' assertiveness is criticized while male's similar behavior is overlooked or praised—demonstrates how non-male individuals are often penalized for exhibiting traits deemed necessary for success in surgery, such as confidence and decisiveness. This bias contributes to the perception that non-male individuals must work harder to be accepted or respected, even when their actions are similar to those of their male peers.

3. What Are Some Barriers That Non-Male Individuals Face in Medical Training, Particularly in Traditionally Male-Dominated Specialties?

- Non-male individuals in medicine often have to delay having children, and disproportionately have to use fertility treatments later in life in order to do so. They deal with sexism and comments that they are inadequate, too weak, don't belong, or sometimes that certain specialties, or residencies are better without them. They are victims to stereotypes, and historically often receive fewer opportunities, fewer role models, less support, and face more obstacles than their male counterparts.

Case Discussion

The case study highlights the many barriers that female medical students and residents face in their training especially when trying to enter specialties that are disproportionately male. Studies have shown that non-male individuals in medicine overall are more likely to experience microaggressions and bias (Anderson et al., 2021) which contribute to physician burnout (Dyrbye, et. al., 2006) and decreased representation of non-male individuals in medicine. This lack of representation directly contributes to non-male individuals' health disparities and poorer health outcomes (Tsugawa, et al., 2017).

Case 2. Sexism in Patient Care

Learning Objectives

1. Discuss how heart disease can present differently in non-male individuals
2. Discuss how non-male individuals' medical concerns are often disregarded, or diagnosis is delayed
3. Discuss how non-male individuals are more commonly to be perceived as having emotional or mental health issues

Case Aim: This case aims to examine how biases against non-male individuals impact patient care and health outcomes.

A 51 year old female patient with presents to her PCP complaining of heart palpitations, chest pain, jaw pain, shoulder pain and anxiety. She apologizes saying "I'm sorry to bother you, but I just haven't been feeling well recently, I've been very stressed out." Her NP treats her for anxiety and depression, prescribes her with anti-inflammatories and checks her thyroid level, and tells her to follow up in 6 weeks. Several days later, the patient goes to the ED with worsening chest pain, jaw pain, and pain radiating down her left arm. She is first told that she has acid reflux and is going to be sent home, but after her son arrives, he insists that she gets an EKG, and she is diagnosed with an NSTEMI.

Case Questions

1. How Might Gender Biases Have Influenced the NP's Decision to Attribute the Patient's Symptoms to Anxiety and Depression, Rather Than Considering the Possibility of a Cardiovascular Issue? Are There Common Stereotypes About Non-Male Individuals' Health That Might Have Shaped This Initial Diagnosis?

- Historically, non-male individuals' health concerns, especially related to emotional states, are more likely to be dismissed as psychological. This might stem from a tendency to view non-male individuals' pain or discomfort through a psychological lens rather than considering physical causes, particularly heart disease, which is more traditionally seen as a male-associated condition. In many cases, non-male individuals' heart attack symptoms are under-recognized or dismissed as "anxiety" or "stress."

2. The Patient Apologized for Seeking Help and Minimized Her Symptoms by Attributing Them to Stress. How Might Societal Expectations for Non-Male Individuals to "Tough It Out" or Not Complain Influence Both the Patient's Self-Reporting and the Clinician's Interpretation of Her Symptoms? How Does the Cultural Expectation for Non-Male Individuals to Be Caregivers and Put Others' Needs First Impact Their Willingness To Seek Care, or Their Perceived Legitimacy of Their Own Health Concerns?

- Societal expectations for non-male individuals to be strong and selfless caregivers often lead them to downplay their symptoms or not seek care until things are very severe. This cultural expectation can influence the way non-male individuals perceive their health concerns, making them feel guilty for "bothering" others, as seen in the patient's apology. These expectations can also cause them to underreport their symptoms, which makes it easier for clinicians to misinterpret their complaints as non-urgent. Non-male individuals may feel hesitant to advocate for themselves when they believe their symptoms will be perceived as exaggerated or overdramatic. In some cultures, non-male individuals are expected to be submissive to males or other leaders.

3. How Does a Historical Underrepresentation of Non-Male Individuals in Clinical Trials and Medical Research Influence the Way Heart Disease Is Diagnosed and Treated in Non-Male Individuals Today? Do You Think That This History Impacts Clinicians' Approach to Diagnosing Heart Disease in Non-Male Individuals?

- Historically, non-male individuals have been underrepresented in clinical trials, and many medical conditions were studied primarily in male populations. As a result, the symptoms and presentations of conditions like heart disease may not have been well understood in non-male individuals . This lack of research can affect the accuracy of diagnosis and treatment in non-male individuals today, as the presentation of symptoms may differ from the "classic" descriptions often used in medical training, which are based on male-dominated studies.

Case Discussion

The case study underscores the difficulty non-male individuals can have when trying to get their medical concerns to be taken seriously. Non-male individuals are often seen as more emotional or anxious, and their physical symptoms may be more readily attributed to psychological causes rather than a serious medical condition like a heart attack. This can lead to missed or delayed diagnoses in non-male individuals, particularly when they present with atypical symptoms.

CONCLUSION

The historical exclusion of non-male individuals from medicine has created a lasting impact on healthcare, reinforcing gender and racial disparities in both medical practice and patient outcomes. Addressing these issues requires structural changes, including greater representation of non-male individuals and Black non-male individuals in medical leadership, policy reforms to eliminate gender bias in research and treatment, and improved mentorship programs for underrepresented physicians. Without these changes, sexism in medicine will continue to undermine patient care and professional equity.

REFERENCES

AAMC. (2021). *Diversity in Medicine: Facts and Figures 2021.* Association of American Medical Colleges.

AAMC. (2022). *The State of Non-male individuals in Academic Medicine.* Association of American Medical Colleges.

Anderson, N., Lett, E., Ngozi Asabor, E., Hernandez, A., Nguemeni Tiako, M. J., Johnson, C., Rizzo, T. M., Latimore, D., Nunez-Smith, M., & Boatright, D. (2021). The association of microaggressions with depressive symptoms and institutional satisfaction among a national cohort of medical students. *Journal of General Internal Medicine, 37*(2), 298–307. DOI: 10.1007/s11606-021-06786-6 PMID: 33939079

Beckford, D., & Johnson, J. (2018). The dual barriers of race and gender in medical professions. *Journal of Black Studies, 49*(5), 549–567.

Bibbins-Domingo, K., & Helman, A. (2022). *Improving Representation in Clinical Trials and Research: Building equity for non-male individuals and underrepresented groups.* The National Academies Press., DOI: 10.17226/26479

Clayton, J. A., & Tannenbaum, C. (2016). Sex and gender reporting in health research: Why it matters. *Journal of the American Medical Association, 316*(18), 1863–1864. PMID: 27802482

Creanga, A. A.. (2017). Racial and ethnic disparities in maternal mortality. *American Journal of Obstetrics and Gynecology, 217*(6), 689–699.

Dyrbye, L. N., Thomas, M. R., Huschka, M. M., Lawson, K. L., Novotny, P. J., Sloan, J. A., & Shanafellt, T. D. (2006). A multicenter study of burnout, depression, and quality of life in minority and nonminority US medical students. *Mayo Clinic Proceedings, 8*(11), 1435–1442. PMID: 17120398

Ehrenreich, B., & English, D. (1973). *Witches, Midwives, and Nurses: A History of Non-male individuals Healers.* Feminist Press.

Greenwood, B. N. (2020). Physician-patient racial concordance and disparities in infant mortality. *Proceedings of the National Academy of Sciences of the United States of America, 117*(35), 21194–21200. PMID: 32817561

Hoffman, K. M. (2016). Racial bias in pain assessment and treatment recommendations. *Proceedings of the National Academy of Sciences of the United States of America, 113*(16), 4296–4301. PMID: 27044069

Human Rights Watch. (2017). "I Want to Be Like Nature Made Me": Medically Unnecessary Surgeries on Intersex Children in the U.S. *Journal of the American Medical Association, 316*(22), 2353-2354.

Lewis, J. A., & Tabacco Mar, R. (2022). Sexism. *Moving Toward Antibigotry,* 175-185.

Mehta, L. S. (2016). Acute myocardial infarction in non-male individuals: A scientific statement from the American Heart Association. *Circulation, 133*(9), 916–947. PMID: 26811316

Morantz-Sanchez, R. (1985). *Sympathy and Science: Non-male individuals Physicians in American Medicine*. University of North Carolina Press.

Nunez-Smith, M. (2010). Institutional culture and minority faculty career success in academic medicine. *Journal of the American Medical Association, 304*(12), 1373–1379.

Office of Disease Prevention and Health Promotion. (n.d.). Social Determinants of Health. *Healthy People 2030*. U.S. Department of Health and Human Services. https://odphp.health.gov/healthypeople/priority-areas/social-determinants-health

Richards, C., Bouman, W. P., & Seal, L. (2016). Intersex, Variations of Sex Characteristics, and DSD: The Need for Change. *Journal of Pediatric Endocrinology & Metabolism, 29*(11), 1263–1268.

Samulowitz, A., Gremyr, I., Eriksson, E., & Hensing, G. (2018). "Brave Men" and "Emotional Non-male individuals ": A theory-guided literature review on gender bias in health care and gendered norms towards patients with chronic pain. *Pain Research & Management, 2018*, 1–14.

Schiebinger, L. (1987). *The history of non-male individuals in medicine.* Signs: Journal of Non-male individuals in Culture and Society, 12(3), 515-531.

Sex. (2025). In *Merriam-Webster.com*. https://www.merriam-webster.com/dictionary/sex

Staats, C., Capatosto, K., Wright, R. A., & Contractor, D. (2015). State of the Science: Implicit Bias Review 2015. Academic Press.

Tsugawa, Y. (2017). Comparison of hospital mortality and readmission rates for Medicare patients treated by male vs. female physicians. *JAMA Internal Medicine, 177*(2), 206–213. PMID: 27992617

Chapter 7
Gender and Sexual Orientation:
Embracing the Intersectionality of Identity

Antoinette Leonard-Jean Charles
https://orcid.org/0009-0002-6283-7730
Antioch University, USA

EXECUTIVE SUMMARY

Gender and sexual orientation are significant aspects of personal identity. Likewise, gender-affirming care is a critical and evolving aspect of modern healthcare, centered on supporting transgender and non-binary (TGNB) individuals aligning their physical and emotional well-being with their gender identity. The chapter explores the principles, practices, and challenges associated with issues of sex, gender, and sexual orientation alongside gender-affirming care, highlighting its transformative potential in reducing health disparities and promoting equity. Key topics include shared definitions of sex, gender, and sexual orientation, current medical policies and practices in puberty suppression, hormone therapy, and surgical options, with a focus on ethical considerations, informed consent, and patient-centered care. The chapter also addresses barriers to accessing care, including systemic discrimination, provider bias, financial constraints, and emphasizes the role of multidisciplinary care teams in overcoming these challenges through the nuanced experiences of individuals.

DOI: 10.4018/979-8-3693-3683-0.ch007

INTRODUCTION

At its core, the Physician Cultural Responsibility framework recognizes that gender is a multifaceted and deeply personal aspect of identity, encompassing an individual internal sense of self, expression, and societal roles. It is distinct from biological sex, which refers to the physical characteristics often assigned at birth, and sexuality, which pertains to romantic, emotional, and sexual attraction. These dimensions do not always align in expected ways, and understanding their independence is fundamental to providing affirming care. Gender-affirming care represents a cornerstone of equitable and inclusive healthcare, addressing the unique needs of transgender and non-binary (TGNB) individuals. Gender-affirming care exists within a healthcare system historically shaped by biases, including sexism, which often reinforces rigid gender norms and binary understandings of sex. These biases not only marginalize transgender and non-binary individuals but also perpetuate disparities in care through implicit assumptions about patient needs and identities.

Gender-affirming care encompasses a broad spectrum of interventions, including medical treatments like hormone therapy and surgical options, psychological support, and social affirmation strategies. Beyond clinical expertise, healthcare providers play a pivotal role in delivering this care with cultural competence, empathy, and an unwavering commitment to fostering safe, inclusive spaces. Recognizing the distinct intersection of gender and sexuality is particularly important, as assumptions and biases can lead to inadequate or inappropriate interventions. For instance, a transgender woman may identify as heterosexual, bisexual, or homosexual, and conflating her gender with her sexual orientation risks alienating her from care.

TGNB (Transgender & Non-Binary) individuals face a unique set of challenges shaped by systemic barriers and social determinants of health. These include stigma, discrimination, economic instability, and inadequate access to affirming healthcare. Such factors contribute to significant disparities in mental and physical health outcomes, with TGNB populations experiencing higher rates of anxiety, depression, substance use, and disordered eating behaviors (Hughto et al., 2017; Rasmussen, 2023). Importantly, studies have shown that access to gender-affirming care is linked to improved mental health outcomes, including reduced suicidality and psychological distress (Almazan & Keuroghlian, 2021; Tordoff et al., 2022).

The absence of affirming care often manifests as various forms of harm. Patients may present with self-harm, substance use, and social withdrawal, frequently stemming from rejection, marginalization, or internalized stigma. For example, Goetz (2023) highlights the prevalence of eating disorders in TGNB (Transgender & Non-Binary) populations, often tied to societal pressures to conform to binary norms. Such behaviors underscore the urgent need for healthcare providers to deliver affirming, patient-centered care that acknowledges TGNB individuals' intersectional challenges.

This chapter seeks to equip healthcare professionals with the knowledge and tools to provide gender-inclusive care. Through a multidisciplinary lens, we will explore the intersections of gender identity, sexuality, and healthcare disparities, emphasizing the critical role of providers in mitigating harm and promoting resilience. By integrating affirming language, understanding the social determinants of health, and fostering therapeutic alliances built on trust and respect, providers can deliver care that affirms the dignity and authenticity of every patient.

Understanding Gender and Sexual Identity: The Foundation of Affirmation

Understanding gender identity serves as the foundational principle of gender-affirming care. It requires recognizing that gender is a deeply personal and multifaceted aspect of human identity, shaped by the intricate interplay of biological, social, and psychological factors. Individuals experience and express their gender in diverse ways, embracing a spectrum that extends beyond binary constructs of male and female. By fostering an environment that embraces gender diversity and inclusivity, healthcare providers can create affirming spaces where individuals feel validated and respected in their authentic identities.

Healthcare providers must also understand how societal norms, stigma, and discrimination influence gender identity development. These external pressures can create significant barriers to exploring and expressing their gender. Providing culturally competent care requires affirming each individual's unique experience, laying the groundwork for therapeutic relationships built on trust, empathy, and mutual respect. This approach empowers individuals and fosters holistic well-being for those seeking gender-affirming care.

Distinguishing Gender and Sexual Identity

The intersection of gender and sexuality is a complex and multifaceted area of study, encompassing behavioral norms, societal expectations, and psychological impacts. A critical component of understanding gender identity is distinguishing it from sexual orientation. Gender refers to an individual's deeply held sense of self, encompassing identity, expression, and societal roles, which may exist on a spectrum beyond the traditional binary of male and female. In contrast, sexuality relates to whom an individual is romantically, emotionally, or sexually attracted to—categories often described as heterosexual, homosexual, bisexual, asexual, and others.

Although gender and sexuality are distinct, societal discourse often intertwines them, leading to misunderstandings. For example, a transgender individual may identify as heterosexual, homosexual, or another orientation, just as a cisgender person might. Conflating these concepts can hinder the provision of affirming and culturally competent care, as assumptions about one's gender identity often lead to incorrect assumptions about one's sexuality.

This distinction is particularly critical in the context of the LGBTQI community and the transgender population's experiences with gender-affirming care. Factors such as healthcare provider knowledge, institutional support, and systemic barriers influence the quality of care and the dynamics of patient-provider interactions. For instance, Hughto et al. (2017) emphasize that healthcare providers play a pivotal role in creating safe and welcoming clinical environments for transgender patients and fostering open communication and trust.

Addressing Mental Health: Supporting Emotional Well-Being

Addressing mental health is a crucial aspect of inclusive care, as individuals navigating gender identity exploration and transition often face unique emotional challenges. Providing comprehensive mental health support is essential to promoting emotional well-being throughout the journey of gender affirmation. Therapeutic interventions, such as individual counseling, group therapy, and support groups, play a vital role in helping individuals navigate the complex emotions, social pressures, and identity-related stressors associated with gender transition.

By integrating mental health support into gender-affirming care, healthcare providers can facilitate resilience, self-acceptance, and holistic well-being for individuals on their journey toward living authentically and affirming their true selves. Several studies have found higher rates of eating disorders among transgender and non-binary (TGNB) individuals who lack access to gender-affirming care (Goetz, 2023; Rasmussen, 2023). For example, one study highlighted the need for integrated, culturally competent eating disorder treatment combined with gender-affirming care, indicating that TGNB individuals who do not receive gender-affirming medical interventions may experience increased eating disorder symptoms and behaviors (Goetz, 2023). Additionally, systematic reviews have documented the increased vulnerability of TGNB individuals to disordered eating behaviors (Rasmussen, 2023).

Access to gender-affirming care, such as hormone therapy and gender-affirming surgeries, has been consistently associated with improved mental health outcomes. Almazan and Keuroghlian (2021) found that these interventions significantly reduce suicidality and self-harm rates. Similarly, a 2022 study revealed that transgender and non-binary youth receiving gender-affirming care had significantly lower odds of suicidality compared to those without such care (Tordoff et al., 2022). The availability of gender-affirming surgeries has also been linked to reduced rates of mental health conditions and psychological distress (Almazan & Keuroghlian, 2021).

By ensuring access to gender-affirming care and integrating mental health services, healthcare systems can address systemic barriers such as discrimination, provider knowledge gaps, and financial constraints (Hughto et al., 2017; Nolan et al., 2020). These efforts not only enhance individual well-being but also affirm the dignity and authenticity of TGNB individuals.

Challenges to Affirming-Care

Transgender individuals frequently encounter barriers to gender-affirming healthcare. Reisner et al. (2015) highlight the importance of comprehensive care models that integrate community assessments, research, and advocacy to establish practical standards of care. These models address systemic challenges such as inadequate provider training and institutional biases, ensuring transgender patients receive the affirming care they require. Moreover, healthcare providers must also understand the societal roles that patients are transitioning into, as these roles can have profound positive or negative effects on their health outcomes.

Despite growing awareness, many medical education programs in the United States and Canada still lack adequate training on transgender health. Nolan et al. (2020) note that this education gap often leaves providers unprepared to address the unique needs of transgender patients. Furthermore, Sengupta (2023) observes that biases and misconceptions among providers can alienate patients and discourage them from seeking care. Without adequate exposure to transgender health during training, medical students—as future physicians—may avoid treating transgender patients altogether (Reddy, 2023).

Loza et al. (2018) underscore the importance of community engagement in developing trans-affirming health services, particularly in underserved areas. Initiatives such as gay-straight alliances improve institutional climates, reducing the victimization of transgender individuals. These efforts highlight the need for healthcare systems to actively involve transgender patients in shaping their care frameworks.

The Role of Knowledge and Attitudes Towards Inclusive and Affirming Care

The quality of interactions between transgender patients and healthcare providers significantly influences health outcomes. Hines et al. (2019) found that many transgender women reported feeling misunderstood during healthcare interactions, leading to feelings of alienation and inadequate care. Mikovits (2022) similarly notes that providers often overlook the social dimensions of gender transitions, focusing solely on medical interventions. This narrow focus neglects the emotional and social aspects essential for comprehensive care.

Gender-affirming care is not solely about medical interventions; it involves understanding the societal, cultural, and systemic factors influencing patient health. Providers must advocate for supportive institutional frameworks and preventive care measures that address these challenges. Community engagement and collaboration with transgender patients in shaping healthcare policies and practices are essential for creating inclusive environments.

Many transgender adults delay or avoid care due to fears of transphobia and discrimination (Seelman et al., 2017). Stroumsa et al. (2019) argue that transphobia—rather than a lack of education—is a significant barrier to effective provider-patient interactions. This highlights the urgent need for targeted training programs to equip healthcare providers with the skills necessary to engage transgender patients respectfully and knowledgeably. Such programs must address biases, foster cultural humility, and prioritize patient autonomy.

By bridging the gaps in education, addressing systemic biases, and fostering affirming provider-patient interactions, healthcare systems can ensure that transgender individuals receive the care they deserve. Affirming care validates individuals' identities and empowers them to thrive, contributing to their overall health and well-being.

Initial Consultation: Building Trust and Understanding

The initial consultation is a pivotal moment in the journey of gender-affirming care, serving as the foundation for building trust and understanding between the healthcare provider and the individual seeking care. The provider establishes a collaborative relationship through open and empathetic communication, acknowledging the individual's unique experiences, needs, and goals. This initial consultation sets the tone for the therapeutic alliance, laying the groundwork for personalized treatment planning and ensuring that the individual feels supported and empowered throughout their journey of gender affirmation.

Interdisciplinary Collaboration: The Role of Healthcare Teams

Interdisciplinary collaboration plays a pivotal role in gender-affirming care, as it brings together a diverse team of healthcare professionals to provide comprehensive support to individuals navigating gender identity exploration and transition. Healthcare teams may include physicians, mental health providers, social workers, nurses, and other specialists working together to tailor treatment plans that are personalized and culturally competent.

Baker and Restar (2022) describe the categories of health services and procedures, including psychological support, hormone therapy, and reconstructive surgeries. Cost and utilization of insurance can be issues during the transition process. Out-of-pocket costs for gender-affirming hormone therapy can be substantial, ranging between $84 to $2,716 in 2010 and from $72 to $3,792 in 2018 (Baker & Restar, 2022). These excessive costs can lead to interruptions in care, leading to emotional and physical harm to the patient. Providers must know which ICD codes to use to ensure health insurance coverage for prescriptions and procedures.

Current Medical Policies and Practices in Gender Transition and Puberty Suppression

The evolving field of transgender healthcare is guided by evidence-based standards that prioritize the mental and physical well-being of transgender (TGNB) and gender-diverse individuals. Current medical practices for gender transition and puberty suppression emphasize individualized, patient-centered care that aligns with the unique needs of each patient. Major medical organizations, such as the World Professional Association for Transgender Health (WPATH) and the Endocrine Society, provide comprehensive guidelines that serve as the foundation for these practices (Vaccaro, 2023; Krebs et al., 2022; Verbeek et al., 2022).

A growing body of research supports the importance of providing affirmative and evidence-based care for TGNB individuals. This includes access to gender-affirming medical interventions, such as puberty blockers, hormone therapy, and gender-affirming surgeries, which have been shown to improve well-being and reduce psychological distress significantly (Austin et al., 2022; Herrmann et al., 2023; Chin et al., 2023; Krebs et al., 2022; Silva et al., 2022; Mills et al., 2022). Puberty blockers, in particular, play a critical role for TGNB youth by temporarily halting the physical changes of puberty, allowing individuals and their families time to explore gender identity and transition options without irreversible developments (Hembree et al., 2017).

Debates and Controversies

Despite the benefits, puberty suppression and other medical interventions for TGNB youth remain subjects of ongoing debate. Critics have raised concerns about potential unintended consequences and the need for further research to understand the long-term effects of these treatments (Elkadi et al., 2023; Jorgensen et al., 2022). Additionally, some have questioned the reliance on gender dysphoria diagnoses as a gatekeeping mechanism, suggesting it may lead to self-fulfilling prophecies or hinder access to care for those who do not fit traditional diagnostic criteria (Elkadi et al., 2023; Ibrahim, 2023).

These debates are further influenced by systemic biases, including sexism, which shape societal and clinical attitudes toward medical interventions for TGNB youth. Sexist assumptions about traditional gender roles can complicate discussions about puberty suppression, with critics often framing these interventions as unnatural or unnecessary disruptions to binary gender norms. Such biases may disproportionately affect access to care for transgender girls, whose desire to align their physical appearance with their identity is often invalidated under the guise of "protecting" traditional femininity. These societal and clinical biases underscore the broader systemic barriers that restrict equitable access to gender-affirming care.

The following section explores the structural inequities and barriers faced by TGNB individuals, highlighting the intersection of systemic discrimination, resource disparities, and societal biases in limiting access to care.

Barriers to Access

Significant barriers persist in accessing gender-affirming care, particularly for marginalized populations. Factors such as lack of insurance coverage, provider bias, and limited availability of specialized services disproportionately impact individuals from low-income backgrounds, rural areas, and communities of color (Chin et al., 2023; Shabalala, 2023; Ingraham et al., 2022). These structural inequities are further compounded by intersecting forms of discrimination, including sexism, transphobia, and racism, which together create unique and often insurmountable obstacles for transgender and non-binary (TGNB) individuals.

Sexism, in particular, intersects with transphobia to reinforce rigid gender norms, resulting in dismissive attitudes toward non-binary identities and other gender expressions that challenge traditional notions of sex and gender. For example, providers may unconsciously apply binary frameworks when addressing patient needs, marginalizing individuals who do not conform to these constructs. Transgender women, in particular, often face compounded biases due to societal expectations of femininity, which influence provider attitudes and may limit access to affirming care. These biases can manifest in delayed or inappropriate care, increased mental health challenges, and diminished trust in the healthcare system.

Recognizing and addressing these intersecting barriers is essential for developing guidelines and best practices that promote equitable and inclusive healthcare. By integrating a framework that acknowledges the pervasive influence of sexism and other systemic inequities, healthcare professionals can better support the diverse needs of TG individuals. The following section outlines evidence-based guidelines and best practices to foster affirming and inclusive care for transgender and non-binary populations.

Guidelines and Best Practices

Leading medical organizations emphasize the importance of individualized care plans that account for age, developmental stage, and caregiver support. The WPATH Standards of Care and Endocrine Society guidelines advocate for multidisciplinary teams comprising endocrinologists, mental health professionals, and primary care providers to deliver coordinated, patient-centered care (Vaccaro, 2023; Krebs et al., 2022; Turban & Brady, 2022). These practices aim to balance the benefits of medical interventions with carefully considering each patient's physical and emotional needs.

The Need for Research and Advocacy

The current medical policies and practices in gender transition and puberty suppression reflect a complex and evolving landscape. While significant progress has been made in affirming the rights and identities of TGNB individuals, ongoing research, policy development, and advocacy are crucial to addressing access barriers and promoting equitable care. Expanding Medicaid and private insurance coverage for gender-affirming interventions, alongside combating provider bias and systemic discrimination, remains a priority for improving health outcomes for TGNB populations (Silva et al., 2022; Shabalala, 2023; Nayar, 2023).

This foundation of care and its associated challenges provide a necessary context for understanding the transformative role of hormone therapy, which builds upon the principles of puberty suppression to further support TGNB individuals in their journey toward affirmation and physical transition.

Hormone Therapy: Enhancing Affirmation and Physical Transition

Hormone therapy is a cornerstone of gender-affirming care, offering transgender and non-binary (TGNB) individuals the opportunity to align their physical characteristics with their gender identity. This medical intervention plays a crucial role in reducing gender dysphoria and enhancing mental and physical well-being by promoting congruence between an individual's internal sense of self and outward appearance.

For transgender men, hormone therapy typically involves testosterone, which induces masculinizing effects such as deepening of the voice, increased muscle mass, redistribution of body fat, and facial and body hair growth. Conversely, transgender women often receive estrogen therapy, which facilitates feminizing effects, including breast development, skin softening, and fat redistribution. In some cases, androgen blockers may be used alongside estrogen to suppress testosterone levels (Shin et al., 2022). These physical changes contribute to gender affirmation, fostering improved self-esteem, resilience, and overall quality of life.

Several studies published within the last few years have highlighted the positive impact of gender-affirming hormone therapy on TGNB individuals' mental health and quality of life. For example, a 2022 study by Tordoff et al. found that TGNB youth receiving gender-affirming care, including hormone therapy, had significantly lower odds of suicidality compared to those who did not receive such care (Tordoff et al., 2022). Similarly, a 2021 study by Almazan and Keuroghlian showed that gender-affirming surgery, which often involves hormone therapy, was associated with reduced rates of mental health conditions and psychological distress (Almazan & Keuroghlian, 2021).

On the other hand, restrictive policies targeting gender-affirming care have been associated with significant detrimental impacts. A 2021 study by Park et al. highlighted the harmful effects of legislation aiming to criminalize gender-affirming care, including hormone therapy and puberty blockers, for TGNB youth (Baker & Restar, 2022). Exposure to news about such restrictive legislation has also been linked to increased anxiety and depression among transgender youth and young adults, as documented by Dhanani and Totton (Hostetter et al., 2022). These findings underscore the need to maintain and expand access to gender-affirming care.

Despite its benefits, hormone therapy requires careful consideration of potential risks and side effects. Testosterone therapy may increase the risk of polycythemia, elevated cholesterol levels, and cardiovascular complications, while estrogen therapy is associated with risks such as venous thromboembolism and changes in liver function (Shin et al., 2022). Regular hormone levels, cardiovascular health, and liver function monitoring are essential to mitigate these risks and ensure patient safety.

Healthcare providers must adopt a patient-centered approach when discussing hormone therapy, ensuring that individuals are well-informed about treatment's potential effects, risks, and benefits. Informed consent is a critical component of gender-affirming care, emphasizing the autonomy of TGNB individuals in making decisions about their healthcare. Providers should also recognize that hormone therapy is not a one-size-fits-all solution; treatment plans must be tailored to the unique needs and goals of each patient.

Efforts to improve access to hormone therapy must address significant structural barriers. The uneven landscape of healthcare coverage for gender-affirming care across states and insurance providers contributes to persistent disparities (Park et al., 2021; Dhanani & Totton, 2023). Advocacy for policy changes, provider education, and integrating gender-affirming care into mainstream healthcare systems are essential for promoting equitable access and improving health outcomes. Major medical organizations, including the World Professional Association for Transgender Health, recognize hormone therapy as the standard of care for TGNB individuals (Falck & Bränström, 2023; Marshall et al., 2022).

To address these challenges, healthcare providers and policymakers must work collaboratively to develop and implement comprehensive, evidence-based guidelines and protocols for the provision of gender-affirming hormone therapy. This includes ensuring that TGNB individuals can access a multidisciplinary team of providers, including endocrinologists, mental health professionals, and primary care physicians, who can deliver coordinated, patient-centered care (Almazan & Keuroghlian, 2021). Expanding Medicaid and private insurance coverage and addressing structural barriers and discrimination will be crucial in promoting equitable access and improving health outcomes for TGNB populations (Masumori et al., 2021).

Hormone therapy is more than a medical intervention; it is a transformative aspect of gender-affirming care that validates the identities of TGNB individuals and fosters their physical, emotional, and social well-being. By providing compassionate, evidence-based, and individualized care, healthcare providers can empower TGNB individuals to thrive authentically.

Overcoming Barriers: Promoting Access and Inclusivity

Many transgender, nonbinary, and gender-diverse (TGNB) individuals face significant obstacles in accessing gender-affirming care due to systemic discrimination, lack of knowledgeable providers, and financial constraints. These barriers not only impede access to essential services but also contribute to adverse health outcomes, exacerbating the physical and mental health disparities experienced by TG populations.

Defining Barriers in Healthcare

Barriers to gender-affirming care are multifaceted and pervasive. Systemic discrimination remains one of the most significant challenges, manifesting as institutional policies, provider biases, and inadequate training in transgender health. For example, providers may lack the necessary knowledge or cultural competence to offer affirming care, resulting in misgendering, inappropriate questioning, or outright refusal of care (Hughto et al., 2017; Nolan et al., 2020). Financial barriers, such as lack of insurance coverage for gender-affirming procedures or hormone therapy, disproportionately affect low-income TGNB individuals, limiting their ability to pursue necessary medical interventions (Krebs et al., 2022; Vaccaro, 2023).

Discrimination is often encountered at multiple levels within the healthcare system. Examples include:

1. Reception and Registration: TGNB patients may experience misgendering or insensitive questioning during check-in, creating an unwelcoming environment.
2. Provider-Patient Interactions: Providers may display biases or rely on outdated practices, such as gatekeeping through gender dysphoria diagnoses, rather than adopting a patient-centered approach (Elkadi et al., 2023).
3. Insurance and Financial Access: Denials of claims for gender-affirming care, restrictive coverage policies, and out-of-pocket costs can create significant financial strain (Austin et al., 2022; Silva et al., 2022).

These barriers discourage preventive care, affirming interventions, and necessary follow-up, leaving patients alienated from the system designed to support their health. Studies show that exposure to such discrimination contributes to fear and mistrust of healthcare systems, increasing the likelihood of delayed or avoided care (Dhanani & Totton, 2023; Hostetter et al., 2022).

Impact on Care and Health Outcomes

The effects of these barriers extend across all levels of healthcare, from preventive services to acute and affirming interventions:

- Preventive Care: Fear of discrimination prevents many TGNB individuals from seeking routine screenings or vaccinations, contributing to undiagnosed conditions and poorer long-term outcomes (Shabalala, 2023).
- Affirming Care: Without knowledgeable providers or supportive environments, patients may abandon their pursuit of gender-affirming interventions, leading to increased dysphoria, mental health challenges, and suicidality (Almazan & Keuroghlian, 2021; Tordoff et al., 2022).
- In emergency or urgent care settings, discriminatory practices or lack of provider competence can exacerbate distress and prevent patients from receiving life-saving interventions.

The Role of the Care Team

A well-structured care team is instrumental in overcoming these barriers and ensuring inclusive, affirming care. The care team should include the following:

- Primary Care Providers: These professionals are central in coordinating care and providing routine and preventive services. Their knowledge of TGNB health needs is crucial for establishing trust and delivering evidence-based care.

- Endocrinologists: Specialists in hormone therapy, endocrinologists ensure the safe administration of hormones and monitor for side effects or complications.
- Mental Health Professionals: Counselors and therapists with expertise in TGNB care provide emotional support, help patients navigate identity-related stressors, and address co-occurring mental health conditions like anxiety or depression (Hembree et al., 2017; Turban & Brady, 2022).
- Social Workers or Case Managers: These professionals assist patients in overcoming logistical challenges, such as accessing insurance coverage, housing, or employment resources.
- Community Advocates: Advocacy groups and peer support networks offer vital resources and foster a sense of belonging for TGNB individuals navigating the healthcare system.

Collaboration among these professionals ensures a holistic, patient-centered approach that addresses the multifaceted needs of TGNB individuals. Multidisciplinary care teams also create a safety net, fostering trust and reducing patients' risk of disengaging from the healthcare system.

Solutions and Advocacy

Solutions and Advocacy promote access and inclusivity; healthcare systems must adopt targeted strategies that address systemic and individual barriers. These include:

1. Provider Education: Comprehensive training on transgender health should be integrated into medical education and continuing professional development to address knowledge gaps and reduce biases (Nolan et al., 2020; Vaccaro, 2023).
2. Policy Advocacy: Expanding insurance coverage for gender-affirming care, addressing restrictive legislation, and standardizing guidelines can reduce financial and legal barriers (Masumori et al., 2021; Baker & Restar, 2022).
3. Institutional Change: Creating inclusive environments, such as gender-neutral restrooms and intake forms with diverse gender options, fosters a sense of safety and respect for TGNB patients.
4. Community Partnerships: Partnering with community organizations and advocacy groups ensures that healthcare systems remain attuned to the evolving needs of TGNB populations and leverage external resources to address gaps (Chin et al., 2023; Shabalala, 2023).

Overcoming barriers to gender-affirming care is essential to promote equity and inclusivity within healthcare systems. By addressing systemic discrimination, enhancing provider education, and fostering multidisciplinary care teams, healthcare systems can create environments where TGNB individuals feel supported, respected, and empowered. The integration of affirming practices improves individual outcomes and fosters a culture of inclusivity that benefits all patients.

Surgical Options: Navigating Decisions and Consent

Surgical interventions are a critical component of gender-affirming care for many transgender and non-binary (TGNB) individuals. These options, which may include chest reconstruction, facial feminization or masculinization, and genital surgeries, provide individuals with the opportunity to align their physical appearance more closely with their gender identity. However, decisions surrounding surgical interventions, particularly for minors, involve complex ethical, legal, and medical considerations.

Decision-Making: Minors vs. Adults

The decision-making process for surgical options varies significantly between minors and adults. Adults, generally defined as individuals over the age of 18, are presumed to have the legal capacity to provide informed consent for medical procedures, including gender-affirming surgeries. This process involves a thorough understanding of the procedure, its risks, benefits, and potential outcomes, ensuring that the individual makes an autonomous decision based on their needs and goals (Turban & Keuroghlian, 2022).

For minors, the decision-making process is more complex and often involves parental or guardian consent in addition to the minor's assent. State laws vary widely in terms of the age at which minors can consent to medical procedures, including those related to gender-affirming care. Some states have enacted laws that allow minors to access certain types of care, such as hormone blockers, without parental consent. In contrast, others impose strict age-related restrictions on all forms of gender-affirming care (Baker & Restar, 2022). This patchwork of legislation creates disparities in access and may leave some minors unable to pursue medically necessary interventions.

In states that allow minors to access gender-affirming care, the involvement of a multidisciplinary care team is critical. These teams, often comprising endocrinologists, surgeons, mental health professionals, and social workers, work collaboratively to assess the minor's readiness for surgery, provide comprehensive counseling, and ensure that the decision aligns with the minor's long-term well-being (Hembree et al., 2017). When parental consent is not attainable, some states permit judicial bypass mechanisms, enabling minors to seek court approval for medically necessary care (Chin et al., 2023).

Defining Age of Consent in Transition Care

The concept of age of consent in transition care differs from its application in other medical contexts. Age of consent generally refers to the legal age at which an individual can independently authorize medical treatments without requiring parental or guardian approval. In gender-affirming care, this age can vary based on the type of intervention. For example, puberty blockers may be accessible to minors as young as 10-12 years old, while surgical interventions are often reserved for older adolescents or adults (Hembree et al., 2017). This tiered approach reflects the varying degrees of permanence and risk associated with different procedures.

Reversal and Detransition

While the majority of individuals who undergo gender-affirming surgeries report high levels of satisfaction and improved quality of life, a subset of individuals may seek reversal or detransition. Reasons for detransitioning are complex and multifaceted, often reflecting changes in gender identity, external pressures, or dissatisfaction with surgical outcomes (Vandenbussche, 2021).

Common factors influencing reversal or detransition include:

- Evolution of Gender Identity: Some individuals may experience shifts in their understanding of their gender over time, prompting a desire to detransition.
- Social and Family Pressures: External factors like familial rejection or societal stigma may compel individuals to reverse their transition.
- Medical Complications or Dissatisfaction: In rare cases, individuals may experience adverse outcomes from surgery, such as scarring or functional limitations, leading to dissatisfaction.

Detransitioning often involves challenges, including navigating the healthcare system to access appropriate care and managing the emotional and social implications. Healthcare providers must approach these situations with empathy, avoid judgment or assumptions, and provide medical and psychological support.

Ethical Considerations in Gender-Affirming Care

Ethical considerations in gender-affirming care are paramount to ensuring the well-being and autonomy of individuals seeking such care. Healthcare providers must uphold the principles of beneficence, non-maleficence, autonomy, and justice. These principles guide the delivery of care that respects individuals' self-identified gender, incorporates affirming language, and provides culturally competent, patient-centered services. Upholding these ethical standards requires a commitment to ongoing education, reflection, and advocacy for the rights and dignity of all individuals, regardless of their gender identity.

Balancing Ethical Principles in Care for Minors and Adults

When working with minors, ethical considerations become even more nuanced, as decisions often involve balancing the autonomy of the individual with the involvement of parents or guardians. Providers must weigh the principles of beneficence (acting in the patient's best interest) and non-maleficence (avoiding harm) while respecting minors' emerging autonomy and capacity to participate in decision-making. Policies must reflect the best available evidence and prioritize the voices and needs of transgender and non-binary (TGNB) individuals, ensuring that care decisions are guided by what is most affirming and beneficial for the patient.

Informed consent is a cornerstone of ethical care for both minors and adults. For adults, the informed consent process should be thorough, transparent, and inclusive, ensuring individuals understand the risks, benefits, and alternatives associated with surgical interventions. For minors, obtaining consent may require additional steps, including parental or guardian involvement and multidisciplinary team assessments, to ensure that decisions are in the minor's best interest and aligned with their long-term well-being.

Addressing Disparities and Advocating for Equitable Access

The disparities in access to surgical options for minors and adults highlight the urgent need for advocacy and policy reforms. Restrictive state laws, lack of insurance coverage, and systemic discrimination create barriers that disproportionately affect marginalized populations. Addressing these disparities requires collaborative efforts among healthcare providers, policymakers, and community organizations to create equitable pathways to care.

Healthcare providers are critical in advocating for policies that reflect evidence-based practices and promote equitable access to care. This includes supporting legislative initiatives to expand insurance coverage for gender-affirming procedures, combatting discriminatory policies, and creating institutional environments prioritizing inclusivity and respect for all patients.

Supporting Patients Through Detransition or Reversal

In rare instances where individuals consider detransition or reversal of surgical interventions, ethical considerations must extend to creating a nonjudgmental and supportive environment. Providers should foster trust and open communication, acknowledging the complexity of these decisions and addressing the patient's medical and psychological needs with empathy. Supporting individuals through detransition aligns with the ethical commitment to autonomy and beneficence, ensuring that care remains patient-centered and affirming, regardless of the individual's trajectory.

Embracing Authenticity and Dignity

Gender-affirming care is a cornerstone of equitable and inclusive healthcare, grounded in recognizing and respecting individuals' diverse identities and lived experiences. Throughout this chapter, we have explored the principles and practices of gender-affirming care, delving into its critical components, including puberty suppression, hormone therapy, surgical options, and the ethical considerations inherent in providing affirming care. These interventions are not merely medical procedures but transformative acts that affirm dignity, reduce disparities, and empower transgender and non-binary (TGNB) individuals to thrive.

The challenges to achieving universal access to gender-affirming care are substantial, encompassing systemic barriers such as discrimination, inadequate provider education, restrictive policies, and financial constraints. Addressing these obstacles requires a collaborative effort among healthcare providers, policymakers, and community advocates. By prioritizing evidence-based practices, enhancing provider training, and advocating for equitable policies, we can dismantle the structural inequities that impede access to care and create environments that foster safety, respect, and affirmation.

Ethical principles such as autonomy, beneficence, non-maleficence, and justice should guide all aspects of gender-affirming care. This requires transparent and thorough informed consent processes, particularly for minors navigating the complexities of transition, as well as a compassionate approach to individuals considering detransition or reversal. Upholding these principles ensures that care remains patient-centered and responsive to each individual's evolving needs and goals.

As healthcare professionals, our role extends beyond the clinical setting. We must advocate for the rights and well-being of TGNB individuals, promoting inclusivity and equity within and beyond healthcare systems. By fostering a culture of respect and affirmation, we honor all individuals' inherent dignity and autonomy, empowering them to live authentically and embrace their true selves.

The following cases illuminate the practical application of gender-affirming care principles, offering insights into this care's complexities, ethical dilemmas, and transformative potential. These real-world scenarios challenge us to deepen our understanding, refine our practices, and reaffirm our commitment to providing compassionate and competent care for all.

CASES

Case 1. 30-Year Transgender Female Lesbian Who Is Considering Reversing Gender Assignment

Learning Objectives

1. Understand the complexities of gender identity exploration and transition, particularly within the context of sexual orientation, through the examination of a case study involving a 30-year-old transgender female lesbian.
2. Recognize the intersectionality of gender identity and sexual orientation and the unique challenges faced by individuals who identify as both transgender and lesbian.
3. Explore the psychological impact of gender dysphoria, social stigma, and internalized shame on the mental health and well-being of transgender individuals, using the case study as a reference point.
4. Discuss the reasons why a transgender individual may consider reversing their gender assignment, including feelings of dissatisfaction, distress, and identity conflict.
5. Examine the ethical considerations surrounding gender assignment reversal, including informed consent, autonomy, and medical necessity, within the case study context.
6. Identify supportive care strategies for transgender individuals considering gender assignment reversal, including counseling, social support, and exploration of alternative treatment options.
7. Discuss the importance of culturally competent care in supporting transgender individuals, particularly those who belong to marginalized communities, such as BIPOC and LGBTQ+ individuals.

8. Recognize the role of community resources, support groups, and advocacy organizations in providing assistance and empowerment to transgender individuals navigating their gender identity journey, using the case study as a reference point.

Case Aim: The case study explores the unique experiences, challenges, and decision-making process of a 30-year-old transgender woman who identifies as a lesbian and is considering reversing her gender assignment. By examining her journey, this case aims to understand the complex interplay of social, psychological, and medical factors influencing her desire for reversal. Central to this exploration is the recognition of how societal pressures, sexism, and internalized stigma may shape her healthcare experiences and decisions.

Jamie is a 30-year-old transgender female who has been living as a woman for several years. Jamie was assigned male at birth but has been identified as female since childhood. Despite undergoing hormone therapy and some gender-affirming surgeries, Jamie expresses dissatisfaction with her current gender identity and experiences distress related to her assigned gender. As a lesbian woman, Jamie grapples with the intersection of her gender identity and sexual orientation, feeling conflicted about her identity within the LGBTQ+ community.

She grew up in a supportive family environment and came out as transgender during her early twenties. While she has found acceptance and support within the transgender community, Jamie struggles to reconcile her gender identity with her sexual orientation as a lesbian. Her experiences of discrimination, social stigma, and internalized shame have contributed to her feelings of isolation and distress.

Case Questions

1. What Are the Individual's Reasons for Considering a Reversal of Her Gender Assignment?

- Taking an extensive history and consulting with psychology is a necessary first step in understanding why the patient is reconsidering sexual identity. Identifying stressors and experiences that may have led patients to newly express dissatisfaction with their current gender identity or experience distress related to their transgender status. They might feel that their assigned gender does not align with their true identity or that they are not entirely comfortable with their transition.

2. How Long Has the Individual Been Living as a Transgender Female, and What Has Been Her Experience During This Time?

- The patient may have been living as a transgender female for a significant period, potentially undergoing hormone therapy and gender-affirming surgeries. Their experiences during this time could include challenges such as discrimination, social stigma, or struggles with acceptance. There may be significant side effects that may contribute to her reconsideration of the process. The provider must know support and social services that may help the patient.

3. Has the Individual Experienced any Significant Challenges or Struggles Related to Her Gender Identity or Transition Process?

- The patient may have faced challenges such as gender dysphoria, difficulties accessing gender-affirming healthcare, or discrimination based on their transgender status. They may also have experienced challenges related to their sexual orientation as a lesbian within the context of their gender identity. Referral to psychology and social services is a necessary step to support patients.

4. How Does the Individual's Sexual Orientation as a Lesbian Intersect With Her Gender Identity and Decision to Reverse Her Gender Assignment?

- The patient's identity as a transgender female lesbian reflects the complexity of identity intersectionality. She is experiencing unique challenges related to navigating both their gender identity and sexual orientation, which could influence their feelings about their gender assignment.

5. What Role Does the Individual's Social Support Network, Including Friends, Family, And Community, Play in Her Decision-Making Process?

- Investigating her support network, including friends, family, and community, may be crucial in their decision-making process. Positive support from loved ones and access to LGBTQ+ affirming spaces may provide validation and encouragement, while lack of support could exacerbate feelings of isolation or distress.

6. Has the Individual Received any Medical or Psychological Assessments or Counseling Regarding Her Desire to Reverse Her Gender Assignment?

- Depending on the level of change, she has undergone medical and psychological assessments to explore their feelings about gender assignment reversal and to assess their mental health status. Counseling and support services may be provided to help them navigate their decision-making process.

7. What Are the Potential Risks and Benefits Associated With Reversing Her Gender Assignment, Both Medically and Psychologically?

- Medical professionals would discuss the potential risks and benefits associated with gender assignment reversal, including surgical procedures, hormone therapy adjustments, and psychological implications. These discussions would provide the individual with comprehensive information to make an informed decision about their healthcare.

8. What Other Treatment Options or Interventions Might Address the Individual's Concerns or Improve Her Well-Being?

- Alternative treatment options or interventions, such as counseling, support groups, or adjustments to hormone therapy, may be explored to address the individual's concerns or improve their well-being

9. How Does the Individual Envision Her Life and Identity Following a Reversal of Her Gender Assignment, and What Role Do Societal Pressures, Sexism, and Traditional Gender Norms Play in Shaping Her Expectations and Decision-Making Process?

- Exploring the individual's goals, aspirations, and vision for her future is essential in understanding her motivations for gender assignment reversal. Societal pressures and sexism, including rigid expectations around femininity and gender roles, may influence her sense of identity and contribute to internalized stigma. By addressing these factors, healthcare providers can help her clarify whether her goals align with her authentic self or are shaped by external influences, ensuring her decisions support her well-being and long-term happiness.

10. What Are the Ethical Considerations Involved in Supporting the Individual's Decision Regarding Her Gender Assignment Reversal, and How Can Healthcare Providers Ensure That Her Autonomy and Dignity Are Respected Throughout the Process?

- Healthcare providers must ensure the individual's autonomy, dignity, and rights are respected throughout decision-making. Ethical considerations may include informed consent, confidentiality, and the principle of nonmaleficence.

Case Discussion

The case of a 30-year-old transgender female lesbian contemplating reversing her gender assignment presents a complex and sensitive situation that requires careful consideration and support. Overall, the case of a transgender female lesbian considering reversing her gender assignment underscores the importance of providing individualized, affirming, and compassionate care that respects her autonomy, dignity, and unique identity journey. By fostering open communication, providing comprehensive support services, and advocating for her rights and well-being, healthcare providers can empower her to make informed decisions about her healthcare and live authentically and confidently.

Transgender women often navigate societal norms and expectations rooted in sexism, such as rigid standards of femininity, beauty, and gender roles. These pressures, compounded by transphobia, can influence feelings of self-worth and identity, contributing to challenges in navigating gender expression and transition decisions. Through a comprehensive examination of her experiences, this case study sheds light on the broader impact of systemic sexism and societal expectations on transgender women, particularly those contemplating transition reversal.

The case emphasizes the importance of affirming, inclusive, and patient-centered healthcare practices that acknowledge and address the influence of sexism and societal norms. By fostering a compassionate and nonjudgmental approach, healthcare providers can better support the autonomy and dignity of transgender individuals navigating complex identities and healthcare decisions.

It is critical to explore her motivations, identity intersectionality, psychological well-being, medical considerations, and ethical and legal implications so that healthcare providers can offer compassionate and individualized support to navigate this challenging decision-making process. By prioritizing patient autonomy, dignity, and well-being, healthcare providers can empower her to make informed decisions about her healthcare journey, ensuring that her unique identity and needs are respected and affirmed.

Fostering a supportive and inclusive healthcare environment where individuals feel validated and empowered to live authentically is essential in promoting holistic well-being and affirming the inherent dignity of all individuals, regardless of their gender identity or sexual orientation. Jorgensen (2023) suggests that the patient's age starts to transition, possibly contributing to regret and detransition. Along with Baker and Restar (2022), the cost and utilization of health insurance can be contributing factors, and the third, in many ways, the most damaging is society.

Jorgensen (2023) discusses two typologies for external and internal detransition. The external forces, such as discrimination, pressure from family, difficulties finding employment, or loss of health insurance, seem to drive the decision to detransition in studies that primarily focused on participants who detransitioned at some point but later reidentified as transgender or gender-diverse (Jorgensen, 2023). The second is internal factors, worsening mental health, or the realization that gender dysphoria was a maladaptive response to trauma, misogyny, internalized homophobia, or pressure from social media and online communities (Jorgensen, 2023).

The provider must be well-versed in local and regional support services, social services, and mental health services. Moreover, the provider must be up to date on ICD coding and follow up with the patient to ensure they have all they need to transition and move forward. Ensuring the patient has the executive functions includes planning, prioritizing, and strategizing to achieve long-term goals and weighing information to make decisions thoughtfully (Jorgensen, 2023).

Case 2. A 10-Year-Old Navigating Gender Identity and Distress

Learning Objectives

1. Recognize the signs of gender dysphoria in children and understand the emotional, psychological, and physical distress it can cause, particularly during the onset of puberty.
2. Identify appropriate immediate and long-term intervention steps to ensure Alex's safety and well-being, including referrals to gender-affirming care specialists.
3. Develop a culturally sensitive and intersectional approach to address the unique challenges faced by BIPOC transgender youth.
4. Understand the healthcare provider's role in fostering a safe, affirming space that supports open communication and trust between the patient, family, and care team.

Case Aim: This case illustrates the critical importance of early intervention, culturally competent care, and multidisciplinary collaboration in supporting transgender youth like Alex. It emphasizes the need for providers to balance immediate safety concerns with long-term affirming care while navigating the intersectionality of cultural, familial, and societal influences.

Alex, a 10-year-old assigned male at birth, confides in his physician during an annual physical exam about his deeply held conviction of being a girl. He shares that he has been experiencing significant distress regarding his gender identity for several years, feeling profound discomfort with his male body and an intense longing to express himself authentically as a girl.

Alex reveals that his distress has worsened as puberty changes begin to occur, heightening his sense of disconnection from his body. In a particularly distressing disclosure, Alex explains that he has attempted to alter his genitalia in secret, motivated by a desire to align his physical body with his gender identity. This alarming behavior reflects the severity of his gender dysphoria and underscores the urgent need for intervention.

Alex attends a diverse public school, where he experiences a supportive environment among his peers. However, he struggles with societal expectations and cultural norms tied to his assigned gender. As a BIPOC individual, Alex faces additional complexities, including navigating cultural and family dynamics that may be less accepting of his gender expression and identity.

Case Discussion Questions

1. What Immediate Actions Should the Physician Take to Ensure Alex's Safety Following His Disclosure of Self-Harm Attempts?

- Immediate safety measures should include addressing Alex's attempts to alter his genitalia in a nonjudgemental manner and by conducting a physical examination to assess any injuries or risks. This can cultivate a safe space within the exam room for Alex to disclose other concerns and to be able to seek help. The physician should also develop a safety plan that includes monitoring for self-harm, close follow up and referrals to mental health professionals with expertise in gender dysphoria. Parents should be included within this plan. Family therapy could be helpful to process.

2. How Can the Physician Initiate a Discussion With Alex's Family to Foster Understanding and Support for His Gender Identity?

- Initiate a family discussion with sensitivity, emphasizing the importance of understanding Alex's feelings and experiences. Provide resources, such as educational materials or referrals to support groups for families of transgender youth, to foster a supportive home environment.

3. What Steps Can the Physician Take to Connect Alex With Mental Health Professionals and Gender-Affirming Care, Including Considerations for Puberty Blockers?

- Refer Alex to a multidisciplinary team, including a pediatric endocrinologist and a mental health professional, for assessment and potential interventions, such as puberty blockers, if clinically appropriate. Discuss the physical changes Alex is experiencing due to puberty and explore the use of puberty blockers (GnRH agonists) to halt further development, allowing him time to explore his gender identity without added distress. Provide age-appropriate education to Alex and his family about how puberty blockers work, their reversibility, and their role in reducing dysphoria (Hembree et al., 2017). Collaborate with school counselors and social workers to create a supportive educational environment.

4. How Can the Physician Address the Cultural and Societal Pressures Alex Faces as a BIPOC Transgender Child?

- Explore the cultural norms and familial expectations Alex faces as a BIPOC transgender child, recognizing how these factors may influence his experiences and needs. Partner with culturally competent organizations or advocates to provide additional support and resources for Alex and his family.

5. What Ethical Considerations Should Guide the Physician in Managing Alex's Care, Including Balancing Confidentiality With the Need for Family Involvement?

- Maintain confidentiality while balancing the need to involve Alex's guardians in his care. Prioritize Alex's autonomy and self-expression, ensuring he feels heard and respected.

Case Discussion

This case highlights the complexities of supporting transgender youth navigating gender dysphoria, particularly as puberty exacerbates distress. Alex, early intervention is critical to ensuring his safety, fostering his mental health, and reducing the long-term risks associated with untreated gender dysphoria, such as anxiety, depression, and suicidality (Tordoff et al., 2022). Puberty hormone blockers, which are reversible medical interventions, represent an essential tool in alleviating the heightened distress Alex is experiencing as his body develops in ways that conflict with his gender identity.

Additionally, cultural sensitivity is paramount, as BIPOC transgender youth often face unique challenges, including stigma within their communities and systemic inequities in accessing affirming care. Providers must adopt an intersectional approach that respects these layers of identity while advocating for equitable access to resources and support. By fostering a collaborative, patient-centered approach, healthcare providers can empower children like Alex to navigate their journeys authentically, surrounded by understanding and affirmation.

Case 3: A Transgender Gay Male Establishing Care

Learning Objectives

1. Recognize the unique healthcare needs of transgender men who identify as gay, with attention to sexual practices, vaccination history, and preventive screenings.
2. Understand the impact of intersectionality on health disparities for mixed-race, transgender, and gay individuals, particularly those who lack access to family health history.
3. Identify systemic barriers to care and develop strategies to overcome these obstacles through advocacy, education, and patient-centered care.
4. Establish evidence-based practices for managing gaps in family health history and uncertain vaccination records.
5. Foster an inclusive and affirming clinical environment that promotes trust, safety, and open communication.

Case Aim: This case highlights the complex and intersectional healthcare needs of a transgender gay male. The case underscores the importance of culturally competent, evidence-based, and affirming care practices by addressing challenges such as limited family health history, vaccination gaps, and systemic barriers. It also guides healthcare providers to enhance their understanding of the broader social and systemic factors influencing patient outcomes.

Jordan, a 35-year-old transgender man who identifies as gay, presents to establish care with a new primary care provider. He is of mixed race and was adopted, which limits his knowledge of his biological family's health history. Jordan recalls receiving the HPV vaccine but is uncertain about other vaccinations. During the visit, he explicitly shares, "I catch, not pitch," clarifying his sexual practices. This disclosure is critical for tailoring comprehensive and affirming care.

Jordan's case reflects the nuanced healthcare needs of transgender men who identify as gay, compounded by systemic barriers, intersectional identity factors, and potential gaps in care arising from inadequate provider education. Navigating these complexities requires a culturally competent, patient-centered approach that considers his sexual orientation, gender identity, and racial background while addressing the structural inequities that may impact his health outcomes

Case Questions

1. What Screening Tests and Routine Preventive Care Are Recommended for a Transgender Man of Jordan's Age and Identity?

- Screening Tests and Routine Preventive Care (Loza et al., 2018): General health screenings: Blood pressure, cholesterol, and glucose levels to screen for hypertension, hyperlipidemia, and diabetes. Cancer screenings: Depending on Jordan's surgical history, Pap smears (if he retains a cervix), chest wall exams (if breast tissue is present), and colorectal cancer screenings should be included. Bone health: Consider bone density testing, particularly if testosterone therapy has been prolonged without concurrent estrogen. STI testing: Comprehensive STI panel, including rectal and pharyngeal swabs for gonorrhea and chlamydia, based on his sexual practices. Mental health screening: Address common concerns in transgender populations, such as depression, anxiety, and minority stress.

2. How Should the Provider Address the Gap in Jordan's Vaccination History, Including Offering Catch-Up Immunizations?

- Addressing Vaccination History (Marshall et al., 2022): Administer age-appropriate vaccinations, including Tdap, influenza, COVID-19, hepatitis A and B, varicella, and zoster vaccines. Consider titers to assess immunity for MMR, varicella, or hepatitis B if documentation is unavailable. Provide education about vaccination guidelines and their role in preventive care for men who have sex with men.

3. What Considerations Should Guide the Provider in Tailoring STI Testing and HIV Prevention Discussions Based on Jordan's Sexual Practices?

- Considerations for Sexual Practices (Mills et al., 2022): Discuss PrEP (pre-exposure prophylaxis) for HIV prevention, given his stated sexual practices. Ensure STI testing aligns with his risks, mainly focusing on rectal and pharyngeal testing. Use affirming language when discussing sexual health, avoiding assumptions, and promoting open dialogue.

4. How Can the Provider Incorporate Jordan's Intersectional Identity Into His Care Plan to Address Potential Systemic Disparities?

- Addressing Intersectionality and Systemic Barriers (Sengupta et al., 2023): Recognize the potential impact of systemic inequities, such as implicit bias and limited access to culturally competent care, on Jordan's health outcomes. Advocate for equity in access to gender-affirming care by connecting Jordan with local LGBTQ+ health organizations and community resources. Explore genetic testing as a tool to address the lack of family health history and assess Jordan's risk for hereditary conditions.

5. What Steps Can the Provider Take to Create a Culturally Competent and Affirming Clinical Environment?

- Creating an Affirming Clinical Environment (Nolan et al., 2020): Use Jordan's correct name and pronouns consistently. Avoid assumptions about his medical or surgical history, instead allowing Jordan to share information on his terms. Implement culturally competent practices, such as inclusive intake forms, gender-neutral language, and visual indicators of LGBTQ+ inclusivity in the clinical space.

Case Discussion

Jordan's case illustrates the intersectional challenges faced by transgender gay men in accessing affirming and comprehensive care (Reisner et al., 2015). A study by Reisner et al. (2015) demonstrates the importance of facilities like this for patients like Jordon. His mixed-race identity, adoption status, and sexual orientation underscore the importance of a nuanced and patient-centered approach. Providers must navigate the absence of family health history by focusing on preventive care, lifestyle risk factors, and genetic screening when appropriate.

Jordan's sexual practices highlight the need for tailored STI testing, discussions about PrEP, and education on the importance of vaccinations. Rouse (2023) discusses the provider's ability to foster an affirming environment and discusses the catches and hoops patients and physicians have to jump through. It is important that the provider use inclusive language, address systemic disparities, and provide care, which is essential to building trust and promoting Jordan's well-being.

This case also reflects broader systemic issues, such as provider knowledge gaps and access barriers, which disproportionately affect LGBTQ+ individuals. Continuous education and advocacy are vital to equipping providers with the skills to deliver inclusive and affirming care. By adopting an intersectional framework and evidence-based practices, healthcare professionals can empower patients like Jordan to thrive in their identities while addressing their unique health needs.

Case 4: A Non-Binary Individual Seeking Hormone Therapy

Learning Objectives

1. Recognize the importance of affirming language and respectful communication in fostering trust with non-binary patients and understand how failing to use preferred identifiers reflects implicit biases and perpetuates sexist behaviors tied to rigid gender norms.
2. Understand the individualized nature of hormone therapy and the need to tailor care to the specific goals of non-binary individuals while acknowledging the influence of societal sexism in dismissing diverse gender identities.
3. Address implicit biases and gaps in provider knowledge about non-binary identities and care needs, emphasizing the role of inclusive practices in combating sexism and fostering equitable care environments.

Case Aim: This case illustrates the potential harm caused by misgendering, dismissive attitudes, and the perpetuation of sexist assumptions in gender-affirming care. It emphasizes the importance of cultural competence, tailored care plans, and respect for non-binary identities in maintaining trust and engagement with healthcare. It also highlights the need to address biases rooted in societal sexism that undermine diverse gender expressions.

Taylor, a 27-year-old non-binary individual, visits a clinic to initiate hormone therapy. Taylor uses they/them pronouns and expresses a desire for low-dose testosterone to achieve subtle masculinization while maintaining certain feminine features. During the appointment, the provider repeatedly misgenders Taylor, referring to them as "she," and dismisses their request for a low-dose regimen, stating, "You need to make a clear decision if you want to transition fully." Taylor leaves the appointment unheard and invalidated, questioning whether to continue seeking care.

Taylor's experience highlights a lack of understanding about non-binary identities and individualized approaches to gender-affirming care, compounded by societal sexism that often assumes rigid gender binaries and dismisses diverse expressions of identity. This dynamic can lead to disengagement from the healthcare system and untreated gender dysphoria, with significant impacts on mental and physical health.

Case Discussion Questions

1. How Should the Provider Have Approached Taylor's Request for Low-Dose Testosterone, and Why Is Individualized Care Critical for Non-Binary Patients?

- Approaching Taylor's Request for Low-Dose Testosterone, let us consider patient-centered approaches: The provider should have listened to Taylor's goals without imposing binary expectations about transition. Non-binary individuals often have unique needs, and a flexible, patient-centered approach is crucial. The provider should explain the options for hormone therapy, addressing the risks, benefits, and potential outcomes of low-dose testosterone. Shared Decision-Making would include collaborating with Taylor to develop a care plan that aligns with their goals and respects their autonomy.

2. What Strategies Can the Provider Use to Consistently Use Affirming Language, Including Correct Pronouns, When Interacting With Non-Binary Patients?

- Speech, tone, verbiage, and body language are vital. Therefore, using Affirming Language by Providers should practice consistently using patients' pronouns and names. Incorporating affirming language in all interactions can foster trust and a sense of safety. Clinics should implement regular training and professional development time on LGBTQ+ inclusivity to ensure all staff understand the importance of using affirming language and avoiding misgendering.

3. How Can the Healthcare System Address Gaps in Provider Education About Non-Binary Identities and Gender-Affirming Care?

- Addressing Provider Education Gaps through Professional Development and Community and Population Engagement. Comprehensive Training Programs: Healthcare systems should provide ongoing education on non-binary identities and gender-affirming care, including hormone therapy. Organizations like the World Professional Association for Transgender Health (WPATH) offer resources to support this. Peer Learning: Encourage providers to learn from colleagues with experience in gender-affirming care or partner with community organizations to enhance cultural competence.

4. What Immediate Steps Can the Provider Take to Rebuild Trust With Taylor After the Negative Experience During the Appointment?

- Once a patient loses trust in the provider or the care system, it is very hard to get it back, but it is not impossible. It is achieved through the provider acknowledging their mistake, apologizing for misgendering, and dismissing Taylor's concerns, demonstrating accountability and a willingness to improve. Offer a follow-up appointment with a commitment to actively listen and provide affirming respectful care. Offer Supportive Resources: Connect Taylor with local LGBTQ+ support groups or patient advocates who can provide additional guidance.

5. How Can Clinics and Healthcare Organizations Create a More Inclusive Environment for Non-Binary and Transgender Patients?

- Creating an Inclusive Environment can look like: Inclusive Policies: Implement intake forms with options for patients to indicate their names, pronouns, and gender identity. Visual Affirmation: Display signage, flags, or other symbols of inclusivity to signal a safe space for LGBTQ+ patients. Community Engagement: Partner with LGBTQ+ organization

6. How Does the Provider's Failure to Use Taylor's Preferred Pronouns Reflect the Influence of Sexism in Healthcare, and What Steps Can Be Taken to Mitigate This Issue in Gender-Affirming Care?

- The provider's failure to use Taylor's preferred pronouns reinforces sexist assumptions that rely on rigid, binary notions of gender tied to biological sex.

This behavior not only disrespects Taylor's identity but also perpetuates the broader societal tendency to marginalize and invalidate non-binary individuals. Such actions undermine trust, contribute to disengagement from care, and exacerbate the disparities faced by transgender and non-binary patients. To mitigate this issue, healthcare providers and institutions must actively combat sexism by fostering environments that respect and affirm diverse gender identities. By recognizing and addressing the role of sexism in these interactions, healthcare systems can improve the quality of gender-affirming care and ensure that all patients feel valued and respected.

- Specific steps include Inclusive Training: Mandate training programs for all staff on gender diversity and the intersection of sexism and healthcare bias. Accountability: Implement policies to address misgendering as a breach of professional conduct. Cultural Shifts: Promote a clinic culture that challenges sexist assumptions by normalizing inclusive practices, such as asking for and consistently using patients' pronouns. Patient Advocacy: Empower patients like Taylor by incorporating feedback mechanisms to report misgendering or other forms of discrimination.

Case Discussion

Failure to respect Taylor's pronouns and dismissing their request for a low-dose hormone regimen undermines their autonomy and erodes trust in the provider. These actions not only dismiss Taylor's non-binary identity but also perpetuate sexism by reinforcing binary gender norms and ignoring the validity of diverse gender expressions. Such experiences contribute to long-term disengagement from care, increased risk of untreated gender dysphoria, and worsening mental health outcomes. Providers must recognize how societal sexism influences these interactions and adopt a patient-centered approach that challenges such biases. This includes using affirming language, acknowledging non-binary identities, and tailoring interventions to align with individual goals while fostering an inclusive and respectful clinical environment.

Case 5: A Lesbian Cisgender Woman with a History of Gender-Based Trauma

Learning Objectives

1. Recognize how sexist assumptions and cultural biases negatively impact the quality of care for lesbian and queer women.

2. Develop trauma-informed practices that account for the intersection of sexual orientation and gender identity with a patient's history of trauma.
3. Understand the unique preventive health needs of lesbian and queer women, including addressing common misconceptions around their risk factors.
4. Foster affirming, inclusive environments that respect diverse identities and avoid perpetuating stereotypes rooted in sexism and heteronormativity.

Case Aim: This case emphasizes the importance of culturally competent and trauma-informed care that addresses the impact of sex, sexism, and cultural biases on patient-provider interactions. It highlights how assumptions rooted in sexist and heteronormative frameworks undermine trust and create long-term barriers to preventive health services for marginalized populations.

Sophia, a 45-year-old cisgender lesbian woman, presents for a routine pelvic exam. She discloses a history of sexual trauma and shares that she is nervous about the exam but understands its importance for preventive care. During the exam, the provider makes inappropriate comments about Sophia's sexual orientation, stating, "You probably do not need this as often since you are not sexually active with men." The provider's assumption not only disregards Sophia's sexual identity but also reflects a sexist attitude rooted in outdated notions that women's health concerns revolve solely around heterosexual relationships.

Sophia feels judged and invalidated, leaving the appointment retraumatized and reluctant to return for future care. This case underscores how sexist assumptions and biases in healthcare intersect with a lack of cultural competence, compounding mistrust and creating barriers to preventive care for lesbian and queer women.

Case Questions

1. How Can the Provider Ensure That Future Interactions With Sophia Are Free of Assumptions Rooted in Sexism or Heteronormativity?

- By adopting affirming communication practices, the provider should use open-ended questions and avoid making assumptions about Sophia's sexual orientation, behavior, or health risks. For example, asking, "What concerns do you have about your sexual or reproductive health?" creates space for Sophia to share her needs without feeling judged. Likewise, providers should undergo regular cultural humility training to recognize and address biases, including those rooted in sexism and heteronormativity. This can ensure more equitable and affirming interactions.

2. How Can the Healthcare System Address and Reduce the Impact of Systemic Sexism and Heteronormativity in Patient-Provider Interactions? What Steps Should the Provider Take to Implement Trauma-Informed Practices That Foster Trust and Create a Safe Clinical Environment for Sophia?

- Empower the Patient to allow Sophia to dictate the pace of the pelvic exam, offering options such as having a chaperone present, using a smaller speculum, or stopping the procedure at any point. The following 3 steps are key: *Validate Concerns-* Acknowledge Sophia's history of trauma and nervousness by affirming her feelings and emphasizing that her comfort and consent are the top priorities. *Explain Each Step-* Provide step-by-step explanations of the procedure, ensuring Sophia feels informed and in control. *Create a Calming Environment-* Offer accommodation, such as a quiet room or sensory modifications (e.g., dimmed lights), to reduce anxiety.

Healthcare leadership can adopt and champion policies that promote inclusivity, equity, and accountability across all levels of the organization. Alongside increasing representation, requiring ongoing training on trauma-informed care, cultural humility, and the intersection of sexism and heteronormativity in healthcare can assist in ensuring providers have the tools to create these spaces. Establishing transparent systems for patients to provide feedback on their care experiences, with pathways for addressing complaints about biases or inappropriate comments can enlighten providers about possible blind spots that impact are.

3. What Preventive Health Screenings and Care Are Essential for Lesbian and Queer Women, Regardless of Their Sexual Orientation or Practices?

- Pelvic Exams and Pap Smears: Routine cervical cancer screenings are necessary for individuals with a cervix, regardless of sexual orientation or sexual activity with men. Breast Cancer Screenings: Regular mammograms based on age and risk factors are critical, particularly for women over 40. STI Testing: Offer STI screenings tailored to Sophia's sexual practices, ensuring the provider discusses risk factors without judgment or assumptions. HPV Vaccination: Recommend the HPV vaccine if Sophia has not received it or completed the series. Mental Health Assessments: Screen for anxiety, depression, and other mental health concerns, particularly given Sophia's history of trauma.

4. How Can the Provider Acknowledge and Repair Harm Caused by Inappropriate Comments While Encouraging Sophia to Return for Future Care?

- The provider should apologize for their inappropriate comment, acknowledge the harm caused, and commit to providing better care. Follow-Up Care Plan: Offer to schedule a follow-up appointment with another provider or ensure Sophia is paired with someone trained in trauma-informed and culturally competent care. Empowerment Through Education: Provide Sophia with resources about LGBTQ+-affirming care and trauma-informed practices, reassuring her that her feedback will improve care quality. Patient Advocacy: Offer access to patient advocacy services or LGBTQ+ support groups to help Sophia feel supported in navigating the healthcare system

Case Discussion

Sophia's experience illustrates how sexist assumptions and heteronormative biases in healthcare create significant barriers for lesbian and queer women. The provider's comment that implied Sophia's sexual health needs are less significant because she is not sexually active with men reflects a broader issue of systemic sexism that reduces women's health concerns to their perceived roles in heterosexual relationships. This not only invalidates Sophia's identity but also perpetuates harmful stereotypes about women's sexuality and risks.

Such interactions exacerbate Sophia's feelings of judgment and traumatization, contributing to her reluctance to engage in future care. Addressing these issues requires providers to actively challenge their biases, adopt inclusive communication practices, and approach all patients' health concerns with respect and cultural competence. Trauma-informed care is particularly critical for individuals with histories of sexual trauma, ensuring that the clinical environment feels safe, validating, and free of judgment.

REFERENCES

Almazan, A., & Keuroghlian, A. (2021). Association between gender-affirming surgeries and mental health outcomes. *JAMA Surgery*, *156*(7), 611. DOI: 10.1001/jamasurg.2021.0952 PMID: 33909023

Austin, A., Holzworth, J., & Papciak, R. (2022). Beyond diagnosis: Gender dysphoria feels like a living hell, a nightmare one cannot ever wake up from. *Psychology of Sexual Orientation and Gender Diversity*, *9*(1), 12–20. DOI: 10.1037/sgd0000460

Baker, K., & Restar, A. (2022). Utilization and Costs of Gender-Affirming Care in a Commercially Insured Transgender Population. The Journal of law, medicine & ethics: A journal of the American Society of Law. *Medical Ethics (Burlington, Mass.)*, *50*(3), 456–470. DOI: 10.1017/jme.2022.87 PMID: 36398652

Baker, K., Wilson, L., Sharma, R., Dukhanin, V., McArthur, K., & Robinson, K. (2021). Hormone therapy, mental health, and quality of life among transgender people: A systematic review. *Journal of the Endocrine Society*, *5*(4), bvab011. Advance online publication. DOI: 10.1210/jendso/bvab011 PMID: 33644622

Bhatt, N., Cannella, J., & Gentile, J. P. (2022). Gender-affirming Care for Transgender Patients. *Innovations in Clinical Neuroscience*, *19*(4-6), 23–32. PMID: 35958971

Block, J. (2023). Gender dysphoria in young people is rising—And so is professional disagreement. *BMJ (Clinical Research Ed.)*, 382. DOI: 10.1136/bmj.p382 PMID: 36822640

. Carswell, J. M., Lopez, X., & Rosenthal, S. M. (2022). The Evolution of Adolescent Gender-Affirming Care: An Historical Perspective. Hormone research in pediatrics, 95(6), 649–656. DOI: 10.1159/000526721

Charter, R., Ussher, J., Perz, J., & Robinson, K. (2021). Negotiating mental health amongst transgender parents in Australia. *International Journal of Transgender Health*, *23*(3), 308–320. DOI: 10.1080/26895269.2021.1875951 PMID: 35799955

Chin, M. G., LaGuardia, J. S., Morgan, K. B. J., Ngo, H., Moghadam, S., Huang, K. X., & Lee, J. C. (2023). *United States health policies on gender-affirming care in 2022. Plastic &Amp.* Reconstructive Surgery. DOI: 10.1097/PRS.0000000000010594

Dhanani, L. Y., & Totton, R. R. (2023). Have You Heard the News? The Effects of Exposure to News About Recent Transgender Legislation on Transgender Youth and Young Adults. *Sexuality Research & Social Policy*, *20*(4), 1345–1359. DOI: 10.1007/s13178-023-00810-6 PMID: 37363351

Elkadi, J., Chudleigh, C., Maguire, A., Ambler, G., Scher, S., & Kozlowska, K. (2023). Developmental pathway choices of young people presenting to a gender service with gender distress: A prospective follow-up study. *Children (Basel, Switzerland), 10*(2), 314. DOI: 10.3390/children10020314 PMID: 36832443

Falck, F., & Bränström, R. (2023). The significance of structural stigma towards transgender people in health care encounters across Europe: Health care access, gender identity disclosure, and discrimination in health care as a function of national legislation and public attitudes. *BMC Public Health, 23*(1), 1031. Advance online publication. DOI: 10.1186/s12889-023-15856-9 PMID: 37259082

Goetz, T., & Wolk, C. B. (2023). Moving toward targeted eating disorder care for transgender, non-binary, and gender-expansive patients in the United States. *International Journal of Eating Disorders, 56*(12), 2210–2222. DOI: 10.1002/eat.24055 PMID: 37638738

. Hembree, W. C., Cohen-Kettenis, P., Gooren, L., Hannema, S. E., Meyer, W. J., Murad, M. H., Rosenthal, S. M., Safer, J. D., Tangpricha, V., & T'Sjoen, G. G. (2017). Endocrine treatment of gender-dysphoric/gender-incongruent persons: An Endocrine Society clinical practice guideline. The Journal of Clinical Endocrinology & Metabolism, 102(11). DOI: 10.1210/jc.2017-01658

Herrmann, L., Barkmann, C., Bindt, C., Fahrenkrug, S., Breu, F., Grebe, J., & Becker-Hébly, I. (2023). Binary and non-binary gender identities, internalizing problems, and treatment wishes among adolescents referred to a gender identity clinic in Germany. *Archives of Sexual Behavior, 53*(1), 91–106. DOI: 10.1007/s10508-023-02674-8 PMID: 37563319

Hines, D., Laury, E., & Habermann, B. (2019). They just do not get me: A qualitative analysis of transgender women's health care experiences and clinician interactions. *The Journal of the Association of Nurses in AIDS Care: JANAC, 30*(5), e82–e95. DOI: 10.1097/JNC.0000000000000023 PMID: 31461741

Holt, N., Hope, D., Mocarski, R., & Woodruff, N. (2023). The often-circuitous path to affirming mental health care for transgender and gender-diverse adults. *Current Psychiatry Reports, 25*(3), 105–111. DOI: 10.1007/s11920-023-01410-2 PMID: 36773177

Hostetter, C., Call, J., Gerke, D. R., Holloway, B. T., Walls, N. E., & Greenfield, J. C. (2022). "we are doing the absolute most that we can, and no one is listening": Barriers and facilitators to health literacy within transgender and nonbinary communities. *International Journal of Environmental Research and Public Health, 19*(3), 1229. DOI: 10.3390/ijerph19031229 PMID: 35162254

Hughto, J., Rose, A., Pachankis, J., & Reisner, S. (2017). Barriers to gender transition-related healthcare: Identifying underserved transgender adults in Massachusetts. *Transgender Health*, *2*(1), 107–118. DOI: 10.1089/trgh.2017.0014 PMID: 29082331

Ibrahim, A., Clarke, J., Beischel, W. J., & van Anders, S. M. (2023). Gender/sex markers, bio/logics, and U.S. identity documents. *Feminism & Psychology*, *34*(1), 132–150. DOI: 10.1177/09593535231193232

Jorgensen, S., Hunter, P., Regenstreif, L., Sinai, J., & Malone, W. (2022). Puberty blockers for gender dysphoric youth: A lack of sound science. *Journal of the American College of Clinical Pharmacy: JAACP*, *5*(9), 1005–1007. DOI: 10.1002/jac5.1691

Jorgensen, S. C. J. (2023). Transition Regret and Detransition: Meanings and Uncertainties. *Archives of Sexual Behavior*, *52*(5), 2173–2184. DOI: 10.1007/s10508-023-02626-2 PMID: 37266795

Kamran, R., Jackman, L., Chan, C., Suk, Y., Jacklin, C., Deck, E., Wietek, N., Stepney, M., Harrison, C., Jain, A., & Rodrigues, J. (2023). Implementation of Patient-Reported Outcome Measures for Gender-Affirming Care Worldwide: A Systematic Review. *JAMA Network Open*, *6*(4), e236425. DOI: 10.1001/jamanetworkopen.2023.6425 PMID: 37010869

Krebs, D., Harris, R., Steinbaum, A., Pilcher, S., Guss, C., Kremen, J., Roberts, S. A., Baskaran, C., Carswell, J., & Millington, K. (2022). Care for transgender young people. *Hormone Research in Paediatrics*, *95*(5), 405–414. DOI: 10.1159/000524030 PMID: 35272283

Lee, J. Y., & Rosenthal, S. M. (2023). Gender-Affirming Care of Transgender and Gender-Diverse Youth: Current Concepts. *Annual Review of Medicine*, *74*(1), 107–116. DOI: 10.1146/annurev-med-043021-032007 PMID: 36260812

Loza, O., Hernandez, P., Calderon-Mora, J., Laks, S., Leiner, M., Reddy, S., Lara, P., & Granados, H. (2018). Developing trans-affirming health services in an underserved area: An intersectional approach. *Transgender Health*, *3*(1), 127–135. DOI: 10.1089/trgh.2018.0011 PMID: 30023431

Marshall, S. A., Stewart, M. K., Barham, C., Ounpraseuth, S., & Curran, G. M. (2022). Facilitators and barriers to providing affirming care for transgender patients in primary care practices in Arkansas. *The Journal of Rural Health*, *39*(1), 251–261. DOI: 10.1111/jrh.12683 PMID: 35644535

Masumori, N., Baba, T., Abe, T., & Niwa, K. (2021). What is the most anticipated change induced by treatment using gender-affirming hormones in individuals with gender incongruence? *International Journal of Urology*, *28*(5), 526–529. DOI: 10.1111/iju.14499 PMID: 33465834

. Meyer, G. (2022). Black transgender women's barriers to gender affirmation in healthcare.. DOI: 10.14293/S2199-1006.1.SOR-.PP4U5UG.v1

Mikovits, J. (2022). "I do not feel like I am a person": Nursing knowledge of transgender care through the lens of transgender people. *Journal of Advanced Nursing*, *78*(9), 3012–3024. DOI: 10.1111/jan.15308 PMID: 35642833

Mills, A., Astle, K., & Frazier, C. (2022). "affirming" journey: Narrative review and practice considerations on gender-affirming care. *Journal of the American College of Clinical Pharmacy: JAACP*, *5*(7), 697–706. DOI: 10.1002/jac5.1621

Moustakli, E., & Tsonis, O. (2023). Exploring hormone therapy effects on reproduction and health in transgender individuals. *Medicina*, *59*(12), 2094. DOI: 10.3390/medicina59122094 PMID: 38138197

Nolan, I., Blasdel, G., Dubin, S., Goetz, T., Greene, R., & Morrison, S. (2020). The current state of transgender medical education in the United States and Canada: Update to a scoping review. *Journal of Medical Education and Curricular Development*, *7*. Advance online publication. DOI: 10.1177/2382120520934813 PMID: 32637641

Puckett, J., Tornello, S., Mustanski, B., & Newcomb, M. (2022). Gender variations, generational effects, and mental health of transgender people about timing and status of gender identity milestones. *Psychology of Sexual Orientation and Gender Diversity*, *9*(2), 165–178. DOI: 10.1037/sgd0000391 PMID: 35983565

Reisner, S., Bradford, J., Hopwood, R., González, A., Makadon, H., Todisco, D., & Mayer, K. (2015). Comprehensive transgender healthcare: The gender affirming clinical and public health model of Fenway health. *Journal of Urban Health*, *92*(3), 584–592. DOI: 10.1007/s11524-015-9947-2 PMID: 25779756

Restar, A., Jin, H., Jarrett, B. A., Adamson, T., Baral, S., Howell, S., & Beckham, S. W. (2021). Characterizing the impact of COVID-19 environment on mental health, gender-affirming services, and socioeconomic loss in a global sample of transgender and non-binary people: A structural equation modeling. *BMJ Global Health*, *6*(3), e004424. DOI: 10.1136/bmjgh-2020-004424 PMID: 33753401

Rouse, M.Jr. (2023). Promoting gender-affirming care: Challenging conflation and embracing complexity. *Policy Insights from the Behavioral and Brain Sciences*, *10*(2), 186–192. DOI: 10.1177/23727322231197148

Seelman, K., Colón-Diaz, M., LeCroix, R., Xavier-Brier, M., & Kattari, L. (2017). Transgender noninclusive healthcare and delaying care because of fear: Connections to general health and mental health among transgender adults. *Transgender Health*, *2*(1), 17–28. DOI: 10.1089/trgh.2016.0024 PMID: 28861545

Sengupta, T., Soni, T., Bolock, A. M., Heisey, S. A., Kuchinski, E. C., Piper, B. J., Joyce, J. M., & Carbe, C. J. (2023). Knowledge, attitudes, and beliefs of medical students toward transgender healthcare: A community-driven initiative. *Cureus*. Advance online publication. DOI: 10.7759/cureus.49992 PMID: 38058529

Shin, S. J., Kumar, A., & Safer, J. D. (2022). Gender-Affirming Surgery: Perioperative Medical Care. Endocrine practice. *Endocrine Practice*, *28*(4), 420–424. DOI: 10.1016/j.eprac.2022.02.007 PMID: 35217191

Silva, K., Nauman, C., Tebbe, E., & Parent, M. (2022). Policy attitudes toward adolescents transitioning gender. *Journal of Counseling Psychology*, *69*(4), 403–415. DOI: 10.1037/cou0000601 PMID: 34968097

Sloan, S., & Benson, J. J. (2021). Toward a conceptual model for successful transgender aging. *Qualitative Social Work: Research and Practice*, *21*(2), 455–471. DOI: 10.1177/1473325021994666

Stroumsa, D., Shires, D., Richardson, C., Jaffee, K., & Woodford, M. (2019). Transphobia rather than education predicts provider knowledge of transgender health care. *Medical Education*, *53*(4), 398–407. DOI: 10.1111/medu.13796 PMID: 30666699

Tordoff, D. M., Wanta, J. W., Collin, A., Stepney, C., Inwards-Breland, D. J., & Ahrens, K. (2022). Mental Health Outcomes in Transgender and Nonbinary Youths Receiving Gender-Affirming Care. *JAMA Network Open*, *5*(2), e220978. DOI: 10.1001/jamanetworkopen.2022.0978 PMID: 35212746

Vaccaro, C., Karageuzian, S. A., & McFadden, E. (2023). The importance of safely prescribing hormones in the transgender community. *Cureus*. Advance online publication. DOI: 10.7759/cureus.44639 PMID: 37799231

Valentine, S. E., Shipherd, J. C., Smith, A. M., & Kauth, M. R. (2021). Improving affirming care for sexual and gender minority veterans. *Psychological Services*, *18*(2), 205–215. DOI: 10.1037/ser0000378 PMID: 31343189

Weingartner, L., Noonan, E. J., Bohnert, C., Potter, J., Shaw, M. A., & Holthouser, A. (2022). Gender-Affirming Care With Transgender and Genderqueer Patients: A Standardized Patient Case. *MedEdPORTAL: the Journal of Teaching and Learning Resources*, *18*, 11249. DOI: 10.15766/mep_2374-8265.11249 PMID: 35664552

WPATH (World Professional Association for Transgender Health). (2022). Standards of Care for the Health of Transgender and Gender Diverse People, Version 8. https://www.wpath.org/soc8

Chapter 8
Intercultural Communication:
An Effective Strategy for the Patient Physician Relationship

S. Srinivasan
https://orcid.org/0009-0002-0179-9849
Department of Humanities and Social Sciences, Graphic Era University, Dehradun, India

R. Vallipriya
https://orcid.org/0009-0008-6692-603X
Department of Physical Science, Institute of Education, India & Tamil Nadu Teacher Education University, Trichy, India

ABSTRACT

The physician-patient relationship (PPR) is a critical element in medical ethics, built on mutual respect, trust, and knowledge. It ensures that physicians meet patient needs, including providing care and education on diagnoses and treatments while creating a working relationship that allows patients to be centered in their care. Intercultural communication is essential for understanding patient perspectives and building trust. However, physician burnout and biases can negatively affect care. This chapter highlights the importance of utilizing intercultural communication to strengthen the physician-patient relationship allowing for better care and health outcomes.

DOI: 10.4018/979-8-3693-3683-0.ch008

INTRODUCTION

The World Medical Association (WMA), in its 2020 Declaration of Cordoba, highlights the significance of the patient-physician relationship. This relationship emphasizes respect for patients' beliefs and autonomy, fostering improved health and well-being. Effective clinical relationships rely on open, honest communication and mutual trust between patients and physicians (Yedidia, 2017). Physicians must provide compassionate, private, confidential, and reliable care, while patients are encouraged to listen and trust their physicians for guidance. These elements collectively enhance the quality of care and health outcomes (Katz, 2002; Murray & McCrone, 2019).

The physician-patient relationship (PPR) is a crucial aspect of medical practice. It encompasses two key elements: knowledge and loyalty. The knowledge to refer to the doctor and patient understanding can make the patient more familiar with their doctor. The loyalty is the patient's understanding of the doctor as an empathetic support for their well-being. PPR can be established by the physician and patient based on their medical needs on a priority basis in various ways, such as regular check-ups, proper diagnosis, and treatment (Harelie et al., 2007).This relationship provides the physician and patient with mutual respect, which can help achieve positive health outcomes and successful treatment results.

The physician-patient relationship (PPR) mainly concentrates on high-quality healthcare and is built on a mutual relationship or understanding, empathy, trust, and confidentiality (Teutsch, 2003). The physician must respect their patient's dignity, safety, and health, which can enhance open communication to improve diagnosis, treatment, and adherence (Cabana et al., 2014). The PPR highlights the physician-patient connection and their trust, which can enable the patient to feel safe and supported. This understanding can address their financial constraints, which may be inadequate for family care (Srinivasan, 2023).

The physician-patient asymmetrical relationship holds due to their medical knowledge. The asymmetry fosters trust. It allows the patient to rely on the physician for truthful information, which can improve the quality of care and support (Pellegrini, 2017; Tucker et al., 2016). Distrust or mistrust arises, affecting the physician-patient collaboration. The physician provides attention and concentration, emphasizing the importance of actively listening to and motivating the patient in a positive way. This can enhance the patient's concern and improve successful outcomes (Nie et al., 2018).

The study revealed that patient-centric care can enhance the relationship between the physician, healthcare workers, and patients. It highlights the need to address effective policies to improve the PPR (Srinivasan et al., 2025). A strong correlation exists between trust and improved health outcomes, including patient satisfaction and treatment adherence (Birkhäuer et al., 2017). A well-maintained PPR ensures comprehensive care, from diagnosis to post-treatment follow-up, fostering better health outcomes and satisfaction (Beckman et al., 1994; Manary et al., 2013; Fuertes et al., 2017; Olaisen et al., 2020).

Four Models of Physician- Patient Relationships

Paternalistic Model

In the parental model (Burke, 1980) or the priestly type of model (Veatch, 1972) physicians provide the appropriate medical treatment for the patient by objectively determining the best treatment (Stone, 1976). The tension between patient autonomy and their well-being, along with the concern for options regarding their health, places the physician's main emphasis on outcomes. The physician acts as the patient's guardian to support and provide a concerned opinion through implementing the best option for the patient.

The Informative Model

The informative model can be called the scientific model (Burke, 1980), the engineering model (Veatch, 1972), or the consumer model. This model's main objective is to provide the physician and patient with relevant information regarding the aspects of medical intervention so that he or she can address the physician in selecting the intervention. The informative model supports a clear distinction between facts and values and assumes the patient lacks facts and are unaware of their conditions.

The Interpretive Model

The third model is the interpretive model which facilitates a physician-patient interaction to elucidate the patient's values and actual wants where the patient can then select available and affordable medical intervention support. The physician provides the patient with information about the nature of conditions and the risk and benefits of possible interventions. According to this model, patient values are not fixed and are unknown. The physician's role is to support the patient in identifying their goals and aspirations of care which can ultimately decide the course of action that best fits the patients' needs.

The Deliberative Model

The deliberative model aims to enhance the interaction between the physician and the patient to help the patient determine their needs. Physicians provide options while patients discusses their known health values and the decision is made collaboratively. This model can enhance patient autonomy as the physician acts as a friend or teacher, helping the patient develop and refine their values while collaborating on the best course of action for treatment.

The Ideal Physician and Patient Relationship

As the physician-patient relationship plays a critical role in health care; it impacts patient outcomes and their satisfaction. Trust and confidence among patients and physicians are essential for feeling comfortable with information and medical advice. Trust and respect then improve communication.

Aligned with the interpretive and deliberative models, good communication is essential for physicians and patients. It actively encourages patients and addresses their concerns and preferences. It can enhance medical care, allowing patients to share appropriate information with practitioners, which can facilitate direct decision-making for health. The mutual relationship ensures confidentiality and collaboration, which can achieve the best possible health outcomes in understanding patient needs, navigating their challenges, collaborating with the physician, and contributing to the overall care and support for patients (Ward, 2018).

The following are benefits of an enriching Physician- Patient Relationship:

- **Enhanced Patient Satisfaction**: To provide the patient with a feeling of comfort and respect enhances the ability to deliver positive healthcare experiences.
- **Better Treatment Adherence**: Patients are more likely to follow regular treatment and prescribed medical conditions when they trust and feel a stronger connection with their physicians.
- **Emotional Support**: Emotional support plays a vital role as the physician provides reassurance and empathy. It can reduce stress and anxiety for patients during diagnosis and treatment.
- **Ethical and Patient-Centered Care**: The patient-centered care approach ensures patient respect, provides confidentiality, and ensures informed consent.
- **Improved Health Outcomes**: The strong relationship between the physician and patient can enhance recovery rates, improve health outcomes, and promote the overall well-being of patients.

- **Shared Decision-Making**: The collaboration between physician and patient can influence preferences in care and decision-making, leading to personalized and effective treatment plans.

The literature emphasizes the relationship between physicians and patients; it includes the importance and challenges, as well as strategies for improvement.

Challenges in the Physician and Patient Relationship

The physician and the patient may have differences in their language and cultural expression that create challenges for the physician-patient relationship. It is stated that fear and anxiety arise in patients due to physicians inability to communicate effectively. This can sometimes be solely due to cultural differences.

It is essential for healthcare settings to understand these cultural differences, as they can influence the quality of care and the outcomes for patients. The intercultural aspect can emphasize that physicians should be aware of patients' values, beliefs, and expectations to provide proper health, illness, and treatment care. Cultural factors such as language, communication style, religious beliefs, and traditions can support the patient's conditions and facilitate treatment for patients who are willing to accept and adhere to medical advice. Physicians can understand patients' cultural differences and provide better care for them. This can lead to more effective communication and respectful care for both parties. Overcoming cultural barriers can reduce biases and provide treatment plans to improve patient satisfaction, thereby reducing health disparities among patients. The relationship involves continuous learning to provide sensitivity to cultural norms and leads to empathetic, inclusive healthcare practices.

Likewise, physicians can find it challenging to balance patient autonomy. Culturally this may vary as some cultural expectations align with the paternalistic and informative models. However, this can be particularly of concern when patients make choices that contradict physician's medical advice. For example, if a patient has concerns about starting treatment for life satisfaction and don't feel heard, this can affect their decision-making regarding additional treatment and sometimes lead to a lack of care (Carrese, 2006).

Additionally, a lack of clear explanations on both sides can negatively affect the quality of interaction (Lewis, 1994). Without this, patients may not feel as though they can make reasonable health care decisions which will impact the physician-patient relationship. There are many patients who complain to the doctors about poor communication rather than a lack of medical knowledge. It can create a breakdown among healthcare providers, affecting their medical practice and leading to medical errors (San & Arranz, 2023).

Keys to Improved Communication Within the Physician-Patient Relationships

Listening, Language, and Word Choice

Effective communication involves the practitioner using clear and simple language to explain appropriate medical terms, diagnosis, and treatment. This can encourage patients to ask questions and clarify their doubts. This also provides space that allows patients to talk and participate in active listening without any interruptions, which can show genuine interest in their concerns. Best practices include-

- **Be Aware of Non-Verbals**: The physician uses their body language, posture, gestures, and facial expressions to support, enhance, and guide the patient by managing spatial distance.
- **Be Aware of Tone:** The physician must use appropriate tone, pitch, pacing, and volume in their voice so that the patient can easily understand them.
- **Be Clear:** To provide information that is accurate, clear, and concise, use simple language that is easy for patients to understand.
- **Use Active Listening:** The physician must encourage the patient to ask questions and avoid interrupting them. Likewise, using methods like describing what was heard can help to clarify that what was intended has been understood.

Empathy, Compassion, and Trust

By expressing validation for the patient's feelings and experiences, the practitioners acknowledge the patient's needs. This can further build trust. Likewise, maintaining patient confidentiality can provide a space for patients to be transparent with their clinicians and get the care they need. This extends so areas of identity that may carry shame or stigma like socioeconomic status. With intercultural communication, physicians can understand patients' family life, economic situation, and coping mechanisms to support patients in providing comprehensive treatment that is easily accessible.

- **Be Nonjudgemental**: To avoid blaming the patient, it is important to maintain a non-judgmental attitude, refraining from judging or stigmatizing the patient. Respectful consideration of the patient's preferences and their needs should be addressed.
- **Be Attentive:** The patient feels respected during the visit and expectations are appropriately managed.

- **Be Discrete:** The physician must maintain the patient's confidentiality and privacy; there is no need to share their personal information.
- **Foster Respectful Interactions:** Ensure all healthcare workers treat patients with kindness and respect, especially those already dealing with physical and mental stress.

Ethical Behavior, Professionalism, and Cultural Sensitivity

Respecting the patient's identity, cultural beliefs, and religious aspects while avoiding biases and assumptions can further reinforce the clinicians goal to ensure patients are well taken care of. When practitioners follow professional ethical standards, such as respecting autonomy, honesty and integrity, just care, this allows for the patients' preferences and values, to be centered in interactions. One example is to use SMART goals created with patients. Patients' choices and values are respected while their care plan reflects their health needs. Their wellbeing becomes primary in interactions.

- **Be Inclusive:** The patient must be involved in the decision-making process, encouraging them to think and make their own decisions.
- **Be Transparent:** The physician must be transparent about the risks to the patients and inform them of the potential challenges.
- **Be Patient:** The physician must give the patient enough time and avoid making them feel ashamed if they make a mistake or repeat something.
- **Provide Patient-Centered Care:** PCC can focus on the patient's social and cultural aspects, addressing the patient's specific needs in an effective way.
- **Promote Advocacy and Support:** To advocate for patient support and provide nutritional and psychological support, it can improve the health outcomes and lead to success.
- **Training on Cultural Humility:** Healthcare providers need training to improve cultural humility, which can enhance intercultural communication, build trust, and improve patient outcomes.

The following ways to improve the cases can examine best practices to improve physicians, bridging cultural aspects to enhance intercultural communication.

CASES

Case 1. Resilience and Advocacy: Building Physician-Patient Trust in TB Care

Learning Objectives

1. To identify patient values and emotions during medical treatment
2. To analyze communication style to cultivate physician-patient relationship
3. To explore cultural considerations of communication in the physician-patient relationship

Case Aim: This case aims to highlight the transformative power of resilience, advocacy, and physician-patient relationships in overcoming health and social challenges. With intercultural communication, patients can feel empowered and supported on their health journey and overcome stigma and isolation.

Mrs. Meena (name changed), is 53 years old. She is a widow and has two children—one daughter and one son. Her son is pursuing a degree in orthopaedics, and her daughter was recently married. When her children were young, her husband passed away, and she was diagnosed with HIV. She has had Tuberculosis (TB) three times. The first time she was diagnosed with TB, she was in disbelief and couldn't accept the diagnosis.

Initially, she visited a private clinic where the physician advised her to undergo a sputum test, which came back positive. The private physician referred her to a government primary health centre (PHC). At the government hospital, the doctor started her treatment immediately. Though the physician was supportive, the behavior of the health staff was harsh, making her feel embarrassed. Over time, as she continued visiting the PHC for fixed dosage combination (FDC) treatments, she built a rapport with the health staff, which became more supportive.

In the beginning, even the physician scolded her for not coming on time for diagnosis, which made her feel worried. However, she became conscious of her health, regularly ate nutritional and protein-rich food, and received a monthly Rs. 500 stipend under the Nikshay Poshan Yojana scheme, though it often arrived late. Despite these challenges, she successfully completed the six-month treatment. During this period, her family avoided her, and she faced stigma, but she managed to overcome these issues.

Her family members and relatives believed she was going to die and even started planning to divide her property. Despite this, she found the courage to complete the treatment successfully. She experienced significant weight loss, a persistent cough, and evening fevers every day. Her family provided her with separate food and utensils, further isolating her. Health workers provided family counselling, but her family members did not change their behavior. However, after she completed the treatment, everyone in her family and her relatives were shocked by her recovery. They were surprised at how she had beaten TB.

She explained that she courageously took her medication regularly, ate well, and persevered despite frequent vomiting and an inability to eat. After her recovery, the physician and health workers helped her find employment. She joined a non-governmental organization (NGO) as a community volunteer.

Meena now has nearly 20 years of experience in community engagement. Her main role and responsibility is to identify highly symptomatic patients and refer them to nearby PHCs or general hospitals. She also creates awareness among vulnerable communities and organizes sensitization events in schools, colleges, and public gatherings. She supports health camps and mobile clinics in identifying symptomatic patients, and the health staff are very appreciative of her work. She feels fulfilled serving in a role similar to that of a health worker, and even the physician encourages her when she refers patients.

With the support of local leaders, she organized nutritional support events for TB patients in treatment. During these events, physicians provided awareness about hygiene, treatment protocols, and best practices. She shares her own story with affected communities, which motivates patients to continue treatment. Her storytelling has impressed the physicians as well.

She participates in all events, including active case finding, TB surveillance, health camps, and patient-provider meetings. Eventually, she became recognized as a "TB Champion." The District TB Officer (DTO) referred to her as an "iron lady" for overcoming TB three times, and her story has inspired many. Now, she works successfully as a TB Champion.

The relationship between a patient and physician, especially when dealing with affected communities from the initial stage, is crucial. It is important to respect the patient's feelings and provide emotional support. Physicians and health workers must understand the real-time situation and act as mentors, offering comprehensive support. This helps patients feel more supported and alleviates their emotional distress.

Case Questions

1. How Can a Physician Establish a Supportive Relationship With a Patient Like Mrs. Meena, Who Initially Feels Embarrassed or Stigmatized by the Healthcare System? What Specific Actions Can a Physician Take to Foster Trust and Empathy in Such Cases?

- The physician should pay attention to her concerns, prioritize patient care, and create an empathetic / non-judgmental atmosphere. Intercultural communication can provide clear education to enhance her decision-making while respecting her cultural aspects, thereby fostering better outcomes. The physician should also emphasize consistent, ongoing support to improve their bond further. This can reduce the patient's feelings of stigma and improve their overall health care experience.

2. How Can Healthcare Providers Demonstrate Cultural Humility When Treating a Patient Like Mrs. Meena, Who May Be Facing Cultural and Social Challenges in Addition to Her Medical Issues? How Can Understanding Her Cultural Background Enhance the Care Process?

- Healthcare workers must acknowledge and respect Mrs. Meena's beliefs, values, and priorities. This can improve her ability to communicate social and cultural challenges / barriers to care. This provides her with the necessary support to reduce those barriers, and leads to effective treatment through therapeutic relationships. This can improve trust and support, leading to successful health outcomes.

3. What Role Does Advocacy Play in Mrs. Meena's Journey to Recovery? How Can Healthcare Professionals Support Their Patients Beyond Just Providing Medical Care, Especially When Dealing With the Stigma Associated With Diseases Like TB and HIV?

- Advocacy can reduce stigma, improve rights, and create awareness programs in the community. Healthcare professionals hear what patients actually need and can bridge the disconnect between organizations, policy makers, leadership and patient experiences. Further, addressing stigma within the community can empower patients with stigmatized diagnoses in their healthcare journey, foster a supportive environment, and improve their psychological well-being and overall health recovery.

4. Mrs. Meena's Resilience in Facing Multiple TB Diagnoses and Stigma Is a Key Aspect of Her Recovery. What Factors Contribute to a Patient's Resilience, and How Can Healthcare Providers Help Cultivate These Factors In Their Patients?

- When the patient has a strong support system, it can improve their coping strategies, boost their confidence, and enhance their hope. Healthcare workers must provide emotional support to the patient and help facilitate expanding patient's support network. This requires understanding of patient's social, religious, and cultural dynamics, encouraging inclusion of social supports and resources, and potentially engaging empathetic discussion of patient's more negative healthcare experiences. This can help build rapport with the patient, improve patient empowerment, and build resilience.

5. How Can Social Support Systems Be Integrated Into Mrs. Meena's Treatment Plan to Help Her Overcome Isolation and Stigma?

- Mrs. Meena's care team should function as an extension of her support network. This includes integrating family involvement, possible involvement in health support groups, community health workers/ community volunteers, and TB Champions as she deems appropriate to support her in reaching recovery.

6. How Important Is Patient Education in Mrs. Meena's Case, particularly Regarding Treatment Adherence and Self-Care Practices? What Strategies Can Be Employed to Ensure That Patients Understand the Importance of Completing Their Treatment Regimen, Even in the Face of Stigma and Personal Challenges?

- Education can enhance their overall patient care. Discussing the importance of completing treatment and dangers of treatment interruptions, especially in the case of TB, may be sufficient to achieve treatment adherence and successful outcomes. However, when potential or actual treatment non-adherence occurs, non-judgmental approaches are crucial to rectify the situation. Determining root cause issues that can be resolved or alternative options can be determined to achieve successful outcomes. Healthcare workers should provide psychological support to ensure the patient receives long-term support for treatment adherence, improve non-compliance, and reduce stigma while overcoming challenges.

7. How Does Stigma Impact Healthcare Outcomes, Particularly for Patients Dealing With Conditions Like TB and HIV? What Steps Can Healthcare Providers Take to Reduce Stigma and Promote Health Equity for Marginalized Patients Like Mrs. Meena?

- Those with stigmatized conditions may be discouraged from seeking treatment, leading to delayed diagnosis and poor treatment adherence. This can result in mental health challenges and a decrease in overall well-being. Healthcare workers should support patients, educate both patients and the general public to reduce stigma, and provide non-judgmental support. This can help to reduce misconceptions from others, advocate for policy changes, and enhance patient care at the systemic level.

Maintaining cultural humility and respect for the patient can improve communication and open avenues for support. Providing support for the patient and attempting to empower the community can reduce some of the stigma can improve health equity for the current patient and future patients.

8. Mrs. Meena's Relationship With the Healthcare Staff Improved Over Time. How Can Healthcare Systems Implement Practices That Ensure Staff Are Sensitive to the Emotional and Psychological Needs of Patients, Especially Those Facing Chronic Illnesses and Stigma?

- The health system should provide regular training for healthcare workers and community volunteers to implement cultural support initiatives, such as promoting empathy, reducing stigma, and creating more effective awareness programs. Processes to reduce healthcare staff burnout would also improve chronic health management, since studies have consistently show negative correlations between burnout and patient outcomes (Garcia, 2019). These interventions can improve the patient's mental health through counseling and stress management. More patient-centered care promotes health equity and improved patient emotional well-being.

9. How Can Physicians and Healthcare Staff Balance Reacting to Patient's Values Surrounding Treatment Not Matching the Expectations of Health Care Workers (e.g., Adherence to Treatment Schedules) With Empathy, Especially When Patients Like Mrs. Meena Are Struggling With the Emotional Burden of Their Illness and the Stigma Attached to It?

- It is important to maintain regular follow up appointments to continue to foster the communication with patients. When patients are unable to continue to or choose not to participate in treatment, physicians and healthcare staff should first listen to patients needs and wants pertaining to continuing treatment. If there are barriers, they should help patients like Mrs. Meena receive the proper resources and/or support to maintain treatment adherence. This may be limited to emotional support and encouragement, or may need to be as expansive as introduction of new services/resources and treatment plan augmentations.

Rather than scolding or disciplining patients for treatment non-adherence, teams must remember that patients have autonomy, even when it doesn't align with the team's values. It is important to maintain open communication and psychological support for patients. When considering treating communicable diseases like TB or HIV, the ethical concerns surrounding patient autonomy and infection control are valid. There may be legal limitations to patients refusing treatment and should be examined based upon each case.

10. Mrs. Meena Eventually Became a TB Champion, Advocating for Others in Marginalized Communities. How Can Physicians and Healthcare Professionals Encourage Patients to Become Advocates for Others, and How Might This Contribute to the Overall Health of the Community?

- Healthcare professionals and physicians can empower patients by providing support through knowledge, emotional support, and offering opportunities to engage with community health services. It can encourage patients like Mrs. Meena to share her experience with the affected TB community. This can reduce stigma, raise awareness, and inspire others through her story. Often this improves patient confidence, which increases their adherence to regular medication and leads to a successful treatment outcome.

Case Discussion

The case study highlights the journey of Mrs. Meena's life, covering multiple aspects of TB diagnosis, her resilience in overcoming adversity, and her transformation into a community advocate. It underscores the critical role of improving physician-patient communication, including cultural aspects of care, to achieve positive health outcomes. The role of intercultural communication is evident from the time Mrs. Meena initially visited health services, where physician scolding caused her emotional distress as she has faced stigma from both her community and family.

One can see that in providing support and enhancing rapport-building to improve her relationship with the healthcare team. Even then there were still challenges to overcome. The health workers provided proper counseling and support to address the family's attitude, but it did not lead to a change in their approach towards her recovery. Likewise, the financial support through the Nikshay Poshan Yojana provided nutritional assistance, which was beneficial for her recovery. However, there were times when the support was not received on time, posing challenges in managing her needs. Being able to communicate these types of barriers are key to patient recovery.

Even though Mrs. Meena faced stigma and isolation, she was able to complete her treatment and her story has inspired others. We see that she currently provides awareness support in the community, patient referral support, and assistance with nutritional services. This demonstrates how the positive impact of communication improved her experience and made a greater contribution to society.

Case 2. Enhancing TB Care Through Physician-Patient Understanding: A Case of Mrs. Kalaiselvi

Learning Objectives

1. Utilize intercultural communication strategies to build rapport with patients
2. Analyze the relationship between physicians and patients
3. Identify the biases and social stigma noted in experiences

Case Aim: The case study aims to explore the physician-patient relationship and how viable understanding, coupled with culturally appropriate care, can enhance patient outcomes and experiences.

Mrs. Kalaiselvi is a 48-year-old woman who completed her 10th grade education. Her husband works as an electrician and takes on microphone set fitting jobs in villages. The family's experience with TB started when her husband was diagnosed with MDR-TB and began treatment. During a medical camp visit for her husband's check-up, Mrs. Kalaiselvi's health status was noticed by the District TB Officer (DTO), who suspected she might also have TB due to her slim and underweight appearance.

Despite initially being misdiagnosed at private hospitals, the DTO's intervention led to a proper X-ray and clinical confirmation of her TB. Both she and her husband underwent treatment simultaneously and successfully completed it, receiving negative final results.

Initially, Mrs. Kalaiselvi sought help from private hospitals, where her symptoms were dismissed, and she was told she did not have TB. This misdiagnosis delayed her treatment and heightened her suffering. At the medical camp, the DTO's recommendation for an X-ray and subsequent CBNAAT test led to immediate treatment initiation. However, the process was not smooth; she faced difficulties such as being unable to produce sputum and experiencing scolding and abusive language from healthcare workers when seeking assistance.

Mrs. Kalaiselvi faced significant stigma from her family and community. Her family members hesitated to interact with her after her diagnosis. Additionally, during the COVID-19 pandemic, many people assumed her symptoms were related to COVID-19, further isolating her. Her husband also faced blame from others when she went to collect her medications, which added to her feelings of embarrassment and mental stress.

Throughout her treatment, the Senior Treatment Supervisor provided regular follow-ups and ensured she received her medication on time. Both she and her husband were given nutritional support, including milk, eggs, and weekly non-vegetarian meals, which were helpful though insufficient. After completing her treatment, Mrs. Kalaiselvi joined an NGO as a community volunteer, where she began supporting other TB patients and advocating for better healthcare practices.

Case Questions

1. How Important Was the District TB Officer's (DTO) Intervention in Mrs. Kalaiselvi's Diagnosis? What Are the Challenges of Diagnosing Conditions in Individuals Who Have Atypical Symptoms?

- If there is question of the diagnosis or patient is not responding to treatment as expected, then additional evaluation is often warranted. Wrong diagnoses can cause delays in care and increased suffering for patients. Furthermore, it can decrease trust between patient and the healthcare system as a whole. This can be reduced by open conversation with patients on the concerns/delay and steps to mitigate the situation going forward.

Medicine is often taught using a set of symptoms or an disease presentation that fits an expectation. However patients don't always fit this norm. Biases, stereotypes, and stigma play a large part in delaying diagnosis with patients deviate from what is expected. Revisiting the differential diagnosis while removing any preconceived notions can assist health care teams in avoiding biases that impact diagnosis.

2. How Can Healthcare Workers Use Communication to Increase Awareness About Stigmatized Conditions, Especially in Communities Where Access to Healthcare May Be Limited? What Strategies Can Be Employed to Educate Families About Prevention and Treatment?

- Healthcare workers can increase awareness about stigma at the community level. They can conduct programs in local / multiple languages and leverage community leaders to share accurate information. Awareness programs on local TV, radio, community centers, social media, posters, pamphlets, and signage wall paintings in public spaces can help reduce stigma and educate populations. Prevention and treatment programs that integrate community spaces and community members can reach people where health care may be limited.

3. How Might Socioeconomic Factors, Such as Occupation and Income, Influence the Likelihood of Contracting Stigmatized Conditions Like TB and the Ability to Access Proper Treatment? How Can Health Care Workers Better Communicate These Risks to Patients Without Stigmatizing Them.

- Lower socio-economic conditions, high-risk occupations, and living in high-density areas will make people more susceptible to various chronic diseases. This is especially true for tuberculosis. If the affected people are provided with immediate medical treatment, it can reduce the TB barriers and improve healthcare outcomes.

4. What Communication Factors Contribute to Treatment Adherence? Which Factors Create Barriers? What Do You Feel Is the Most Difficult in Balancing This?

- Open, non-judgmental, and empahetic communication provide support for better treatment adherence. However, when patients feel judged, scoleded, or unheard this can strain their relationship with medicine and could potentially create barriers for patients to seek care, even in the future. Use this as an opportunity to reflect on your beliefs surrounding treating patients. Some questions to ask yourself may include- How will I respond when patients cannot or do not wish to follow the treatment plan? What beliefs of mine will be challenged in these scenarios?

5. Considering Mrs. Kalaiselvi and Her Husband Live in a Rural Setting, What Unique Challenges Do Rural Populations Face in Accessing Timely Culturally Relevant Care? How Can Healthcare Systems Better Serve These Communities?

- Access to care is often very different in rural settings. The geographical location of health care settings often leaves rural communities more isolated. Typically, there are fewer health care facilities, less or no ancillary clinical services (laboratory, imaging, surgical, etc.), access to health professionals or health professionals with advanced training may be impaired, and specialty providers may not be available or are only available with longer commutes. Tertiary services for more severe cases are even further removed in rural settings. These barriers can delay care. Sociocultural factors may further limit the ability to travel to get to the additional care settings when needed. Healthcare workers can provide support through mobile health services, telemedicine, and training for healthcare workers in these areas. Policy level changes can ensure proper health facilities in these communities remain or are built.

6. How Might Mrs. Kalaiselvi's Cultural Background, Education Level, and Family Dynamics Influence Her Approach to Healthcare? How Can Healthcare Providers Be More Sensitive to These Factors When Treating Patients in Similar Situations?

- Mrs. Kalaiselvi's social and cultural background, along with her understanding of the goals of treatment shape her approach to care. In these situations, it is important for healthcare workers to provide additional support to ensure proper treatment is reached. Steps should also be taken to ensure these are respecting patient's cultural beliefs and needs. The healthcare professional may need to explain clinical information in different ways and pause discussion to ensure patient is understanding the clinical information present.

Case Discussion

The case study of Mrs. Kalaiselvi underscores the significance of anti-oppressive healthcare practices, cultural humility, and effective advocacy in addressing systemic barriers and social stigma faced by TB patients. Her journey highlights the transformative impact of compassionate care, respectful physician-patient relationships, and culturally sensitive communication on improving health outcomes and restoring patient dignity. Mrs. Kalaiselvi's case also highlights the importance of anti-oppressive practices in healthcare. Her initial encounters with dismissive private healthcare providers and the disrespect she faced at the PHC underscore the need for healthcare workers to address power dynamics and provide compassionate care. The DTO can ensure improved health outcomes and provide instructions without any barriers to ensure proper, timely diagnosis and real-time treatment for affected patients.

Healthcare workers provide proper care and support for patients, respecting their dignity and self-respect to improve their social and cultural contexts. Mrs. Kalaiselvi's past experience reflects that they lacked empathy and had poor communication from the healthcare workers, which deterred the patients from seeking care. The DTO has provided an attitude for the patient that can improve successful positive treatment outcomes. Mrs. Kalaiselvi's story emphasizes the need for the healthcare system to adopt anti-oppressive practices to improve patient advocacy and provide cultural care and support. This will not only improve the successful health outcome, but it can also enhance dignity and increase trust, which supports the healthcare process.

CONCLUSION

The physician-patient relationship plays a vital role in improving healthcare, which can lead to better patient satisfaction, meeting their service and support needs. Using intercultural communication can improve treatment adherence and overall health outcomes through centering care to patients needs. This fosters stronger bonds and trust with health care teams.

The cases above highlight the benefits of practicing the best practices of intercultural communication as well as the risks of poor communication. Both patients benefitted when their specific needs were incorporated in their care plans. Likewise, both patients were harmed by poor communication by health care workers. When patients feel supported by team members care can tailored to meet patients where they are and overcome barriers that contribute to health disparities.

REFERENCES

Beckman, H. B., Markakis, K. M., Suchman, A. L., & Frankel, R. M. (1994). The doctor-patient relationship and malpractice: Lessons from plaintiff depositions. *Archives of Internal Medicine, 154*(12), 1365–1370. DOI: 10.1001/archinte.1994.00420120093010 PMID: 8002688

Birkhäuer, J., Gaab, J., Kossowsky, J., Hasler, S., Krummenacher, P., Werner, C., & Gerger, H. (2017). Trust in the health care professional and health outcome: A meta-analysis. *PLoS One, 12*(2), e0170988. DOI: 10.1371/journal.pone.0170988 PMID: 28170443

Burke, G. (1980). Ethics and medical decision-making. *Primary Care, 7*(4), 615–624. DOI: 10.1016/S0095-4543(21)01416-0 PMID: 6908085

Cabana, M. D., Slish, K. K., Evans, D., Mellins, R. B., Brown, R. W., Lin, X., Kaciroti, N., & Clark, N. M. (2014). Impact of physician asthma care education on patient outcomes. *Health Education & Behavior, 41*(5), 509–517. DOI: 10.1177/1090198114547510 PMID: 25270176

Carrese, J. A. (2006). Refusal of care: patients' well-being and physicians' ethical obligations:"but doctor, I want to go home". *Journal of the American Medical Association, 296*(6), 691–695. DOI: 10.1001/jama.296.6.691 PMID: 16896112

Fuertes, J. N., Toporovsky, A., Reyes, M., & Osborne, J. B. (2017). The physician-patient working alliance: Theory, research, and future possibilities. *Patient Education and Counseling, 100*(4), 610–615. DOI: 10.1016/j.pec.2016.10.018 PMID: 27773600

Garcia, C. L., Abreu, L. C., Ramos, J. L. S., Castro, C. F. D., Smiderle, F. R. N., Santos, J. A. D., & Bezerra, I. M. P. (2019). Influence of Burnout on Patient Safety: Systematic Review and Meta-Analysis. *Medicina (Kaunas, Lithuania), 55*(9), 553. DOI: 10.3390/medicina55090553 PMID: 31480365

Hareli, S., Karnieli-Miller, O., Hermoni, D., & Eidelman, S. (2007). Factors in the doctor–patient relationship that accentuate physicians' hurt feelings when patients terminate the relationship with them. *Patient Education and Counseling, 67*(1-2), 169–175. DOI: 10.1016/j.pec.2007.03.010 PMID: 17448620

Katz, J. (2002). *The silent world of doctor and patient*. Jhu Press. https://www.google.co.in/books/edition/The_Silent_World_of_Doctor_and_Patient/x1DNCNNX8AIC?hl=en&gbpv=1&dq=Patients+can+listen+to+physicians+provide+guidance+and+truest+for+the+obligations+it+is+outcome+assessment+in+the+better+health+conditions.&pg=PR9&printsec=frontcover

Lewis, J. R. (1994). Patient views on quality care in general practice: Literature review. *Social Science & Medicine*, *39*(5), 655–670. DOI: 10.1016/0277-9536(94)90022-1 PMID: 7973865

Manary, M. P., Boulding, W., Staelin, R., & Glickman, S. W. (2013). The patient experience and health outcomes. *The New England Journal of Medicine*, *368*(3), 201–203. DOI: 10.1056/NEJMp1211775 PMID: 23268647

Murray, B., & McCrone, S. (2015). An integrative review of promoting trust in the patient–primary care provider relationship. *Journal of Advanced Nursing*, *71*(1), 3–23. DOI: 10.1111/jan.12502 PMID: 25113235

Nie, J. B., Cheng, Y., Zou, X., Gong, N., Tucker, J. D., Wong, B., & Kleinman, A. (2018). The vicious circle of patient–physician mistrust in China: Health professionals' perspectives, institutional conflict of interest, and building trust through medical professionalism. *Developing World Bioethics*, *18*(1), 26–36. DOI: 10.1111/dewb.12170 PMID: 28922547

Olaisen, R. H., Schluchter, M. D., Flocke, S. A., Smyth, K. A., Koroukian, S. M., & Stange, K. C. (2020). Assessing the longitudinal impact of physician-patient relationship on functional health. *Annals of Family Medicine*, *18*(5), 422–429. DOI: 10.1370/afm.2554 PMID: 32928758

Pellegrini, C. A. (2017). Trust: The keystone of the patient-physician relationship. *Journal of the American College of Surgeons*, *224*(2), 95–102. DOI: 10.1016/j.jamcollsurg.2016.10.032 PMID: 27773776

San, L., & Arranz, B. (2023). Effective patient-physician communication in the era of neuropsychopharmacology. *European Neuropsychopharmacology*, *71*, 1–2. DOI: 10.1016/j.euroneuro.2023.02.007 PMID: 36867984

Srinivasan, S. (2023). Elderly TB patients in India: Situation Analysis, Tuijin Jishu/Journal of Propulsion Technology, Vol. 44 No. 6 (2023), 364-367. DOI: 10.52783/tjjpt.v44.i6.3140

Srinivasan, S. (2025). Patient-Centric Care in Tuberculosis Management: Addressing Challenges and Improving Health Outcomes. In *Convergence of Population Health Management, Pharmacogenomics, and Patient-Centered Care* (pp. 265-282). IGI Global. DOI: 10.4018/979-8-3693-3260-3.ch012

Stone, A. A. (1976). *Mental Health and Law: A System in Transition*. Jason Aronson.

Teutsch, C. (2003). Patient–doctor communication. *Medical Clinics*, *87*(5), 1115–1145. https://www.medical.theclinics.com/article/S0025-7125(03)00066-X/abstract PMID: 14621334

Tucker, J. D., Wong, B., Nie, J. B., & Kleinman, A. (2016). Rebuilding patient–physician trust in China. *Lancet, 388*(10046), 755. DOI: 10.1016/S0140-6736(16)31362-9 PMID: 27560268

Veatch, R. M. (1972). Models for ethical medicine in a revolutionary age. *The Hastings Center Report, 2*(3), 5–7. DOI: 10.2307/3560825 PMID: 4679693

Ward, P. (2018). Trust and communication in a doctor-patient relationship: A literature review. *Journal of Healthcare Communications, 3*(3), 36. DOI: 10.4172/2472-1654.100146

Yedidia, M. J. (2007). Transforming doctor-patient relationships to promote patient-centered care: Lessons from palliative care. *Journal of Pain and Symptom Management, 33*(1), 40–57. DOI: 10.1016/j.jpainsymman.2006.06.007 PMID: 17196906

Chapter 9
Stigma:
Intersection of Oppression and Medicine

Nassim Lamine Louail
Mercy St. Rita's Medical Center, USA

EXECUTIVE SUMMARY

Oppression surrounding multiple areas of patient identity have been used to stigmatize patient needs and outcomes. This creates barriers to care and impacts health outcomes. This chapter will explore the stigmatization of diverse patients through the lens of pain management. Patients can often have complex pain concerns alongside intersectional stigma which impacts patient-centered care and collaborative decision-making. Equal pain management policies can help stigmatized populations eliminate inequities. Supporting patients with pain from underrepresented groups requires intersectional policy and practice, addressing sociocultural reasons of health disparities among these groups, and integrating an understanding of ethnicity, gender, sexual orientation, ability, age, and socioeconomic status into healthcare practice. By implementing these strategies and promoting patient engagement, individuals with chronic pain can receive the care, support, and validation that is needed to facilitate pain relief regardless of their identity.

INTRODUCTION

Stigma is a concept compounded by intersectionality and it acknowledges that individuals can simultaneously face multiple forms of oppression like racism, sexism, ableism, and classism. For example, marginalized communities such as racial and ethnic minorities, LGBTQ+ individuals, and those with disabilities may experience a combination of stigmatization in addition to their chronic pain (Hobson, 2022).

DOI: 10.4018/979-8-3693-3683-0.ch009

This overlapping stigma not only further marginalizes individuals living with pain but also contributes to health disparities. The intersection of oppression and stigma in pain patients within the healthcare and medicine system in the United States is a multifaceted issue that requires careful examination.

Throughout history, pain has been a subject of interest and curiosity, leading to diverse interpretations influenced by cultural beliefs and social contexts. Ancient civilizations attributed pain to phenomena beyond the scope of natural explanations or disruptions in bodily equilibrium while traditional Chinese medicine linked it to disruptions in Qi energy flow. These cultural perspectives shaped approaches to pain management and the development of medical practices. Currently, there is a substantial portion of the population that experiences chronic pain. characterized by persistent pain lasting over three months without an apparent anatomical or neurophysiological origin (Katz et al., 2015). However, individuals with chronic pain face not only physical symptoms but also stigma and oppression, intensifying their suffering and hindering access to adequate healthcare and support (Perugino et al., 2022). Different cultures and periods have offered diverse interpretations and understandings of pain, influenced by their unique beliefs, values, and social contexts. Examining these historical perspectives provides valuable insights into the perception, treatment, and societal stigmatization of pain.

Stigma in the context of chronic pain refers to the negative evaluation and judgment that individuals with chronic pain experience, resulting in their rejection, discrimination, and exclusion from various aspects of society (Perugino et al., 2022). This stigma can manifest through viewing pain as a psychological issue or invalidating one's experiences (Ruddere & Craig, 2016). Blame may also be attributed to those experiencing pain. It should be noted that the stigmatization experienced by individuals with chronic pain is not only perpetuated by societal attitudes but can also be internalized by individuals living with chronic pain, leading to feelings of shame, self-blame, and social isolation (Perugino et al., 2022).

The healthcare system plays a vital role in the experiences of individuals with chronic pain. However, it is important to acknowledge that healthcare settings can also contribute to perpetuating stigma and oppression. Research has demonstrated that healthcare providers may hold biased attitudes toward patients with chronic pain, resulting in disparities in the assessment, treatment, and management of their pain (Craig, 2019). Additionally, structural factors such as systemic racism and socioeconomic inequalities further compound these disparities by limiting marginalized populations' access to quality healthcare (Johnson, 2022). Understanding how oppression and stigma intersect for individuals with chronic pain is crucial for addressing their unique challenges and promoting equitable and compassionate healthcare practices.

This analysis aims to shed light on the complex dynamics of oppression and stigma faced by individuals with chronic pain. This understanding can inform healthcare providers, policymakers, and researchers in developing policies that prioritize equitable and patient-centered care for those living with chronic pain. The healthcare system can work towards a more inclusive, compassionate, and responsive system that adequately addresses the needs of all individuals, regardless of their circumstances.

Stigma and Oppression in Healthcare Settings

The presence of stigma and oppression within healthcare settings can exert a substantial influence on the experiences of individuals with chronic pain, ultimately intensifying their distress and impeding their ability to obtain suitable medical treatment. Extensive research has yielded significant findings pertaining to the multifaceted nature of stigma and discrimination experienced by those living with chronic pain. These studies have contributed to a deeper understanding of the various obstacles they confront within healthcare systems.

One sign of stigma in healthcare settings is the tendency to label pain as a disease or a mental disorder. Healthcare personnel frequently exhibit suspicion or doubt towards those experiencing pain, ascribing their agony to psychological reasons rather than acknowledging the underlying physiological basis of their disease. The absence of validation and suitable therapy exacerbates the perpetuation of stigmatization pertaining to chronic pain. For instance, research conducted by Stringer et al. (2015) has demonstrated that physicians may exhibit a reluctance to engage in physical contact or examination of patients suffering from chronic pain, primarily because of misconceptions and biases.

Moreover, persons afflicted with chronic illnesses such as Ehlers-Danlos Syndrome exemplify the interplay between stigma and the healthcare system. The lack of awareness and expertise regarding Ehlers-Danlos Syndrome (EDS) among medical professionals often poses challenges for individuals with this condition in obtaining an accurate diagnosis and suitable therapy (Katz et al., 2015). As a result, individuals may encounter emotions characterized by irritation, invalidation, and an increased sense of stigmatization. This exhibits the necessity for healthcare practitioners to possess comprehensive knowledge regarding uncommon medical diseases such as Ehlers-Danlos syndrome and to adopt a pain treatment approach that is characterized by compassion and empathy (Sing et al., 2020).

People who live with chronic pain are at risk of being marginalized due to the increasing prevalence of pain management practices that are based on the medical model. Perugino et al. (2022) argue that the biological approach, which prioritizes the identification of precise anatomical or neurophysiological factors, may fail to fully acknowledge the intricate and multidimensional characteristics inherent in chronic pain. Consequently, individuals whose medical issues do not align with this framework may encounter difficulties in accessing complete and efficacious healthcare. The process of medicalization might also give rise to the belief that pain is exclusively a physical matter, thereby neglecting the psychological and social dimensions of pain encounters (Ruddere & Craig, 2016).

The perceptions and encounters of patients suffering from chronic pain are influenced by several social and cultural elements present in healthcare environments. Systemic biases and structural inequalities can contribute to the presence of stigma and prejudice experienced by marginalized communities, such as racial and ethnic minorities (Anderson & Lane, 2023). Previous studies have provided evidence of discrepancies in pain management and treatment results that are influenced by race and ethnicity, emphasizing the significance of addressing these injustices within healthcare systems (Perrot, 2019). For example, persons diagnosed with sickle cell disease, a medical ailment that predominantly impacts individuals of African descent, frequently encounter social stigma and discriminatory treatment as a result of prevailing beliefs and biases (Bediako et al., 2014).

Adopting a comprehensive approach to effectively tackle the challenges of stigma and oppression within healthcare environments is crucial. This involves enhancing healthcare personnel's awareness and delivering educational initiatives regarding the fine details of chronic pain and the varied experiences encountered by those coping with pain. The implementation of culturally sensitive and patient-centered care methods has the potential to mitigate the adverse effects of stigma and discrimination on patients' overall well-being and treatment outcomes (Ashtari & Taylor, 2023). The promotion of diversity and inclusivity within the healthcare staff has been identified to enhance the provision of equitable and responsive care for underrepresented communities (Stangl et al., 2023).

When attempting to cultivate a healthcare environment that is characterized by compassion and support for patients experiencing chronic pain, it is important to recognize and confront the stigmatization they encounter. Through a comprehensive analysis of the diverse manifestations of stigma and oppression in the context of pain treatment, coupled with a thoughtful examination of the intersectional experiences of individuals within this population, it becomes possible to enhance the inclusivity and efficacy of healthcare provision. Promoting awareness, education, and policy changes that prioritize equitable and compassionate pain management for all individuals, irrespective of their intersecting identities and conditions, necessitates collaboration among healthcare professionals, researchers, advocacy groups, and patients themselves (Hausmann et al., 2020).

Stigma and Oppression in Pain Management

The negative attitudes and social stigma experienced by individuals seeking pain relief have significant implications for their management of chronic pain. Stigmatization, particularly concerning the use of cannabis as a treatment option, can create barriers to accessing appropriate care and limit patients' options for effective pain management. Despite evidence supporting the efficacy of medical cannabis in relieving pain, its association with recreational drug use and legal restrictions contributes to its continued stigmatization (Ruddere & Craig, 2016). Consequently, healthcare providers may be hesitant to discuss or recommend cannabis as a viable treatment choice, thereby hindering access to potentially beneficial therapies for patients experiencing chronic pain.

Individuals with specific chronic diseases, such as sickle cell disease, often encounter unique challenges when it comes to pain management due to the stigma associated with their condition. Sickle cell disease is a genetic blood disorder characterized by episodes of severe pain called vaso-occlusive crises. Stigma related to this disease can manifest in various ways, including healthcare providers questioning the severity of these painful episodes or attributing them to seeking drugs (Craig, 2019). This stigma can contribute to insufficient pain management and hinder timely access to appropriate care for individuals living with sickle cell disease.

Pain management for the elderly population presents specific difficulties as they often encounter stigma and ageism, which can hinder their access to appropriate pain relief. Older adults may have additional health conditions and multiple medication use, complicating pain management and increasing the potential for adverse reactions to pain medications (Katz, 2015). Moreover, healthcare providers' ageist preconceptions and biases may result in the disregarding or insufficient treatment of pain in older adults, thus contributing to a lack of acknowledgment and inadequate treatment of pain within this demographic group. Serious concerns can be brushed off as simply a part of aging, delaying accurate diagnosis and treatment. This is also seen in populations with differing abilities. Biases held by health care workers can impact patient care through the assumptions about quality of life and pain management, leading to poorer health outcomes.

Stigma also exists surrounding care for women. There are large health disparities between men and women, and it may stem from the historical exclusion of women from medical research. This exclusion has led to a lack of understanding and awareness of women’s specific health issues including pain responses. As a result, women's pain is often not taken seriously, and their medical needs are often not fully addressed. Concerns are often noted to be psychosomatic and emotional rather than having an organic cause delaying care and impacting outcomes.

The convergence of stigma and pain management is further illustrated in the experiences of individuals with chronic illnesses such as Ehlers-Danlos Syndrome. The intricate nature of EDS combined with healthcare providers' limited awareness can result in skepticism, doubt, and insufficient pain treatment for those afflicted by this condition (Camerota, 2023). The stigmatization associated with EDS can worsen the difficulties encountered by patients when seeking an accurate diagnosis and receiving proper care.

Stigma within healthcare disproportionately affects patients with substance use disorders (SUDs), reflecting broader themes of oppression in medicine. This stigma is often rooted in societal biases that frame addiction as a moral failing rather than a chronic health condition, resulting in inadequate care for these patients. Healthcare providers may consciously or unconsciously view individuals with SUDs as manipulative or undeserving of empathy, leading to disparities in pain management and overall treatment. These biases perpetuate systemic inequities, leaving patients marginalized and vulnerable to undertreatment, misdiagnosis, or outright dismissal of their concerns. Research highlights how this stigmatization creates a cycle of oppression: patients with SUDs frequently avoid seeking medical care due to fear of judgment, further exacerbating their health conditions (Brondani et al., 2017).

The structural barriers within the healthcare system, such as limited access to addiction treatment programs and restrictive pain management policies, amplify the struggles faced by these patients (Zwick et al., 2020). The intersection of stigma and systemic oppression mirrors broader societal patterns of neglect for marginalized groups, often reinforcing cycles of poverty, poor health, and criminalization. Addressing these issues requires not only provider education to combat bias but also policy reforms that prioritize harm reduction and equitable access to care. Without these changes, the healthcare system risks perpetuating injustice, leaving vulnerable populations to suffer at the due to the effects of stigma and inadequate medical treatment.

Dealing with the negative perceptions and biases in pain management requires a comprehensive approach. Healthcare professionals should be well-informed about various treatment options, including medical cannabis, and encouraged to have open and non-judgmental conversations with patients regarding their preferences for managing pain. Additionally, efforts should be made to increase awareness and reduce prejudice surrounding specific chronic illnesses like sickle cell disease and EDS, so that individuals suffering from these conditions can receive the necessary care and support they require. Subsequent sections will delve deeper into how stigma and oppression are evident in pain management, and discuss the obstacles faced by patients seeking appropriate care and potential strategies for addressing these issues. By recognizing and tackling stigma while promoting patient-centered approaches to pain care, we can strive toward fairness in healthcare delivery.

Theoretical Frameworks for Understanding Intersectionality and Stigma

It is important to understand the various experiences faced by chronic pain patients who are members of several marginalized groups via the lens of intersectionality, a notion initially proposed by Kimberlé Crenshaw (Katz et al., 2015). The concept of intersectionality acknowledges that individuals may experience many and interconnected types of oppression due to the intersection of their social identities, including but not limited to race, gender, sexuality, disability, age, and socioeconomic status. An individual who is confronted with persistent suffering, and who self-identifies as belonging to both a racial minority group and the LGBTQ+ community, may encounter increased levels of social disapproval and prejudice because of the intersectionality of these several dimensions of their identity. By adopting an intersectional framework, a more comprehensive understanding can be achieved regarding the interconnections and impacts of different systems of oppression on persons navigating experiences of suffering.

These theoretical frameworks provide a robust foundation for examining the intersection of oppression and stigma among those who are undergoing pain. Through the utilization of these conceptual frameworks, a deeper understanding of the intricate nature of stigma and its impact on those experiencing chronic pain can be achieved. Research findings indicate that individuals who have chronic pain and identify as belonging to racial and ethnic minority groups may encounter heightened levels of stigma and discrimination because of systemic prejudices and structural inequalities (Hausmann et al., 2020). The presence of intersectional stigma has the potential to exacerbate the marginalization experienced by individuals who suffer from chronic pain, hence perpetuating health inequities.

Understanding the convergence of chronic pain and mental health disorders introduces an additional stratum of intricacy to the encounters of individuals suffering from pain. The co-occurrence of chronic pain with depression and anxiety is prevalent, and the negative societal perception of mental health might exacerbate the difficulties encountered by persons in their pursuit of pain relief (Katz et al., 2015). The convergence of chronic pain and the stigmatization of mental health can result in heightened levels of psychological distress, social seclusion, and act as a barrier to obtaining suitable healthcare services.

We can learn to develop a more complete comprehension of the intersectionality between health-related stigma and chronic pain and consider the experiences of those who are afflicted with HIV and the stigma that relates to it. Individuals who are afflicted with HIV frequently encounter significant levels of social stigma, which can be even further intensified when combined with chronic pain. The presence of intersectional stigma has apparent consequences for both the physical well-being and emotional health of individuals, as well as their overall quality of life.

The experiences encountered by those suffering from pain and certain chronic illnesses serve to underscore the interconnectedness of stigma and oppression. Individuals diagnosed with hypermobile Ehlers-Danlos Syndrome (EDS) have distinct obstacles in the realm of pain treatment because of healthcare practitioners' limited awareness and comprehension of the disorder (Malfait et al., 2021). The co-occurrence of chronic pain, joint hypermobility, and Ehlers-Danlos Syndrome (EDS) can lead to skepticism, disbelief, and insufficient pain management among persons affected by this disorder. An illustrative example is provided by a case study that examined the experiences of a 34-year-old individual with hypermobile Ehlers-Danlos syndrome (EDS) and persistent discomfort. The commencement of this journey occurred in adolescence when the individual began to encounter regular occurrences of joint dislocations and fatigue. Over the course of time, the intensity of the pain escalated significantly, exerting a profound influence on their day-to-day activities and overall state of health. Regrettably, Sarah faced numerous challenges in locating suitable medical care for her ailment (Gunendran & Dwarakanath, 2023). This example serves as a demonstration of the complex struggles encountered by individuals with Ehlers-Danlos Syndrome (EDS) and chronic pain.

Individuals diagnosed with fibromyalgia, a persistent pain disorder, frequently encounter doubt and skepticism from healthcare practitioners because of the absence of concrete diagnostic indicators (Perrot, 2019). This is further compounded by sexism as the concerns of women are often ignored or attributed to mental health concerns. This phenomenon can lead to patients experiencing feelings of invalidation and frustration, hence exacerbating their pain experience. This statement underscores the challenges encountered by those diagnosed with fibromyalgia in accessing adequate assistance and pain management, primarily due to a dearth of comprehension and the presence of societal stigma surrounding their condition.

The firsthand accounts of individuals suffering from chronic illnesses and experiencing agony often undermine the relationship between stigma and injustice. Individuals diagnosed with hypermobile Ehlers-Danlos Syndrome (EDS) have distinct obstacles in the realm of pain management because of healthcare practitioners' limited awareness and comprehension of the disorder (Ruddere & Craig, 2016). The co-occurrence of chronic pain, joint hypermobility, and Ehlers-Danlos syndrome (EDS) can give rise to skepticism, disbelief, and suboptimal pain treatment among persons affected by this disorder. These problems exemplify the way individuals afflicted with diverse chronic illnesses encounter overlapping manifestations of stigma and discrimination throughout their process of pain management. The presence of stigma and discrimination faced by individuals diagnosed with sickle cell disease and fibromyalgia underscores the necessity for healthcare personnel to possess comprehensive knowledge regarding these disorders and adopt a compassionate and understanding approach towards pain management. Likewise, the obstacles encountered by individuals with EDS underscore the significance of enhancing awareness and comprehension among healthcare practitioners to guarantee suitable healthcare for this demographic.

To effectively address the complex problems experienced by individuals suffering from chronic diseases and chronic pain, it's important to adopt a comprehensive and inclusive approach that considers the intersecting factors that contribute to their unique circumstances. It is imperative for healthcare practitioners to acknowledge and authenticate the varied experiences and necessities of these patients, so guaranteeing that healthcare is customized to address their individualized needs. This includes the promotion of awareness and education of these conditions, the implementation of patient-centered care practices, and the mitigation of prejudices and misconceptions that lead to stigma and discrimination.

Through the recognition and resolution of the complicated obstacles encountered by individuals suffering from pain across various chronic illnesses, healthcare practitioners and policymakers can strive to cultivate a more impartial and patient-centric framework for pain management. The promotion of awareness, education, and policy changes that prioritize equitable and compassionate pain management for all individuals, irrespective of their intersecting identities and conditions, necessitates collaboration among healthcare professionals, researchers, advocacy groups, and patients themselves.

Intersectionality and the Experience of Pain Patients

When chronic pain coexists with mental health conditions, it adds another layer of complexity to the experiences of these patients. Chronic pain is frequently associated with depression and anxiety, thus compounding the challenges that individuals face when seeking appropriate management for their condition (Katz et al., 2015). The convergence of chronic pain and the stigmatization surrounding mental health can contribute to heightened psychological distress, social isolation, and obstacles in accessing appropriate care.

The encounters of individuals with chronic diseases further highlight how stigma intersects with oppressive forces. For example, those living with hypermobile Ehlers-Danlos Syndrome face unique hurdles when it comes to managing their pain due to a lack of awareness and understanding from healthcare professionals (Anderson & Lane, 2023). The combination of chronic pain, joint hypermobility, and EDS often leads to skepticism, disbelief, and insufficient management methods for individuals affected by this condition (Malfait et al., 2021). The intersection of oppression and stigma in pain patients within the healthcare system in the United States creates a complex set of challenges that must be addressed.

Taking a comprehensive and inclusive approach is essential in addressing the intersecting experiences of individuals with chronic pain. It is crucial for healthcare providers to acknowledge and validate the diverse identities and lived experiences of pain patients, ensuring that their treatment is customized to address their individual requirements. This includes being mindful of the unique challenges faced by individuals who have multiple marginalized identities and providing culturally sensitive and inclusive care that addresses these intersections. Additionally, it is important to integrate mental health support into pain management strategies to address both the stigma surrounding mental health conditions as well as their intersectionality with chronic pain. This involves destigmatizing mental health issues, promoting access to appropriate services for mental well-being, and recognizing how physical and psychological aspects are interconnected within the context of managing pain (Adhikary et al., 2023).

To promote fairness and inclusivity in pain care, healthcare providers and policymakers need to acknowledge and tackle the complex challenges faced by individuals with chronic pain. This can be achieved through various strategies, including interventions aimed at diminishing stigma and discrimination, integrating intersectionality into healthcare policies and practices, as well as incorporating integrative medicine to address the unique needs of pain patients (Craig et al., 2019; Roberts-West et al., 2023; Vogel et al., 2021). By implementing these strategies, we can strive towards a future where individuals with chronic pain receive the care, support, and validation they deserve, free from the burden of intersectional stigma.

Strategies for Addressing Intersectional Stigma in Pain Patients

One promising avenue for reducing stigma in pain patients is through initiatives that promote principles of diversity and inclusion across all aspects of healthcare delivery (Stringer et al. 2015). This can involve creating a healthcare environment that is welcoming and inclusive for individuals from diverse backgrounds, ensuring culturally sensitive care practices, and promoting diversity in the healthcare workforce. By embracing diversity and inclusivity, healthcare systems can foster an environment that values and respects the unique experiences and needs of pain patients.

In addition, it is crucial to incorporate an intersectional approach into healthcare policies and practices to address the specific needs of pain patients who belong to multiple marginalized groups. This entails acknowledging and addressing the social factors that contribute to health disparities among these individuals (Perugino et al., 2022). By considering intersecting factors such as race, gender, sexuality, disability, and socioeconomic status, healthcare systems can develop more customized and effective strategies for managing pain. For example, implementing policies that prioritize equitable access to pain management resources and services can help mitigate the disparities faced by marginalized communities (Ruddere & Craig, 2016).

The prioritization of patient-centered care and shared decision-making as means of addressing the complex intersectional stigma experienced by individuals with pain is crucial. This approach entails actively involving patients in their treatment plans, respecting their autonomy, and considering their unique preferences and values (Anderson & Lane, 2023). By encouraging patients to actively participate in their healthcare journey, healthcare providers can help mitigate the negative effects of stigma and discrimination while fostering more positive experiences within the healthcare system. Incorporating integrative medicine approaches, which involve combining conventional medical treatments with complementary therapies, can be instrumental in meeting the needs of patients experiencing pain. These approaches acknowledge the comprehensive and multidimensional nature of pain experiences and prioritize a holistic approach to pain management (Craig et al., 2019). By integrating complementary therapies such as acupuncture, mindfulness-based practices, and physical therapy, integrative medicine offers additional strategies for patients to effectively manage their symptoms while enhancing their overall well-being.

Furthermore, addressing intersectional stigma in pain patients requires ongoing education and training for healthcare providers. This includes increasing awareness and understanding of the unique challenges faced by individuals with intersecting marginalized identities, as well as providing tools and resources to promote culturally sensitive and inclusive care practices (Sing et al., 2020). By equipping healthcare providers with the knowledge and skills to address intersectional stigma, healthcare systems can foster a more supportive and inclusive environment for pain patients.

It is vital to adopt a comprehensive and inclusive approach that exhibits the understanding of intersectional stigma in pain patients. This approach should involve interventions at the individual, healthcare system, and policy levels. By reducing stigma, ensuring equitable access to care, and integrating patient-centered and integrative approaches, healthcare providers and policymakers can contribute to the development of a more compassionate and fair pain care system. It is important to acknowledge and confront the distinct obstacles experienced by pain patients with intersecting marginalized identities to create a healthcare system that is supportive, responsive, and inclusive for all individuals living with chronic pain.

Stigma remains a significant in healthcare and affects patients of all demographics and conditions. This case series explores how stigma impacts individuals, particularly by gender, race, socioeconomic status and the historical marginalization of certain groups in the medical system. From the dismissal of women's pain to the racial biases in pain management and the societal neglect of those with addiction, these cases show how stigma is a form of oppression in medicine. Women reporting pain are often met with skepticism, told they're being too emotional or given inadequate care at critical moments like reproductive health procedures or chronic pain management (Bever, 2022). Racial disparities make these challenges worse, as seen with patients of color, especially Black women who are often assumed to have less pain tolerance or are seeking medical care for nefarious reasons.

The intersection of stigma and systemic inequities is also seen in the broader crisis of "deaths of despair" where untreated physical and mental pain is contributing to rising mortality rates. These cases show the bidirectional relationship between physical pain and despair, and the need for full and unbiased care. Across all the stories, common themes emerge: the psychological and physical suffering patients endure because of medical dismissal, the historical exclusion of marginalized groups from research and the importance of self-advocacy in overcoming these systemic barriers. By addressing these issues this series hopes to help us understand how stigma not only compromises individual care but also perpetuates broader health inequities and demands urgent systemic change to achieve equity and compassion in medicine.

CASES

Cases 1-4. From heart disease to IUDs: How doctors dismiss women's pain (Bever, 2022)

Learning Objectives

1. Analyze the differences in care women experience when presenting with a medical issue.
2. Describe the psychological and physical struggles individuals may face when seeking treatment.

Case Aim: The dismissal of women's pain by healthcare professionals is a pervasive and deeply troubling issue. This case storyline explores the experiences of several women who have faced significant challenges in receiving appropriate care for their pain.

1. Reproductive Health Complaints

A woman, experienced excruciating pain during the insertion of an intrauterine device (IUD). As she cried out and begged the doctor to stop, her pleas were ignored, exemplifying the disregard for women's pain in reproductive health concerns and procedures. Similarly, another patient, opted for an epidural during an excruciating 33-hour labor. Despite the supposed pain relief, she felt every contraction and cramp intensely, but her complaints were dismissed by her medical team.

2. Racial Disparities in Pain Management

A Black patient suffering from a sickle cell disease pain crisis meticulously prepared herself before visiting the emergency room, fearing she would be dismissed as a drug seeker. She arrives only to have to advocate for her pain plan to be enacted. It takes 2 hours and speaking with 3 different physicians before someone looked into her chart and found the treatment plan from her hematologist. The physician then still consults the hematology team prior to starting her on any medication for her pain.

3. Psychological Dismissal, Old Age, and Chronic Pain

A 68-year-old woman from Tampa endured chronic pain from arthritis, degenerative disk disease, and spinal stenosis. She was in obvious distress and her pain was often attributed to psychological causes, reflecting a widespread tendency to label women as emotional. After her inner thighs become numb, she was seen in the emergency room and underwent emergency surgery to address the compression of her spine.

4. Psychological Dismissal, Childhood, and Chronic Pain

A 27 year old woman, starting from her teens, experienced debilitating joint pain. She was told by numerous doctors that her pain was all in her head and dismissed when repeatedly voicing her concerns. Over the years, she was diagnosed with GERD, Crohn's Disease, POTs and migraine headaches. After having several pelvic bone dislocations, a postpartum hemorrhage, and prolonged wound healing with a C-section, a physician was concerned that something else might be occurring. She was finally diagnosed with hypermobile Ehlers-Danlos syndrome undermining the years of neglect and misdiagnosis.

Case Questions

1. What systems can we adopt to make sure patients are heard?

- *We can deploy several systems such as patient advocacy programs. These programs can assist patients in communicating their concerns and needs effectively. The use of patient feedback mechanisms by using surveys and feedback forms to gather patients' experiences and acting on this data can help guide improvement in care. Staff training on active listening and empathy can also help healthcare professionals better understand and respond to patients' concerns.*

2. How can we take women that are dealing with pain more seriously?

- *Taking women's pain more seriously involves utilizing comprehensive and unbiased pain assessment tools. This includes using the most up-to-date resources such as pre-test probability criteria for certain conditions that may be influenced by gender. It is important to educate healthcare providers about the historical biases and the importance of validating women's pain experiences. Advocating for women in research will help ensure that women are adequately represented in clinical trials and medical studies to understand their specific pain responses and needs.*

3. How should pain concerning reproductive health be approached?

- *Pain concerning reproductive health should be approached with:*
    - *Pre-procedure Counseling: Discussing potential pain and discomfort thoroughly before procedures like IUD insertions and any other concerns or expectations.*
    - *Adequate Pain Management Plans: Developing individualized pain management plans alongside your provider that include options for pain relief during and after procedures.*
    - *Empathy: Actively listening to and acknowledging the pain experiences of patients, while avoiding dismissal of their complaints.*

4. Should the pain tolerance of an individual dictate the type of care they receive?

- *Pain tolerance should not dictate the type of care received. Each individual's pain should be taken seriously and managed according to their specific needs. This ensures that those with lower pain tolerance receive adequate relief and those with higher tolerance are not overlooked.*

5. How should pain be measured in different individuals?

- *Pain should be measured using multifaceted pain scales. This can be achieved by employing scales that include numeric ratings, visual analogs, and descriptive terms to capture a comprehensive picture of the patient's pain. Individual pain diaries encourage patients to document the intensity, duration, and nature of their pain. Ensuring regular follow-up with a provider and conducting regular pain assessments to track changes and adjust treatment plans accordingly can aid in personalizing treatment.*

6. Should pain scales be adjusted based on certain factors such as age and gender?

- *Pain scales should be calibrated to account for age, gender, and other relevant factors. Utilizing different scales for children, adults, and the elderly to account for developmental and cognitive differences. It is also important to encourage the use of gender-sensitive tools to recognize that men and women may report and experience pain differently, ensuring a more accurate assessment.*

7. How can patients feel heard when describing pain symptoms?

- *Active Listening: Medical professionals should practice active listening, giving patients ample time to describe their symptoms without interruption.*
- *Empathetic Communication: Providers should validate patients' feelings and concerns, using empathetic language and body language.*
- *Patient-Centered Care: Involving patients in their treatment plans and decision-making processes to ensure their voices are central to their care.*

8. What type of systemic changes can be made to address the varying perceptions of pain in different individuals?

- *Systemic changes can include mandatory bias training on recognizing and countering biases related to gender, race, and age in pain management. Policy reforms can be discussed regarding policies that standardize pain assessment and management across all demographics. Research and investment in research are also crucial to understand how different demographics experience pain and adjusting clinical guidelines accordingly.*

9. What type of education can providers obtain that would aid in the perception of pain in patients?

- *Providers can benefit from Continuous Medical Education (CME). These courses focus on pain management, gender and racial biases, and patient communication. Interactive sessions such as workshops or seminars that explore the latest research and strategies in effective pain management can aid individuals to feel included in their care journey and be more involved. Simulation training is also available for many procedures and treatments, which can give the patient and provider more confidence when tackling the individual's concerns.*

10. What kind of resources should be provided with patients who feel like they haven't been heard?

- *Patient Advocacy Services: Organizations or personnel dedicated to supporting patients in navigating the healthcare system.*
- *Support Groups: Peer support groups where patients can share experiences and strategies for advocating for themselves. This allows patients to communicate with others who can relate to their struggles and concerns.*
- *Educational Resources: Information that has been peer-reviewed on how to effectively communicate pain and symptoms to healthcare providers and what to expect from medical consultations.*

Case Discussion

Addressing the dismissal of women's pain in the medical field requires a multifaceted approach, including systemic changes, enhanced education for providers, and better support for patients. By implementing standardized assessment protocols, training healthcare professionals to recognize and counteract biases, and ensuring patients feel heard and validated, we can work towards a more equitable and effective healthcare system. These steps will help bridge the pain gap, ensuring all patients receive the compassionate and comprehensive care they deserve

Case 5. Physical pain causes despair

Learning Objectives:

1. Assess the negative impacts of pain on an individual or population.
2. Evaluate different societal factors such as the economy and employment status can affect individuals and populations suffering from pain.

Case Aim: This case sheds light on the relationship between untreated physical pain, mental health struggles, and the stigma that perpetuates inadequate care.

A 47 year old gay, transman presented to a new primary care physician after a recent hospitalization. He has been battling chronic pain for the last 17 years after a motorcycle accident which has also left him with a colostomy bag and extensive facial scarring. He notes feeling fulfilled in life until the accident. Shortly afterwards he began to experience intense abdominal, back, and joint pain, terrible nightmares, disturbed sleep, immense sadness, fear of leaving his home, panic attacks, and thoughts that he would have been better off dead rather than surviving the accident. He was diagnosed with chronic pain, depression, and PTSD at that time. He tried therapy and medications for the depression and PTSD which only helped the PTSD. After his surgeries, physicians were not willing to continue to treat his pain with opioids.

His chronic pain is still unmanaged which has left him on partial disability as SSI maintains that he can work part time. His depressive symptoms have led to a divorce, isolation from his support system, as well as loss of his employment, good credit rating, home and car. He tried self-medicating with marijuana, then alcohol, and most recently Xanax that he purchased from the internet. He was rushed to the hospital, barely breathing, necessitated and connected with a new medical team including referrals to psychiatry, psychology, and a new primary care physician.

Case Questions

1. How can physical pain lead to despair?

- *Physical pain can lead to despair by significantly worsening mental health. Physical pain can exacerbate mental discomfort, anxiety, and depression, while mental health issues can manifest as physical pain. This interplay creates a vicious cycle where each condition aggravates the other, leading to increased suffering and a higher risk of substance abuse and mortality. Chronic pain can disrupt sleep, reduce quality of life, and limit daily functioning, which can contribute to feelings of hopelessness and depression. Additionally, the stress of managing ongoing pain can lead individuals to substance abuse as a form of self-medication, further deepening their sense of despair.*

In this case, we see the patient's acute injury led to chronic pain and mental health concerns which have impacted all areas of his life.

2. How can despair lead to physical pain?

- *Despair can manifest as physical pain through the psychosomatic effects of mental distress. Stress, anxiety, and depression can trigger physical symptoms, including headaches, muscle pain, and gastrointestinal issues. These symptoms can become chronic, creating a feedback loop where mental anguish leads to physical discomfort, which in turn exacerbates mental health problems. We can see this manifested in the case above.*

3. What is the role of opioids in pain management?

- *Opioids play a significant role in the relationship between pain and despair. Proper assessment and management is needed to treat pain while preventing poor outcomes. Appropriate dosing and management can provide patients with chronic pain relief, allowing them to improve their quality of life and outlook.*

While prescribed to manage pain, opioids can also lead to addiction and increased sensitivity to pain over time. This paradoxical effect means that although opioids provide temporary relief, they can heighten pain and contribute to the cycle of despair in the long run. This is by increasing dependency and the risk of overdose.

These concerns are compounded by stigma associated with patient identity. The patient in this case was young, gay, and transgender when his journey with chronic pain began. Stereotypes about drug use in these populations may have contributed to physicians reluctance to adequately treat his pain.

4. How can pain be assessed and properly managed? Why are some American physicians challenging the use of self-reported pain assessments?

- *Many pain assessments exist including those for acute pain and recording pain over time. Self-reported pain is subjective and can vary widely between individuals. Thus some physicians note these scales can make it difficult to assess accurately and worry about over-prescribing opioids. Inconsistencies in data collection methods and a lack of standardized measures can also complicate accurate history gathering and pain data which can result in inappropriate pain management strategies and policies. This highlights the need for comprehensive pain management and mental health support. Better understanding physical pain at a larger scale and destigmatizing pain management practices can lead to managing individual patients pain better and improving health disparities.*

Case Discussion

According to, Macchia (2023), the period between February 2021 and February 2022 marked a devastating chapter in America's ongoing battle with "deaths of despair," with 110,000 lives lost to drug-related incidents. This tragic statistic is more than just a number; it reflects a growing trend fueled by economic instability, mental health challenges, and pervasive hopelessness. Physical pain plays a critical role in this system.

Research showed that physical pain significantly worsens mental discomfort and anxiety, leading to sleep disturbances and a heightened risk of depression. Psychological stressors such as job-related stress, social discrimination, familial tensions, and adverse childhood experiences further contribute to the prevalence of physical pain, creating a cyclical pattern that is hard to break. This interplay between physical and mental anguish is clearly illustrated in the opioid crisis, where substance abuse not only dulls the pain temporarily but ultimately rewires the brain to become more sensitive and less tolerant to pain. This further perpetuates the cycle of addiction and despair. Likewise, a global study involving 146 countries revealed a significant correlation between high unemployment rates and increased reports of physical pain. This finding shows the profound impact of economic downturns on physical well-being. It suggests that financial stress can manifest physically, leading to greater physical discomfort and profound mental distress.

The relationship between despair and pain is bidirectional. Physical pain can lead to despair by exacerbating mental health issues, reducing quality of life, and driving individuals towards substance abuse as a form of self-medication. Conversely, despair can manifest as physical pain, with mental stress and anxiety triggering physical symptoms and increasing the perception of pain. This intricate relationship highlights the importance of addressing both physical and mental health in tandem to effectively combat the rise in deaths of despair.

The role of opioids can become an issue both as a treatment for pain and a contributor to addiction. Physicians and policymakers need to find the fine balance between the need for pain management with the risks of substance abuse. This balance is crucial in developing strategies that can reduce the burden of both physical pain and mental despair. Recording and monitoring pain data is vital for understanding and addressing this crisis. However, challenges such as subjective self-reporting, varying pain thresholds, and potential biases must be addressed to ensure accurate and useful data. Effective monitoring can inform better pain management practices and policy decisions, ultimately helping to reduce deaths of despair.

CONCLUSION

Development efforts which are concerned with increasing diversity and inclusivity in all healthcare sectors can be seen as potential ways of reducing the stereotypes towards people living with severe pain such as those who suffer from genetic diseases or traumatic injuries among others. This is one of the more promising avenues for eliminating stigma. This can involve establishing culturally responsive care practices, fostering diversity in the healthcare staff, and providing a healthcare atmosphere that is friendly and inclusive for persons from a variety of backgrounds. It is possible for healthcare institutions to cultivate an atmosphere that honors and respects the unique experiences and requirements of pain patients with an openness to diversity and inclusivity.

An intersectional approach into the policies and practices of the healthcare industry is quite important to cater to the requirements of patients suffering from pain who are members of more than one underrepresented group. This involves recognizing the societal factors that contribute to health inequalities among these populations and taking action to alleviate those concerns. The potential for exponential growth is possible for healthcare systems to establish more individualized and efficient solutions for the management of pain if they consider the different factors such as race, gender, sexual orientation, disability, and socioeconomic position. For instance, the implementation of policies that give priority to equitable access to pain management resources and services can assist in mitigating the disparities that are experienced by communities who are marginalized.

It's crucial to provide patient-centered care and collaborative decision-making the utmost priority as a means of tackling the complicated intersectional stigma that people who endure pain are subjected to. This strategy involves patients being actively involved in the development of their respective treatment plans, patients' autonomy being respected, and the patients' individual preferences and values being taken into consideration. The negative impacts of stigma and prejudice can be mitigated, and more positive experiences can be fostered within the healthcare system, if medical professionals encourage patients to take an active role in their own medical care and treatment throughout the course of their treatment. It may be possible to better satisfy the requirements of individuals who are experiencing pain by using integrative medicine approaches. These approaches might involve integrating conventional medical treatments with alternative therapies. The complex nature of pain experiences is considered by these techniques, which places more emphasis on taking a holistic approach to pain management. Integrative medicine provides patients with extra methods for efficiently managing their symptoms while boosting their general well-being. These additional tactics are made possible by the integration of complementary therapies such as acupuncture, mindfulness-based practices, and physical therapy.

Addressing intersectional stigma in pain patients requires ongoing education and training for healthcare providers. This includes increasing awareness and understanding of the unique challenges faced by individuals with intersecting marginalized identities, as well as providing tools and resources to promote culturally sensitive and inclusive care practices. By equipping healthcare providers with the knowledge and skills to address intersectional stigma, healthcare systems can foster a more supportive and inclusive environment for pain patients.

In conclusion, addressing intersectional stigma in pain patients requires a comprehensive and inclusive approach that encompasses interventions at various levels. It's important to acknowledge and confront the well-defined obstacles experienced by pain patients with intersecting marginalized identities to create a healthcare system that is supportive. This can lead to more responsive and inclusive care for all individuals living with chronic pain. By implementing these strategies, we can strive towards a future where individuals with chronic pain receive the care, support, and validation they deserve.

REFERENCES

Adhikary, D., Barman, S., & Ranjan, R. (2023). Internet-based cognitive behavioural therapy for individuals with depression and chronic health conditions: A systematic review. *Cureus*. Advance online publication. DOI: 10.7759/cureus.37822 PMID: 37213982

Anderson, L., & Lane, K. (2023). Hypermobile ehlers-danlos syndrome/hypermobility spectrum disorders in older women: A feasibility study. *Musculoskeletal Care*, *21*(3), 741–748. Advance online publication. DOI: 10.1002/msc.1747 PMID: 36864687

Ashtari, S., & Taylor, A. (2023). Patients with rare diseases and the power of online support groups: Implications for the medical community. *JMIR Formative Research*, *7*, e41610. DOI: 10.2196/41610 PMID: 37707878

Bediako, S., Lanzkron, S., Diener-West, M., Onojobi, G., Beach, M., & Haywood, C.Jr. (2014). The measure of sickle cell stigma: Initial findings from the improving patient outcomes through respect and trust study. *Journal of Health Psychology*, *21*(5), 808–820. DOI: 10.1177/1359105314539530 PMID: 24997169

Bever, L. (2022, December 13). Women's pain often is dismissed by doctors. Washington Post. https://www.washingtonpost.com/wellness/interactive/2022/women-pain-gender-bias-doctors/

Bowleg, L., Malekzadeh, A., Mbaba, M., & Boone, C. (2022). Ending the hiv epidemic for all, not just some: Structural racism as a fundamental but overlooked social-structural determinant of the us hiv epidemic. *Current Opinion in HIV and AIDS*, *17*(2), 40–45. DOI: 10.1097/COH.0000000000000724 PMID: 35102051

Brondani, M. A., Alan, R., & Donnelly, L. (2017). Stigma of addiction and mental illness in healthcare: The case of patients' experiences in dental settings. *PLoS One*, *12*(5), e0177388. DOI: 10.1371/journal.pone.0177388 PMID: 28531176

Bulgin, D., Asnani, M., Vorderstrasse, A., Royal, C., Pan, W., & Tanabe, P. (2021). Stigma and quality of life in adults with sickle cell disease in jamaica and the united states. *Psychology Health and Medicine*, *28*(5), 1133–1147. DOI: 10.1080/13548506.2021.2019808 PMID: 34957879

Camerota, F., Mariani, R., Cordiano, G., Di Trani, M., Lodato, V., Ferraris, A., Pasquini, M., & Celletti, C. (2023). The language of pain in the hypermobile ehlers–danlos syndrome: Metaphors as a key to understanding the experience of pain and as a rehabilitation tool. *Brain Sciences*, *13*(7), 1042. DOI: 10.3390/brainsci13071042 PMID: 37508973

Cole, E. (2009). Intersectionality and research in psychology. *The American Psychologist*, *64*(3), 170–180. DOI: 10.1037/a0014564 PMID: 19348518

Craig, K., Holmes, C., Hudspith, M., Moor, G., Moosa-Mitha, M., Varcoe, C., & Wallace, B. (2019). Pain in persons who are marginalized by social conditions. *Pain*, *161*(2), 261–265. DOI: 10.1097/j.pain.0000000000001719 PMID: 31651578

Geter, A., Herron, A., & Sutton, M. (2018). Hiv-related stigma by healthcare providers in the united states: A systematic review. *AIDS Patient Care and STDs*, *32*(10), 418–424. DOI: 10.1089/apc.2018.0114 PMID: 30277814

Geter, A., Herron, A., & Sutton, M. (2018). Hiv-related stigma by healthcare providers in the united states: A systematic review. *AIDS Patient Care and STDs*, *32*(10), 418–424. DOI: 10.1089/apc.2018.0114 PMID: 30277814

Hart, T., Sharvendiran, R., Chikermane, V., Kidwai, A., & Grace, D. (2021). At the intersection of homophobia and racism: Sociocultural context and the sexual health of south asian canadian gay and bisexual men. *Stigma and Health*. Advance online publication. DOI: 10.1037/sah0000295

Hausmann, L., Jones, A., McInnes, S., & Zickmund, S. (2020). Identifying healthcare experiences associated with perceptions of racial/ethnic discrimination among veterans with pain: A cross-sectional mixed methods survey. *PLoS One*, *15*(9), e0237650. DOI: 10.1371/journal.pone.0237650 PMID: 32881940

Hobson, J., Gilstrap, S., Owens, M., Gloston, G., Ho, M., Gathright, J., Dotson, H. F., White, D. M., Cody, S. L., Justin Thomas, S., & Goodin, B. (2022). Intersectional hiv and chronic pain stigma: Implications for mood, sleep, and pain severity. *Journal of the International Association of Providers of AIDS Care*, *21*, 232595822210779. DOI: 10.1177/23259582221077941 PMID: 35200070

Horrigan, B., Lewis, S., Abrams, D., & Pechura, C. (2012). Integrative medicine in america—-how integrative medicine is being practiced in clinical centers across the united states. *Global Advances in Health and Medicine : Improving Healthcare Outcomes Worldwide*, *1*(3), 18–52. DOI: 10.7453/gahmj.2012.1.3.006

Johnson, C. (2022). Conquering the health disparities of structural racism. *Journal of Public Health Management and Practice*, *28*(Supplement 1), S15–S17. DOI: 10.1097/PHH.0000000000001431 PMID: 34797256

Katz, J., Rosenbloom, B., & Fashler, S. (2015). Chronic pain, psychopathology, and dsm-5 somatic symptom disorder. *Canadian Journal of Psychiatry*, *60*(4), 160–167. DOI: 10.1177/070674371506000402 PMID: 26174215

Macchia, L. (2023, January 30). Rising Physical Pain Is Linked to More 'Deaths of Despair.' Scientific American. https://www.scientificamerican.com/article/rising physical-pain-is-linked-to-more-deaths-of-despair1/

MacSorley, R., White, J., Conerly, V., Walker, J., Lofton, S., Ragland, G., Davey, D. B., & Robertson, A. (2014). Pain assessment and management strategies for elderly patients. *Home Healthcare Nurse, 32*(5), 272–285. DOI: 10.1097/NHH.0000000000000065 PMID: 24802598

Malfait, F., Colman, M., Vroman, R., Wandele, I., Rombaut, L., Miller, R., & Syx, D. (2021). Pain in the ehlers–danlos syndromes: Mechanisms, models, and challenges. *American Journal of Medical Genetics. Part C, Seminars in Medical Genetics, 187*(4), 429–445. DOI: 10.1002/ajmg.c.31950 PMID: 34797601

Meghani, S. (2011). Corporatization of pain medicine: Implications for widening pain care disparities. *Pain Medicine, 12*(4), 634–644. DOI: 10.1111/j.1526-4637.2011.01074.x PMID: 21392249

Muntinga, M., Krajenbrink, V., Peerdeman, S., Croiset, G., & Verdonk, P. (2015). Toward diversity-responsive medical education: Taking an intersectionality-based approach to a curriculum evaluation. *Advances in Health Sciences Education : Theory and Practice, 21*(3), 541–559. DOI: 10.1007/s10459-015-9650-9 PMID: 26603884

Perrot, S. (2019). Fibromyalgia: A misconnection in a multiconnected world? *European Journal of Pain (London, England), 23*(5), 866–873. DOI: 10.1002/ejp.1367 PMID: 30663833

Perugino, F., Angelis, V., Pompili, M., & Martelletti, P. (2022). Stigma and chronic pain. *Pain and Therapy, 11*(4), 1085–1094. DOI: 10.1007/s40122-022-00418-5 PMID: 35930220

Roberts-West, L., Gravatt, A., Guest, N., Hunt, A., Siddique, L., & Serbic, D. (2023). A comparison of social exclusion towards people with depression or chronic back pain. *British Journal of Pain, 17*(3), 267–280. DOI: 10.1177/20494637221148337 PMID: 37342396

Ruddere, L., & Craig, K. (2016). Understanding stigma and chronic pain: A-state-of-the-art review. *Pain, 157*(8), 1607–1610. DOI: 10.1097/j.pain.0000000000000512 PMID: 26859821

Ryan-Ndegwa, S., Zamani, R., & Akrami, M. (2021). Assessing demographic access to hip replacement surgery in the united kingdom: A systematic review. *International Journal for Equity in Health, 20*(1), 224. Advance online publication. DOI: 10.1186/s12939-021-01561-9 PMID: 34641862

Santiago-Rodriguez, E., Rivas, C., Maiorana, A., Pérez, A., Erguera, X., Johnson, M., Christopoulos, K. A., Marquez, C., & Sauceda, J. (2021). Unpacking the "backpack of shame": Exploring intersections of stigma among latinx people living with hiv in san francisco, ca. *Cultural Diversity & Ethnic Minority Psychology*, *27*(4), 630–637. DOI: 10.1037/cdp0000487 PMID: 34410754

Schatman, M. (2011). Pain and corporatization: More special interests, more disparities, more vulnerability. *Pain Medicine*, *12*(4), 632–633. DOI: 10.1111/j.1526-4637.2011.01092.x PMID: 21463473

Sing, S., Peters, R., Syurina, E., Irwanto, I., Naniche, D., & Zweekhorst, M. (2020). Intersectionality and health-related stigma: Insights from experiences of people living with stigmatized health conditions in indonesia. *International Journal for Equity in Health*, *19*(1), 206. Advance online publication. DOI: 10.1186/s12939-020-01318-w PMID: 33176809

Stangl, A., Atkins, K., Leddy, A., Sievwright, K., Sevelius, J., Lippman, S., Veras, M. A., Zamudio-Haas, S., Smith, M. K., Pachankis, J. E., Logie, C. H., Rao, D., Weiser, S., & Nyblade, L. (2023). What do we know about interventions to reduce intersectional stigma and discrimination in the context of hiv? a systematic review. *Stigma and Health*, *8*(3), 393–408. DOI: 10.1037/sah0000414

Stringer, K., Turan, B., McCormick, L., Durojaiye, M., Nyblade, L., Kempf, M., Lichtenstein, B., & Turan, J. (2015). Hiv-related stigma among healthcare providers in the deep south. *AIDS and Behavior*, *20*(1), 115–125. DOI: 10.1007/s10461-015-1256-y PMID: 26650383

Syed, M., & McLean, K. (2015). Understanding identity integration: Theoretical, methodological, and applied issues. *Journal of Adolescence*, *47*(1), 109–118. DOI: 10.1016/j.adolescence.2015.09.005 PMID: 26522883

Telusca, N., Gaisey, J., Woods, C., Khan, J., & Mackey, S. (2022). Strategies to promote racial healthcare equity in pain medicine: A call to action. *Pain Medicine*, *23*(7), 1225–1230. DOI: 10.1093/pm/pnac057 PMID: 35412639

Vogel, M., Choi, F., Westenberg, J., Cabanis, M., Nikoo, N., Nikoo, M., Hwang, S. W., Somers, J., Schütz, C. G., & Krausz, M. (2021). Chronic pain among individuals experiencing homelessness and its interdependence with opioid and other substance use and mental illness. *International Journal of Environmental Research and Public Health*, *19*(1), 5. DOI: 10.3390/ijerph19010005 PMID: 35010263

Zwick, J., Appleseth, H., & Arndt, S. (2020). Stigma: How it affects the substance use disorder patient. *Substance Abuse Treatment, Prevention, and Policy*, *15*(1), 50. DOI: 10.1186/s13011-020-00288-0 PMID: 32718328

Appendix: Additional Resources

The following is a collection of additional resources to supplement classroom experiences as well as further personal edification. Chosen by experts, these resources offer text or written documents for reading as well as multimedia options to assist in reaching a variety of learning styles and accessibilities. Validated curricular resources have been recommended for classroom activities and additional supports.

Chapter 1: Physician Cultural Responsibility: Teaching a New Way to Practice

Physician cultural responsibility encompasses five pillars: cultural humility, Anti-oppression, Advocacy, Intercultural Communication, and Self-awareness and reflection. The resources provided will incorporate best practices from these areas in hopes of encouraging further learning, both in the classroom and through self-study.

Written Texts

1. *The MONROE Method: A Methodology on Navigating Race, Oppression, and Equity in Medical Education Through Physician Cultural Responsibility* by Christen Johnson, MD, EdD, MPH, FAAFP, ProQuest Dissertations and Theses Global, 2023. This resource provides the theoretical background of physician cultural responsibility and best practices for implementation. A mixed-methods study of implementation is also presented to describe the success of this method.
2. *Nonviolent Communication: A Language of Life* by Marshall Rosenberg, Puddle Dancer Press, 2015. Rosenberg presents a method for using language to effectively convey what one is feeling or needing while honoring the humanity of everyone in the conversation. This resource can help cultivate improved communication skills that focus on connection rather than judgment.

3. *Self-Compassion* by Kristin Neff, PhD, 2015. Dr. Neff explores how compassionate inner dialogue can lessen judgment. In Physician Cultural Responsibility, this can assist with self-awareness, self-reflection, and coping with difficult discussions and realizations.
4. *Reflections on a Well-Traveled Path: Self-awareness, mindful practice, and relationship-centered care as foundations for medical education* by S. Dobie, Academic Medicine 82(4), 2007. This resource explores the necessity of self-awareness in medical training. Dr. Dobie highlights the benefits of integrating a deeper awareness of the self and mindful existence within medical practice and patient care.
5. *Narrative Intersectionality in Caring for Marginalized or Disadvantaged Patients* by M. Blackie, et.al, Academic Medicine, 94(1), 2019. Dr. Blackie emphasizes the power of narratives in medical education. This resource can assist in supporting the use of narrative medicine within the classroom.

Additional Resources

1. *Physician Cultural Responsibility: A Path to Better Outcomes for Patients, students, and Physicians* by Christen Johnson, MD, EdD, MPH, FAAFP, dipABLM (in print, 2025)
2. *Who is the "Self" in Self-Aware: Professional self-awareness from a critical theory perspective* by M. Kondrat, Social Service Review. The University of Chicago, 1999.
3. *Becoming a white antiracist: A practical guide for leaders, educators and activists* by S. Brookfield & M. Hess, Sterling, VA: Stylus Publishers, 2021.
4. *Empowering Students by Developing Their Intercultural Communication Competence: A two-way process* by C. Briguglio, Educate, advocate, empower, 2006.
5. *Teaching Intercultural Communication: ICT resources and best practices* by S. Chiper, Procedia Social and Behavioral Sciences, 93, 2012.
6. *Opportunity and Life-Long Health Outcomes: A review of the effects and solutions of hypersegregation on health disparities* by C. Johnson. Core Scholar, Wright State University, 2017.
7. *Racial Microaggressions in Everyday Life* by Sue et. al., American Psychologist, 2007.
8. *Becoming Active Bystanders and Advocated: Teaching Medical Students to respond to Bias in the clinical setting* by York et. al., Academic Medicine, 2021.
9. *Community-Engaged Lifestyle Medicine: Building Health Equity Through Preventive Medicine Residency Training* by J. Krishnaswami, et al. American Journal of Preventative Medicine 55, 2018.

Multimedia Resources

1. **Right To Be Bystander Training** (https://righttobe.org/training/bystander-intervention-training/) Aligned with the pillar of advocacy, these resources yield an opportunity to teach learners what to do when they are faced with oppressive situations in medicine. Studies have shown that bystander training heavily influences workplace culture and experiences for staff and patients in medicine.
2. **Back to Basics: An A-Z of Anti-Oppressive Practice by Siobhan Maclean** (Youtube: https://www.youtube.com/watch?v=G1bnOCc64jM) This resource gives an overview of the components of anti-oppression through a very foundational video webinar.
3. **Cross-Cultural Communication by Pellegrino Riccardi** (TED Talk: https://www.youtube.com/watch?v=YMyofREc5Jk) This video provides a reflective view of intercultural communication through an evaluation of the perception of the self and others.
4. **Cultural Humility by Dr. Juliana Mosley** (TED Talk: https://www.youtube.com/watch?v=Ww_ml21L7Ns) Dr. Mosley provides a cursory overview of cultural humility in this resource come the lens of strength in one's own identity. This can help learners to better conceptualize the impact of culture on their medical practice and their personal/professional development.
5. **Moving Beyond Cultural Competency to Practicing Cultural Humility by Unbound Medicine** (Youtube: https://www.youtube.com/watch?v=ClRdMi2tyRM) In this resource, Tiffany Gibson explains culture and ties the understanding of culture to the development of cultural humility. This can help learners to differentiate culture from other aspects of inclusive practice and highlight additional considerations for patient-centered care.

Additional Resources

1. **5D's of Bystander Intervention by Asian Americans Advancing Justice** (Youtube: https://www.youtube.com/watch?v=ASkX2O9zB24&list=PLShboSEeEaPQ5JKO6L9DG78V8AcXyZjZh)
2. **Anti-Oppressive Practice by Melissa Taylor** (Youtube: https://www.youtube.com/watch?v=gNcoiXKVYfA)

Support for Curricular Planning and Activities

1. **American Board of Family Physicians Starfield Summit** (https://www.starfieldsummit.com/) This resource comes from multiple convention sessions aimed at improving health equity. This can be useful for activities and individual study materials.
2. **American Academy of Family Physicians Anti-racism: Tools for Change** (https://www.aafp.org/cme/all/health-equity/anti-racism.html#:~:text=Bridge%20care%20gaps%20by%20breaking,with%20patients%20from%20varied%20backgrounds) This curricular activity allows individual study that provides continuing medical education. While the framework in this activity is not the Physician Cultural Responsibility Framework, the activity strongly relies on self-reflection.

Chapter 2: Bias: Understanding and Addressing Disparities in Patient Care Across Multiple Demographics

This chapter aims to give learners a deeper understanding of how implicit and structural biases impact patient care and offer strategies for reducing disparities. This approach ensures that learners can critically engage with the topic from both theoretical and applied perspectives, fostering the use of physician cultural responsibility and ethical decision-making in clinical practice. Likewise the resources below provide additional learning about bias and ways that we can overcome them.

Written Texts

1. *Health disparities in the United States: Social Class, Race, Ethnicity, and the Social Determinants of Health* by D. Barr, Johns Hopkins University Press, 2019. This source provides a foundational analysis of how social determinants contribute to disparities in U.S. healthcare, contextualizing the broader impact of bias in medical education and practice.
2. *Why are health disparities everyone's problem?* By L. Cooper, L, Johns Hopkins University Press, 2021. This book highlights systemic inequities in healthcare and provides a compelling rationale for why addressing bias in medical education is essential for achieving health equity.
3. *Mind Over Prejudice: An Implicit Bias Training in Medical Education Using Cognitive Bias Modification* by C. Hsu, *J Grad Med Educ*. 2023. Hsu's work examines cognitive strategies to counteract implicit bias in medical education, supporting the call for structural competency training in curricula.

4. *Implicit bias in health professions: From recognition to transformation* by J. Sukhera, *Academic Medicine*, 2020. This text supports transformative learning theory, like Physician Cultural Responsibility as as a tool to implement learning activities that counteract bias in patient interactions and improve equitable healthcare delivery.
5. *An Intersectional Approach to Understanding Barriers to Healthcare for Women* by S. Vohra-Gupta, et al., *Journal of Community Health, 2023.* This article highlights the compounded effects of intersectional bias in healthcare, supporting the necessity for inclusive medical training frameworks.

Multimedia Resources

1. **Researching unconscious bias in health care by Michelle van Ryn, Ph.D.** (YouTube: https://www.youtube.com/watch?v=igf3telOA5E) This video delves into research on unconscious bias in medical interactions, offering insights into mitigating its effects on healthcare delivery.
2. **How to overcome our biases? Walk boldly toward them by V. Myers** (TED Talk: https://www.ted.com/talks/verna_myers_how_to_overcome_our_biases_walk_boldly_toward_them) This TED Talk examines implicit bias and actionable steps to address it, making it relevant for healthcare professionals aiming to foster equitable care.
3. **Project implicit** (https://implicit.harvard.edu/implicit/) This resource is instrumental in helping medical professionals recognize and mitigate their own biases. It is a widely recognized tool for measuring implicit biases.
4. **Mind Bugs by Mahzarin R. Banaji** (Ted Talk: https://www.youtube.com/watch?v=AFEaCFFsM2U) Dr. Banaji, a pioneer in implicit bias research, discusses cognitive biases and their impact, reinforcing the importance of addressing unconscious prejudices in medicine.
5. **Overcoming cultural stereotypes by CookRoss, inc.** (YouTube: https://www.youtube.com/watch?v=MDw68BQxKEk) This video highlights how cultural stereotypes impact interpersonal interactions, reinforcing the importance of awareness and training in medical education to mitigate biases.
6. **Everyday Bias: Identifying and navigating unconscious judgments by Howard Ross** (YouTube. https://www.youtube.com/watch?v=v01SxXui9XQ) Howard Ross explores unconscious bias and its pervasive influence, offering practical strategies relevant to addressing bias in medical decision-making and patient care.

Support for Curricular Planning and Activities:

1. **Association of American Medical Colleges Diversity, equity, and inclusion competencies across the learning continuum** (https://store.aamc.org/diversity-equity-and-inclusion-competencies-across-the-learning-continuum.html) This AAMC resource outlines DEI competencies essential for structuring equitable medical education and integrating bias-free training models
2. **American Academy of Family Physicians Implicit Bias Training Facilitator Guide.** (https://www.aafp.org/dam/AAFP/documents/patient_care/health_equity/implicit-bias-training-facilitator-guide.pdf?refID=renewbs) This facilitator guide offers structured approaches for implementing implicit bias training in medical curricula, enhancing awareness and accountability in clinical practice

Chapter 3: Intersectionality: Where Identities Collide

This chapter explores how intersectionality, including race, gender, disability, religion, and age, contributes to discriminatory practices that impact health outcomes. The resources provide additional context into each of the aforementioned topics in the hopes of challenging biases, facilitating meaningful discussion, and encouraging ideas of how we can improve health equity for patients.

Written Texts

1. *The Association Between Racial Microaggressions and Depressive Symptoms: A Cross-Sectional Analysis by M.* Aquino and M. Budescu, Psi Chi Journal of Psychological Research, 2021. Explores the psychological impact of racial microaggressions, emphasizing how these subtle yet pervasive forms of discrimination contribute to mental health disparities in marginalized communities.
2. *Legacies of Ableism and the Pursuit of Disability Justice in Medicine by A.* Banerjee, The Lancet, 2025. Examines the historical and ongoing challenges of ableism in medicine, advocating for disability justice as a necessary framework for equitable healthcare practices.
3. *Midwives' and Other Perinatal Health Workers' Perceptions of the Black Maternal Mortality Crisis in the United States by* M. Craft-Blacksheare and P. Kahn, 2022. Highlights the perspectives of perinatal health workers on the disproportionate maternal mortality rates among Black women, underscoring systemic racism and the need for culturally competent care.

4. *How do ageism, death anxiety and aging anxiety among medical students and residents affect their attitude towards medical care for older patients: a systematic review* by E. J. Draper, et. al., BMC Medical Education, 2024. Investigates how biases against aging influence medical education and provider attitudes toward elderly patients, impacting their care and overall health outcomes.
5. *Promoting Health Care Equity: The Instrumentality of Medicare and Medicaid in Fighting Ableism within the American Health Care System* by E. Earl, Seton Hall Law Review, 2023. Analyzes how Medicare and Medicaid policies have historically addressed, or failed to address, healthcare access issues for disabled individuals, providing a legal perspective on health equity.
6. *A Bioarchaeological Study of African American Health and Mortality in the Post-Emancipation U.S. South.* By M. Franklin and S. M. Wilson, American Antiquity, 2020. Provides a historical perspective on racial disparities in health by examining skeletal remains, offering insights into the long-term effects of systemic racism on African American health outcomes.
7. *Addressing the National Crisis Facing Black and Latina Women, Birthing People, and Infants: The Maternal and Child Health Equity Summit* by M. Krishnamoorthi, et. al., Obstetrics & Gynecology, 2023. Discusses the findings of a national summit addressing racial disparities in maternal and infant health, providing policy recommendations and strategies for improvement.
8. *Do race, neglect, and childhood poverty predict physical health in adulthood? A multilevel prospective analysis* by V. Nikulina and C.S. Widom, Child Abuse & Neglect, 2014. Examines the long-term health consequences of childhood poverty, neglect, and racial disparities, emphasizing the role of early-life experiences in shaping adult health outcomes.
9. *Born on the Wrong Side of the Tracks: Exploring the Causal Effects of Segregation on Infant Health* by H. Vu, et. al., Journal of Health Economics, 2024. Investigates how residential segregation affects infant health, linking systemic inequities in housing and neighborhood conditions to disparities in birth outcomes.
10. *Intersectionality in Clinical Medicine: The Need for a Conceptual Framework* by Y. Wilson, et. al., The American Journal of Bioethics, 2019. Calls for the integration of intersectionality into clinical medicine, providing a conceptual framework to address disparities and improve culturally responsive care.

Multimedia Resources

1. **Intersectionality – The Interconnectedness of Class, Gender, Race and Other Types of Vulnerability by Somnath Saha, MD, MPH** (Youtube: https://www.youtube.com/watch?v=tJI08-qsMUw) This short video supplies a graphic representation of intersectionality to assist in conceptualization. This may also

be incorporated within an activity for students to follow along in real-time, gauging their intersectionality.

2. **The Urgency of Intersectionality by Kimberle Crenshaw** (YouTube: https://www.youtube.com/watch?v=akOe5-UsQ2o) This video featuring the originator of the theory of intersectionality highlights how individuals can have multiple forms of exclusion as well, emphasizing how it manifests in prejudice and discrimination
3. **On the Pulse, Episode 22: From Ableism to Disability Advocate by Dr. Bonnie Swenor** (YouTube: https://youtu.be/9_yN6iyT6QY?si=USiLlUOpiN66rkA2) This auditory-only video features Dr. Bonnie Swenor of the Johns Hopkins School of Nursing talks about her personal experience with a disability and how that propelled her into a career in disability equity research and advocacy.
4. **Addressing Ageism in Medicine by Jesse Katz, MD** (YouTube: https://www.youtube.com/watch?v=PrrOd0UA3ZA) This is a part of the Geriatric Grand Rounds by Gerontology and Geriatrics fellow Jesse Katz at the University of Washington. With scenarios and discussion, it highlights bias in medicine against ageing adults.
5. **Religion and Medicine: a Dialogue with Health Care Providers on Navigation Religious Diversity** (YouTube: https://www.youtube.com/watch?v=agO6qm1V9rQ) Although Western medical practices today are shaped more by science, religious views still strongly influence many people and what they expect from caregivers. As a result, religious literacy and the skills of dialogue are essential for medical caregivers. Join us for a dialogue centered on the relationship between religion and medicine and hear our panelists' experiences navigating diverse religious orientations among their patients.

Additional Resources

1. **Racism, Sexism and Unconscious Bias by Denise Rodgers MD** (Youtube: https://www.youtube.com/watch?v=Z6Gy4xVmhYo)
2. **Why Rural Matters by Frederick Chen MD, MPH** (Youtube: https://www.youtube.com/watch?v=AY0UWkkDQj8)
3. **Immigrant Populations by Michael Rodriguez, MD, MPH** (Youtube: https://www.youtube.com/watch?v=tUUtRf8e9dw)

Support for Curricular Planning and Activities

1. **Disability and Ableism in Medicine: A Curriculum for Medical Students** (https://www.mededportal.org/doi/10.15766/mep_2374-8265.11073#:~:text=Educationa%20Objectives,address%20ableist%20norms%20and%20practices)

This curriculum offers future physicians opportunities to engage critically with issues related to disability and to consider strategies to improve care for this population, medical education can play a role in addressing our healthcare system's failures to adequately serve patients with disabilities. The curriculum is built on the structural competency curriculum published on *MedEdPORTAL* by Joshua Neff and colleagues.

2. **Issues of Poverty by Southern Poverty Law Center** (https://www.learningforjustice.org/classroom-resources/lessons/issues-of-poverty) "Issues of Poverty" is comprised of four lessons with two overarching goals. First, the lessons aim to help students understand that poverty is systemic and rooted in economics, politics, and discrimination. Second, the lessons provide evidence to show that poverty, far from being random, disproportionately affects Americans who have traditionally experienced oppression—African Americans, Latinos, immigrants, and children.

Chapter 4. Socioeconomic Status: Challenges From Medicaid Spend-Down to Information Technology Issues

This chapter investigates the multifaceted impact of socioeconomic status (SES) on healthcare access, quality, and outcomes. These resources emphasize systemic inequities and provide curricular and clinical strategies to dismantle structural barriers, supporting future healthcare professionals in delivering equitable, informed, and accessible care.

Written Texts

1. *Structural racism and health inequities in the USA: Evidence and interventions* by Z. D. Bailey, et. al., The Lancet, 2017. This article provides critical insights into how structural racism exacerbates socioeconomic disparities in health outcomes, reinforcing discussions on systemic barriers in healthcare.
2. *The social determinants of health: It's time to consider the causes of the causes* by P. Braveman and L. Gottlieb, Public Health Reports, 2014. This foundational article explores how socioeconomic determinants shape health outcomes, reinforcing the chapter's discussion on systemic barriers to care.
3. *Social causes of health and disease* by W. C. Cockerham, Polity Press, 2021. This book explores the intersection of socioeconomic factors and health, illustrating the broader societal implications of medical inequities.

4. *Estimated deaths attributable to social factors in the United States* by S. Galea, et. al., American journal of public health, 2011. This study quantifies the impact of social determinants on mortality, providing empirical evidence on the effects of socioeconomic disparities in healthcare.
5. *Achieving population health in accountable care organizations* by K. Hacker and D. K. Walker, American journal of public health, 2013. This article examines the role of policy interventions in mitigating socioeconomic disparities, supporting recommendations for systemic reforms in the chapter.
6. *The social psychology of class and classism* by B. Lott, American Psychologist, 2012. This resource provides an overview of class and classism. This is helpful in assisting students in identifying different experiences that one may have and thus considering questions they may not have asked before and beliefs that may be challenged by this reality.
7. *Communities in Action: Pathways to Health Equity* by The National Academies of Sciences, Engineering, and Medicine, The National Academies Press, 2017. This book provides a comprehensive review of community-driven efforts to address health inequities, aligning with discussions on access to care and resource distribution.
8. *Essentials of the U.S. health care system* by L. Shi and D. A. Singh, Jones & Bartlett Learning, 2020. This text provides an overview of the structural components of the U.S. healthcare system and illustrates systemic barriers to access and affordability for low-income populations.
9. *The inner level: How more equal societies reduce stress, restore sanity, and improve everyone's well-being* by R. Wilkinson and K. Pickett, Allen Lane, 2018. This book examines the psychological and social impact of economic inequality, emphasizing how socioeconomic disparities shape overall well-being and health.
10. *How are income and wealth linked to health and longevity?* by S. H. Woolf, et. al., The Urban Institute, 2015. This study examines the relationship between economic stability and health outcomes, supporting discussions on wealth accessibility and healthcare affordability.

Multimedia Resources:

1. **Social inequalities in health by National Institutes of Health (NIH).** (YouTube: https://www.youtube.com/watch?v=roAQHn5rEoQ) This NIH video provides an in-depth analysis of how social and economic disparities influence health outcomes, reinforcing the chapter's discussion on structural inequalities and access to care

2. **Medicaid & CHIP: Health coverage for low-income Americans by KFF (Kaiser Family Foundation)** (YouTube: https://youtu.be/f9NUCvrrRz4?si=rfx3MCqpX8otH4M2) This video explains Medicaid policies and challenges, complementing the chapter's focus on spend-down policies and payer laws.
3. **The poverty clinic: Healing the long-term effects of childhood adversity** (TEDTalk: https://youtu.be/95ovIJ3dsNk?si=yZTOpZadJStvRB3Y) This TEDx Talk explores the relationship between socioeconomic status and health outcomes, reinforcing discussions on resource scarcity and long-term health consequences.
4. **Health disparities and technology: Bridging the digital divide by the Association of American Medical Colleges** (https://aamc.elevate.commpartners.com/products/advancing-health-equity-through-telehealth-aamc-learning-series) This webinar series highlights disparities in healthcare access due to technological barriers, relevant to the chapter's discussion on IT issues in healthcare accessibility.

Support for Curricular Planning and Activities:

1. **Access to Health Services by Healthy People 2030** (https://odphp.health.gov/healthypeople/priority-areas/social-determinants-health/literature-summaries/access-health-services) This government resource provides a detailed overview of the objectives for Healthy People alongside data. This can be used for additional learning as well as projects incorporating data-driven insights into policy changes and systemic reforms needed to address socioeconomic disparities.
2. **SPENT** (https://playspent.org/) SPENT is a virtual poverty simulation giving learners the opportunity to see how difficult it can be to live at or below the poverty line. We acknowledge that this resource cannot fully portray the experiences of those living at or below the poverty line however, it can assist learners who have never been exposed to think critically about matters of socioeconomic status.

Chapter 5. Race: The Implications of Historical Oppression on Healthcare

This chapter explores how historical oppression, systemic racism, and racially biased medical practices have shaped contemporary healthcare inequities. Drawing from interdisciplinary sources, these resources offer a holistic view for understanding how racial constructs were embedded into the foundations of medicine and continue to influence clinical decision-making, provider-patient relationships, and institutional practices as well as ways to mitigate this impact.

Written Texts

1. *Medical Apartheid,* By Harriet Washington, Doubleday, 2006. This book explores the historical, ethical, and social impacts of racism in in medical experimentation and expansion in the US.
2. *Medical Bondage: Race, Gender, and the Origins of American Gynecology* By Deidre Cooper Owens, University of Georgia Press, 2017 This resource details the experiments of Dr. James Marion Sims, who exploited females who were enslaved as test subjects which acts as an essential case study.
3. *Hidden in Plain Sight — Reconsidering the Use of Race Correction in Clinical Algorithms* by D.A. Vyas, et. al., New England Journal of Medicine, 2020. This resource presents an overview of race corrections in a variety of medical specialties impacting diagnosis and treatment of disease which contributes to racial health disparities.
4. *Black and Blue*, By John Hoberman, University of California Press, 2012. This book discusses the historical background of racism in medicine and discusses how racism impacts the treatment of different organs and specialties. It also has a chapter about educating against racism in medical schools.
5. *Race and Medicine in Nineteenth- and Early Twentieth-Century America* By Todd L. Savitt, Kent State University Press, 2007. This resource provides a compilation of articles detailing the historical background of race and medicine during times of slavery, including experimentation on slaves, diseases disproportionately affecting Black Americans during the time, and medical education of Black physicians.

Additional Resources

1. *Levels of Racism: A Theoretic Framework and a Gardener's Tale* by Camara Phyllis Jones, MD, MPH, PhD, American Journal of Public Health, 2000.
2. *Me and White Supremacy: Combat Racism, Change the World, and Be a Good Ancestor* by L. Saad, Sourcebooks, 2020.
3. *Conquering the Health Disparities of Structural Racism* by Christen Johnson, MD, MPH, Journal of Public Health Management and Practice, 2021.
4. *White Privilege: Unpacking the Invisible Knapsack* By Peggy McIntosh, 1989.
5. *The psychology of American Racism* by Roberts & Rizzo, The American Psychologist 76(3), 2021.
6. *Antiracism: An Introduction* by Zamalin, New York University Press, 2019.

7. *Systemic racism and US health care* by J. Feagin and Z. Bennefiled, Social Science and Medicine, 2013.
8. *Structural racism and supporting black lives role of health professionals* by R. Hardeman, et. al., New England Journal of Medicine, 2016.
9. *A 'Forgotten History' Of How The U.S. Government Segregated America* by T. Gross, National Public Radio, 2017.

Multimedia Resources

1. **Clinical Problem Solvers: Antiracism in Medicine Episode 1** (Podcast: https://clinicalproblemsolving.com/2020/08/25/episode-120-antiracism-in-medicine-series-episode-1-racism-police-violence-and-health/) This podcast is a series about racism in medicine. The first episode addresses structural racism and how that impacts clinical practice.
2. **The Problem with Race-Based Medicine by Dorothy Roberts** (TedTalk: https://www.youtube.com/watch?v=KxLMjn4WPBY) This resource provides an overview of how race can impact the diagnosis and treatment of disease.
3. **How Racism makes us sick by David Williams** (Ted Talk: https://www.youtube.com/watch?v=VzyjDR_AWzE) This Ted Talk discusses ways that discrimination may impact health, including implicit bias and social determinants of health
4. **Maintaining Cultural Humility by CookRoss, Inc.** (Youtube: https://www.youtube.com/watch?v=NLCSOZuhdJk) This short video explains the concept of cultural humility, which is one of the pillars of Physician Cultural Responsibility.

Support for Curricular Planning and Activities:

1. **Teaching About Racism in the Context of Persistent Health and Healthcare Disparities: How Educators Can Enlighten Themselves and Their Learners Toolkit Society of Teachers of Family Medicine** (https://health.uconn.edu/faculty-development/wp-content/uploads/sites/69/2016/12/stfm_toolkit.pdf) This resources provides a framework of how to teach about race, aligned with Physician Cultural Responsbilitiy, with activities that can be used in education about racism.
2. **Twelve Tips for Implementing and Teaching Anti-racism Curriculum in Medical Education by M. Racic, Medical Teacher 2023.** (https://doi.org/10.1080/0142159X.2023.2206534) This resource provides guidance and practical tips for curriculum development surrounding topics of race and racism.

Chapter 6. Sex: Enduring Invisibility and Its Impact on Healthcare

The selected written texts explore the historical exclusion of women from medical education and practice, the continued underrepresentation of women in leadership roles, and biases in research that have led to gaps in diagnosing and treating female patients. These resources also examine the long-term health consequences of gender bias, highlighting disparities in pain management, reproductive healthcare, and clinical decision-making.

Written Texts

1. *The Yentl Syndrome and Women's Cardiovascular Health: The Gender Bias in Medical Treatment* by C. N. Bairey Merz, et. al., Circulation, 2017. Examines how gender bias in cardiology has led to misdiagnosis and undertreatment of heart disease in women.
2. *The Fibromyalgia Story: Medical Authority and Women's Worlds of Pain* by K.K. Barker, Temple University Press, 2011. Examines how gendered perceptions of pain conditions, such as fibromyalgia, have led to delays in diagnosis and treatment for women.
3. *Disparities in Women's Health Research Funding: A Call for Equity in Biomedical Research Priorities* by V. L. Bonham, et. al., Journal of Health Politics, Policy, and Law, 2021. Analyzes the gender gap in biomedical research funding and its impact on healthcare advancements for women's health.
4. *Invisible Women: Data Bias in a World Designed for Men* by C. Criado-Perez, Abrams Press, 2019. Investigates how gender bias in medical research has led to gaps in understanding women's health, from underrepresentation in clinical trials to misdiagnosis of conditions affecting women.
5. *Gender Medicine: The Groundbreaking New Science of Gender- and Sex-Based Diagnosis and Treatment* by M. Glezerman, Abrams Press, 2016. Explores how sex-based physiological differences should inform medical treatment and clinical guidelines.
6. *Gender Bias in Medicine* by K. Hamberg, Women's Health, 2008. Investigates implicit biases in medical training and practice that lead to differential treatment of male and female patients.
7. *Racial Bias in Pain Assessment and Treatment Recommendations, and False Beliefs About Biological Differences Between Blacks and Whites* by K.M. Hoffman, et. al., Proceedings of the National Academy of Sciences, 2016. Highlights how both racial and gender biases influence pain management, leading to disparities in treatment and patient outcomes.

8. *Biological Sex, Gender, and Women's Health: Implications for Research, Clinical Practice, and Policy* by L. Klein and R. Correa-de-Araujo, Journal of Women's Health, 2020. Discusses the necessity of incorporating sex-based differences in medical research and clinical practice to ensure equitable healthcare outcomes.
9. *Bibliometric Analysis of Global Research Output on Gender Bias in Medicine (2000–2020)* by W. M. Sweileh, Journal of Global Health, 2021. Reviews research trends on gender bias in healthcare, highlighting key themes and gaps in the literature.
10. *Sexism in Medical Education: The History and Impact of Women's Exclusion from Medicine* by J. Wainer and J. Carline, Journal of Women's Health, 2010. Provides historical context on the exclusion of women from medical education, examining how institutional barriers shaped the gender disparities seen in medicine today.

Additional Resources

1. *Unwell women: Misdiagnosis and Myth in a Man-Made World* by E. Cleghorn, Penguin Press, 2021.
2. *The pain gap: How Sexism and Racism in Healthcare Kill Women* by A. Hossain, Simon and Schuster, 2021.

Multimedia Resources

1. **Gender bias creates a culture of disbelief for female patients by Colene Arnold** (Ted Talk: https://www.youtube.com/watch?v=U1XvFSoUhWI) Explores how gender bias affects patient care and outcomes, providing insights into recognizing and mitigating these biases in clinical settings.
2. **How HerMD's Dr. Somi Javaid is Revolutionizing Women's Healthcare by The Pain Gap Podcast** (Podcast: https://www.youtube.com/watch?v=lMEp1pTwFuw) Podcast Host and directed by the author of Pain Gap which examines the Inequities and inequalities in diagnostic, care and treatment of gender and race in the US
3. **Advancing women's health equity by Dr. Veena Babu** (Ted Talk: https://www.youtube.com/watch?v=Fv_o11Th18Q) Discussing Pain Management in Women Menses and Society expectations.
4. **Seasoned Women's Health Matters by Vanessa Hill** (Ted Talk: https://www.youtube.com/watch?v=1EslC_HEJMw) This resource discusses women's health in the view of ageism.

Support for Curricular Planning and Activities

1. **GWIMS Toolkits by the Association of American Medical Colleges** (https://www.aamc.org/career-development/affinity-groups/gwims/toolkit) This toolkit provides numerous resources for curricular planning.
2. **Health Equity Curricular Toolkit by the American Academy of Family Physicians** (https://www.aafp.org/family-physician/patient-care/the-everyone-project/health-equity-tools.html) Provides 14 modules including resources on sexism in patient care.

Chapter 7. Gender and Sexual Orientation: Embracing the Intersectionality of Identity

These texts, studies, and multimedia sources can be helpful in academic settings, navigating the healthcare system, and supporting marginalized communities. These resources provide essential insights into provider bias, systemic discrimination, and the structural barriers that affect equitable care, reinforcing the importance of affirming, multidisciplinary, and policy-driven healthcare solutions.

Written Texts

1. *Sex and gender in neurodevelopmental conditions* by S. Bölte, et. al, Nature reviews, 2023. This peer-reviewed article explores the impact of sex (binary or otherwise) on the patient and its manifestation of illness. Demonstrate that sex, gender, and sexuality can impact multiple facets of health and illness.
2. *Three essays on the theory of sexuality: The 1905 Edition* by S. Freud, Verso Books, 2017. These essays explore early theoretical ideological frameworks of sexuality and identity. Providing historical context for contemporary understanding/misunderstanding of gender and sexual orientation.
3. *How the Clinic Made Gender: The Medical History of a Transformative Idea* by S. Eder, University of Chicago Press, 2022. An investigation of how clinical institutions have historically shaped concepts of gender, shedding light on the medicalization and pathologization of identity.
4. *Clinician's guide to LGBTQIA+ care: Cultural Safety and Social Justice in Primary, Sexual, and Reproductive Healthcare* by R. LAc, et. al., Springer Publishing Company. 2021. A guide centered on cultural humility and justice in clinical practice, offering a structural competency approach to LGBTQIA+ healthcare.

5. *Clinical practice guidelines for transsexual, transgender, and gender diverse minors* by A. Moral-Martos, et al., Annals of Pediatrics, 2022. Provides ideas for Clinical guidelines that provide age-specific, evidence-based recommendations for affirming care and promoting health outcomes for gender-diverse youth.
6. *Bodies in Doubt: An American History of Intersex* by E, Reis, JHU Press, 2021. This is a historical text that explores the treatment and perception of intersex bodies in the U.S., highlighting how medicine has enforced binary understandings of sex and gender.
7. *Transgender history* by S. Stryker, Seal Press, 2008. This accessible chronicle outlines key events and movements in transgender history, illuminating the socio-political struggles that have shaped medical and social understandings of gender identity.
8. *Black on both sides: A Racial History of Trans Identity* by C. R. Snorton, University of Minnesota Press, 2017. An exploration of the intersection of race and gender through a historical lens, demonstrating how trans identity is racialized within medical and cultural discourse.
9. *Lesbian, gay, bisexual, and transgender healthcare: A Clinical Guide to Preventive, Primary, and Specialist Care* by K. Eckstrand and J. M. Ehrenfeld, Springer Books, 2016. A clinical guide offers evidence-based practices for delivering inclusive care to LGBTQIA+ populations, making it essential for promoting health equity through affirming medical education.
10. *This book is gay* by J. Dawson, Sourcebooks Fire, 2021. This book demystifies LGBTQIA+ identities and experiences for young audiences, reinforcing the need for inclusive educational practices and curricula.

Multimedia Resources

1. **AACAP SOGIIC Resource Center** (https://www.aacap.org/AACAP/Member_Resources/SOGIIC/SOGIIC.aspx) Provides curated tools and position statements to support clinicians and educators addressing the mental health needs of LGBTQ+ youth.
2. **The Fenway Institute - LGBTQIA+ Health Education Center** (https://www.lgbtqiahealtheducation.org/resources/type/collection/) Offers clinical and community-based learning modules to advance culturally competent LGBTQIA+ care.
3. **CHC Gender Identity & Sexuality Resource Library.** (https://www.chconline.org/resourcelibrary/gender-identity-sexuality-resources/) A youth-focused library of articles, toolkits, and videos for supporting inclusive discussions on gender and sexual orientation.

4. **VNACJ LGBTQ Center for Health & Wellness** (https://lgbtqhealthcenter.org/) Serves as a model for patient-centered care, addressing health disparities through advocacy, education, and direct services.
5. **AAMC LGBTQ+ Health Videos** (https://www.aamc.org/about-us/equity-diversity-inclusion/lgbt-health-resources/videos) Provides faculty development materials and educational videos that promote equity and inclusion in LGBTQ+ medical education.

Support for Curricular Planning and Activities

1. **The Safe Zone Project** (https://thesafezoneproject.com/activities/) This resource offers interactive training modules and discussion-based activities designed to promote LGBTQIA+ inclusion in educational and clinical environments. It supports competency-based learning and fosters cultural humility among healthcare providers.
2. **Advocates for Youth** (https://www.advocatesforyouth.org/) This platform provides evidence-based resources and youth-centered advocacy tools to promote inclusive sexual health education, making it a vital curricular asset for addressing gender and sexual orientation through an intersectional and justice-focused lens.

Chapter 8. Intercultural Communication: An Effective Strategy for the Patient-Physician Relationship

Intercultural communication can reduce misinterpretation and miscommunication between physicians and patients. This enhances patient outcomes, trust, and health equity. The following resources assist in cultivating the communication skills to treat every patient equitably.

Written Texts

1. *Patient-Physician Communication in Intercultural Settings: An Integrative Review* by M. Alkhamees and I. Alasqah, Heliyon. 2023. This resource provides an overview of best practices and challenges in patient-physician communication across different cultural backgrounds.
2. *Cross-Cultural Patient Counseling and Communication in the Integrative Medicine Setting: Respecting the Patient's Health Belief Model of Care* by E. Ben-Arye, et. al., Current psychiatry reports,2024. This article provides a valuable perspective on cross-cultural communication in integrative medicine

by emphasizing the importance of respecting patients' health belief models in clinical interactions.

3. *Teaching Intracultural and Intercultural Communication: A Critique Suggested Method* by D. DeVoss, et. al., Journal of Business and Technical Communication. 2002. This resources explores methods for teaching and applying intercultural communication skills in professional and healthcare settings.
5. *Physician Cultural Competence and Patient Ratings of the Patient-Physician Relationship* by K. Paez, et. al., Journal of General Internal Medicine, 2009. The authors investigate how physician cultural competence directly impacts patient satisfaction and trust.
6. *The Role of Language in Effective Communication in the Medical Field: A Study of Doctor-Patient Interaction* by S. Rahmawati, et. al., APEBSKID International Conference on Multidisciplinary Studies. 2024. This study examines the role of language and linguistic barriers in shaping effective physician-patient interactions.
7. *Cultural diversity in health and illness* by R. Spector, Pearson. 2017. This is a foundational text that examines the impact of cultural beliefs, values, and practices on health, illness, and healthcare delivery which impact communication..
8. *Diversity in Clinical Practice: A Practical & Shame-Free Guide to reducing cultural offenses & Repairing Cross-Cultural relationships* by L. Fisher, PESI Publishing, Incorporated, 2021. This resource offers a pragmatic approach to navigating cultural differences in healthcare settings. This resource emphasizes self-awareness, cultural humility, and strategies for addressing and repairing missteps in cross-cultural interactions, making it highly relevant to the chapter's focus on intercultural communication.
9. *Health Equity, Diversity, and Inclusion: Context, controversies, and solutions: Context, Controversies, and Solutions* by P. R. Rose, Jones & Bartlett Learning, 2020. This text provides a comprehensive analysis of the systemic factors influencing healthcare disparities, including cultural, racial, and socioeconomic barriers to equitable patient care.

Multimedia Resources:

1. **Intercultural communication in healthcare by TargetHIV** (YouTube: https://www.youtube.com/watch?v=IcnViEfqTJ) This resource offers an outline of multiple areas of identity and ways to be culturally aware within patient interactions.
2. **Communication with patients of different cultures by Nursing Surgery Group 4** (YouTube: https://www.youtube.com/watch?v=XRrcGODv6ik) This resource provides a good overview of basic intercultural communication skills

within a relatable learner centered source. Alternatively this can be used as a possible example for a learning activity.

3. **Psychosocial and Cultural considerations for providing healthcare to immigrant and refugee populations by M. Santana** (Podcast: https://clinicalproblemsolving.com/2023/05/02/episode-285-anti-racism-in-medicine-series-episode-21-psychosocial-and-cultural-considerations-for-providing-healthcare-to-immigrant-and-refugee-populations/) This podcast describes multiple considerations for patient interactions with those from immigrant and refugee populations including the impacts of trauma.
4. **Understanding health experiences and values in order to address social determinants of health by Nancy Pandhi, MD, MPH, PhD.** (YouTube: https://www.youtube.com/watch?v=OQXJ0iDS2SY) This presentation describes the necessity of centering patient interactions around patient values which is critical in intercultural communication.
5. **Patient communication: cultural and healthcare by Christine Von Raesfeld** (YouTube: https://www.youtube.com/watch?v=zl95VMCoDP8) This video provides a patient account of the importance of intercultural communication and what can happen without it.

Support for Curricular Planning and Activities:

1. **Cross Cultural Education for Medical Students by the Association of American Medical Colleges** (https://www.aamc.org/media/20856/download#:~:text=The%20intent%20of%20a%20cultural,members%20of%20the%20medical%20community) This AAMC resource provides framework for evaluating cross-cultural experiences with communication in medical training.
2. **Think Cultural Health** (https://thinkculturalhealth.hhs.gov/education) This resource offers training modules on cultural humility and effective communication strategies for healthcare professionals.

Chapter 9. Stigma: Intersection of Oppression and Medicine

This chapter examines how intersectional oppression contributes to the stigmatization of pain management, creating barriers to equitable patient care. By integrating evidence-based research, real-world case studies, and multimedia resources, these additional materials provide a deeper understanding of how bias, policy, and systemic structures shape disparities in pain treatment across diverse patient identities.

Written Texts

1. *A historical review of pain disparities research: Advancing toward health equity and empowerment* by S. Q. Booker, et al. Nursing Outlook, 2023. This article explores historical trends in pain disparities research, providing a foundation for understanding the systemic nature of inequities in pain management.
2. *Toward the Social Communication Model of Pain* by K. D. Craig, In Vervoort, T., et al. (Eds.), Social and Interpersonal Dynamics in Pain, Springer, 2018. This book chapter examines the role of social communication in pain perception, reinforcing how stigma influences patient-provider interactions.
3. *Bias in Musculoskeletal Pain Management and Bias-Targeted Interventions to Improve Pain Outcomes: A Scoping Review* by B. Eze, et al. Orthopedic Nursing, 2022. This scoping review highlights implicit biases in musculoskeletal pain treatment, identifying interventions to improve outcomes for marginalized populations.
4. *The Pain Gap: How Sexism and Racism in Healthcare Kill Women* by A. Hossain, Simon and Schuster, 2022. This book explores how gender and racial biases impact pain management, contributing to disparities in medical treatment.
5. *Pain and Prejudice: How the Medical System Ignores Women—and What We Can Do About It* by G. Jackson, Greystone Books, 2021. This book investigates systemic gender biases in healthcare, particularly in the context of pain management and medical decision-making.
6. *Social Determinants and Consequences of Pain: Toward Multilevel, Intersectional, and Life Course Perspectives* by F.P. Kapos, et al., Journal of Pain, 2024 This article examines social determinants of pain, emphasizing the need for an intersectional approach to understanding disparities.
7. *The History of Pain* by R. Rey, Harvard University Press. (1995) This historical analysis provides insight into evolving perspectives on pain and its medicalization over time.
8. *Sitting Pretty: The View from My Ordinary Resilient Disabled Body* by R. Taussig, HarperOne. 2020 This memoir highlights lived experiences of chronic pain and disability, providing a patient-centered perspective on stigma in healthcare.
9. *The Body Keeps the Score: Brain, Mind, and Body in the Healing of Trauma* by B.A. Van Der Kolk, Penguin Books. 2015 This book explores how trauma affects pain perception, linking psychological and physiological responses to stigma in medicine.
10. *Disability Visibility: First-Person Stories from the Twenty-First Century* by A. Wong, Vintage. 2020. This anthology provides firsthand narratives of individuals with disabilities, shedding light on the intersection of pain, identity, and healthcare disparities.

Multimedia Resources

1. **Dancing through the pain of Ehlers-Danlos Syndrome by Attitude** (YouTube: https://www.youtube.com/watch?v=-ba4OC1FqBY) This video highlights the challenges of living with chronic pain conditions, emphasizing the resilience of patients navigating stigma in medical settings.
2. **The Bias Behind Your Undiagnosed Chronic Pain by S. DeCaria** (TED Talk: https://www.ted.com/talks/sheetal_decaria_the_bias_behind_your_undiagnosed_chronic_pain) This TED Talk examines how stigma contributes to undiagnosed and undertreated chronic pain, particularly among marginalized populations.
3. **Interdisciplinary Panel Discussion: Racial/Ethnic Disparities in Pain Management by Michigan Pharmacy** (YouTube: https://www.youtube.com/watch?v=eLGnpdZp19s) This panel discussion explores stigmatization of racial and ethnic disparities in pain management, incorporating perspectives from multiple healthcare disciplines.
4. **We Are Visible - Trailer 1** (Vimeo. https://vimeo.com/349770539) This documentary trailer provides insight into the lived experiences of individuals with disabilities, reinforcing themes of medical bias and accessibility barriers.

Support for Curricular Planning and Activities

1. **Pain Care and Disparities in Under-Served, Under-Resourced Populations by AAPM Education Center** (https://www.pathlms.com/aapm/courses/20484) This educational resource focuses on pain management in underserved populations, offering frameworks for reducing disparities in care.
2. **ASA-AAOS Pain Alleviation Toolkit** (https://www.asahq.org/advocacy-and-asapac/advocacy-topics/pain-medicine-talking-points/the-pain-toolkit) This toolkit provides clinicians with strategies to improve pain treatment equity and reduce bias in medical decision-making.

Compilation of References

AAMC. (2021). *Diversity in Medicine: Facts and Figures 2021*. Association of American Medical Colleges.

AAMC. (2022). *The State of Non-male individuals in Academic Medicine*. Association of American Medical Colleges.

AAMC. (2024, March 22). *EDUCATE Act Introduced by Rep. Greg Murphy, M.D.* AAMC. https://www.aamc.org/advocacy-policy/washington-highlights/educate-act-introduced-rep-greg-murphy-md

AAMC. (n.d.). *Figure 11. Percentage of U.S. medical school matriculants planning to practice in an underserved area by race/ethnicity, academic year 2018-2019*. AAMC. https://www.aamc.org/data-reports/workforce/data/figure-11-percentage-us-medical-school-matriculants-planning-practice-underserved-area-race

AARP. (2020, May). *Caregiving in the U.S.* Retrieved from AARP: https://www.aarp.org/content/dam/aarp/ppi/2020/05/executive-summary-caregiving-in-the-united-states.doi.10.26419-2Fppi.00103.003.pdf

Adhikary, D., Barman, S., & Ranjan, R. (2023). Internet-based cognitive behavioural therapy for individuals with depression and chronic health conditions: A systematic review. *Cureus*. Advance online publication. DOI: 10.7759/cureus.37822 PMID: 37213982

ADHS. (2021). *Leading Causes of Death and Health Disparities Among The American Indian and Alaska Native Population in Arizona*. Arizona Department of Health Services Interventions.

Adults Who Report Not Having a Personal Doctor/Health Care Provider by Race/Ethnicity. (2022). KFF.

Allen, J. O., & Sikora, N. (2023). Aging Stigma and the Health of US Adults Over 65: What Do We Know? *Clinical Interventions in Aging*, *18*, 2093–2116. DOI: 10.2147/CIA.S396833 PMID: 38116457

Almazan, A., & Keuroghlian, A. (2021). Association between gender-affirming surgeries and mental health outcomes. *JAMA Surgery*, *156*(7), 611. DOI: 10.1001/jamasurg.2021.0952 PMID: 33909023

American Council on Aging. (2024, January 26). *Spending Down Assets to Become Medicaid Eligible for Nursing Home / Long Term Care*. Retrieved from American Council on Aging: https://www.medicaidplanningassistance.org/medicaid-spend-down/

Anderson, L., & Lane, K. (2023). Hypermobile ehlers-danlos syndrome/hypermobility spectrum disorders in older women: A feasibility study. *Musculoskeletal Care*, *21*(3), 741–748. Advance online publication. DOI: 10.1002/msc.1747 PMID: 36864687

Anderson, N., Lett, E., Ngozi Asabor, E., Hernandez, A., Nguemeni Tiako, M. J., Johnson, C., Rizzo, T. M., Latimore, D., Nunez-Smith, M., & Boatright, D. (2021). The association of microaggressions with depressive symptoms and institutional satisfaction among a national cohort of medical students. *Journal of General Internal Medicine*, *37*(2), 298–307. DOI: 10.1007/s11606-021-06786-6 PMID: 33939079

Ashtari, S., & Taylor, A. (2023). Patients with rare diseases and the power of online support groups: Implications for the medical community. *JMIR Formative Research*, *7*, e41610. DOI: 10.2196/41610 PMID: 37707878

Association of American Medical Colleges. (2018). *Figure 18. Percentage of all active physicians by race/ethnicity, 2018*. AAMC. https://www.aamc.org/data-reports/workforce/interactive-data/figure-18-percentage-all-active-physicians-race/ethnicity-2018

Austin, A., Holzworth, J., & Papciak, R. (2022). Beyond diagnosis: Gender dysphoria feels like a living hell, a nightmare one cannot ever wake up from. *Psychology of Sexual Orientation and Gender Diversity*, *9*(1), 12–20. DOI: 10.1037/sgd0000460

Baker, K., & Restar, A. (2022). Utilization and Costs of Gender-Affirming Care in a Commercially Insured Transgender Population. The Journal of law, medicine & ethics: A journal of the American Society of Law. *Medical Ethics (Burlington, Mass.)*, *50*(3), 456–470. DOI: 10.1017/jme.2022.87 PMID: 36398652

Baker, K., Wilson, L., Sharma, R., Dukhanin, V., McArthur, K., & Robinson, K. (2021). Hormone therapy, mental health, and quality of life among transgender people: A systematic review. *Journal of the Endocrine Society*, *5*(4), bvab011. Advance online publication. DOI: 10.1210/jendso/bvab011 PMID: 33644622

Barnum, M. (2017, July 12). *Do school vouchers 'work'? As the debate heats up, here's what research really says*. Retrieved May 31, 2023, from Charlkbeat: https://www.chalkbeat.org/2017/7/12/21108235/school-choice-vouchers-system-pros-and-cons-research/

Bauer, B. (2023, October 19). *How to Avoid the Medicare Part D Donut Hole*. Retrieved from National Council on Aging: https://www.ncoa.org/article/how-to-avoid-the-medicare-part-d-donut-hole

BBC. (2014). *Ethics: a general introduction*. Retrieved from What is ethics?: https://www.bbc.co.uk/ethics/introduction/intro_1.shtml

Beavis, A. S. W., Hojjati, A., Kassam, A., Choudhury, D., Fraser, M., Masching, R., & Nixon, S. A. (2015). What All Students in Healthcare Training Programs Should Learn to Increase Health Equity: Perspectices on postcolonialsm and the health of Aboriginal peoples in Canada. *BMC Medical Education*, *15*(155), 155. DOI: 10.1186/s12909-015-0442-y PMID: 26400722

Beckford, D., & Johnson, J. (2018). The dual barriers of race and gender in medical professions. *Journal of Black Studies*, *49*(5), 549–567.

Beckman, H. B., Markakis, K. M., Suchman, A. L., & Frankel, R. M. (1994). The doctor-patient relationship and malpractice: Lessons from plaintiff depositions. *Archives of Internal Medicine*, *154*(12), 1365–1370. DOI: 10.1001/archinte.1994.00420120093010 PMID: 8002688

Bediako, S., Lanzkron, S., Diener-West, M., Onojobi, G., Beach, M., & Haywood, C.Jr. (2014). The measure of sickle cell stigma: Initial findings from the improving patient outcomes through respect and trust study. *Journal of Health Psychology*, *21*(5), 808–820. DOI: 10.1177/1359105314539530 PMID: 24997169

Berkman, N. D., Sheridan, S. L., Donahue, K. E., Halpern, D. J., & Crotty, K. (2011). Low health literacy and health outcomes: An updated systematic review. *Annals of Internal Medicine*, *155*(2), 97–107. DOI: 10.7326/0003-4819-155-2-201107190-00005 PMID: 21768583

Berthold, H. K., Gouni-Berthold, I., Bestehorn, K. P., Böhm, M., & Krone, W. (2008). Physician gender is associated with the quality of type 2 diabetes care. *Journal of Internal Medicine, 264*(4), 340–350. DOI: 10.1111/j.1365-2796.2008.01967.x PMID: 18397244

Betancourt, J. R., Green, A. R., Carrillo, J. E., & Ananeh-Firempong, O.II. (2003). Defining Cultural Competence: A practical framework for addressing racial/ethnic disparities in health and health care. *Public Health Reports, 118*(4), 293–302. DOI: 10.1016/S0033-3549(04)50253-4 PMID: 12815076

Bever, L. (2022, December 13). Women's pain often is dismissed by doctors. Washington Post. https://www.washingtonpost.com/wellness/interactive/2022/women-pain-gender-bias-doctors/

Bhakta, N. R., Bime, C., Kaminsky, D. A., McCormack, M. C., Thakur, N., Stanojevic, S., Baugh, A. D., Braun, L., Lovinsky-Desir, S., Adamson, R., Witonsky, J., Wise, R. A., Levy, S. D., Brown, R., Forno, E., Cohen, R. T., Johnson, M., Balmes, J., Mageto, Y., & Burney, P. (2023). Race and Ethnicity in Pulmonary Function Test Interpretation: An Official American Thoracic Society Statement. *American Journal of Respiratory and Critical Care Medicine, 207*(8), 978–995. DOI: 10.1164/rccm.202302-0310ST PMID: 36973004

Bhatt, N., Cannella, J., & Gentile, J. P. (2022). Gender-affirming Care for Transgender Patients. *Innovations in Clinical Neuroscience, 19*(4-6), 23–32. PMID: 35958971

Bibbins-Domingo, K., & Helman, A. (2022). *Improving Representation in Clinical Trials and Research: Building equity for non-male individuals and underrepresented groups*. The National Academies Press., DOI: 10.17226/26479

Birkhäuer, J., Gaab, J., Kossowsky, J., Hasler, S., Krummenacher, P., Werner, C., & Gerger, H. (2017). Trust in the health care professional and health outcome: A meta-analysis. *PLoS One, 12*(2), e0170988. DOI: 10.1371/journal.pone.0170988 PMID: 28170443

Blackie, M., Wear, D., & Zarconi, J. (2019). Narrative Intersectionality in Caring for Marginalized or Disadvantaged Patients. *Academic Medicine, 94*(1), 59–63. PMID: 30134270

Blakemore, E. (2019, June 27). *How the GI Bill's Promise Was Denied to a Million Black WWII Veterans*. HISTORY. https://www.history.com/news/gi-bill-black-wwii-veterans-benefits

Block, J. (2023). Gender dysphoria in young people is rising—And so is professional disagreement. *BMJ (Clinical Research Ed.)*, 382. DOI: 10.1136/bmj.p382 PMID: 36822640

Bond, R. M., Gaither, K., Nasser, S. A., Albert, M. A., Ferdinand, K. C., Njoroge, J. N., Parapid, B., Hayes, S. N., Pegus, C., Sogade, B., Grodzinsky, A., Watson, K. E., McCullough, C. A., & Ofili, E. (2021). Working Agenda for Black Mothers. *Circulation: Cardiovascular Quality and Outcomes*, *14*(2), e007643. Advance online publication. DOI: 10.1161/CIRCOUTCOMES.120.007643 PMID: 33563007

Boroumand, S., Stein, M. J., Jay, M., Shen, J. W., Hirsh, M., & Dharamsi, S. (2020). Addressing the health advocate role in medical education. *BMC Medical Education*, *20*(28), 1–5. DOI: 10.1186/s12909-020-1938-7 PMID: 32000759

Bowleg, L., Malekzadeh, A., Mbaba, M., & Boone, C. (2022). Ending the hiv epidemic for all, not just some: Structural racism as a fundamental but overlooked social-structural determinant of the us hiv epidemic. *Current Opinion in HIV and AIDS*, *17*(2), 40–45. DOI: 10.1097/COH.0000000000000724 PMID: 35102051

Bradley, K. (2022). *The Socioeconomic Achievement Gap in the US Public Schools*. Retrieved from Ballard Brief: https://ballardbrief.byu.edu/issue-briefs/the-socioeconomic-achievement-gap-in-the-us-public-schools

Brandon, D. T., Isaac, L. A., & LaVeist, T. A. (2005). The legacy of Tuskegee and trust in medical care: Is Tuskegee responsible for race differences in mistrust of medical care? *Journal of the National Medical Association*, *97*(7), 951–956. PMID: 16080664

Braveman, P. A., Cubbin, C., Egerter, S., Williams, D. R., & Pamuk, E. (2010). Socioeconomic disparities in health in the United States: What the patterns tell us. *American Journal of Public Health*, *100*(S1), 186–196. DOI: 10.2105/AJPH.2009.166082 PMID: 20147693

Bremen, J. M. (2023, December 14). *Will Pay Increases Exceed Inflation In2024?* Retrieved from Forbes: https://www.forbes.com/sites/johnbremen/2023/12/14/will-pay-increases-exceed-inflation-in-2024/?sh=233bb2c72266

Briguglio, C. (2006). *Empowering students by developing their intercultural communication competence: A two-way process. Educate, advocate, empower*. ISANA International Education Association Inc.

Brondani, M. A., Alan, R., & Donnelly, L. (2017). Stigma of addiction and mental illness in healthcare: The case of patients' experiences in dental settings. *PLoS One*, *12*(5), e0177388. DOI: 10.1371/journal.pone.0177388 PMID: 28531176

Brookfield, S. D., & Hess, M. E. (2021). *Becoming a White antiracist: A practical guide for educators, leaders, and activists*. Stylus Publishing.

Bulgin, D., Asnani, M., Vorderstrasse, A., Royal, C., Pan, W., & Tanabe, P. (2021). Stigma and quality of life in adults with sickle cell disease in jamaica and the united states. *Psychology Health and Medicine*, *28*(5), 1133–1147. DOI: 10.1080/13548506.2021.2019808 PMID: 34957879

Burke, G. (1980). Ethics and medical decision-making. *Primary Care*, *7*(4), 615–624. DOI: 10.1016/S0095-4543(21)01416-0 PMID: 6908085

Cabana, M. D., Slish, K. K., Evans, D., Mellins, R. B., Brown, R. W., Lin, X., Kaciroti, N., & Clark, N. M. (2014). Impact of physician asthma care education on patient outcomes. *Health Education & Behavior*, *41*(5), 509–517. DOI: 10.1177/1090198114547510 PMID: 25270176

California Healthcare Foundation. (2018). *Listening to Black Mothers in California ISSUE BRIEF*. https://www.nationalpartnership.org/our-work/resources/health-care/maternity/listening-to-black-mothers-in-california.pdf

Cambridge Dictionary. (2025). *Meaning of ethic in English*. Retrieved from Cambridge Dictionary: https://dictionary.cambridge.org/us/dictionary/english/ethic

Camerota, F., Mariani, R., Cordiano, G., Di Trani, M., Lodato, V., Ferraris, A., Pasquini, M., & Celletti, C. (2023). The language of pain in the hypermobile ehlers–danlos syndrome: Metaphors as a key to understanding the experience of pain and as a rehabilitation tool. *Brain Sciences*, *13*(7), 1042. DOI: 10.3390/brainsci13071042 PMID: 37508973

Campbell, C. M., & Edwards, R. R. (2012). Ethnic differences in pain and pain management. *Pain Management*, *2*(3), 219–230. DOI: 10.2217/pmt.12.7 PMID: 23687518

Carrese, J. A. (2006). Refusal of care: patients' well-being and physicians' ethical obligations:"but doctor, I want to go home". *Journal of the American Medical Association*, *296*(6), 691–695. DOI: 10.1001/jama.296.6.691 PMID: 16896112

Cartwright, S. (1851). Diseases and Peculiarities of the Negro Race. *De Bow's Review, 1*(2).

Casanova-Perez, R., Apodaca, C., Bascom, E., Mohanraj, D., Lane, C., Vidyarthi, D., Beneteau, E., Sabin, J., Pratt, W., Weibel, N., & Hartzler, A. L. (2022). Broken down by bias: Healthcare biases experienced by BIPOC and LGBTQ+ patients. *AMIA ... Annual Symposium proceedings.AMIA Symposium,2021*, 275–284.

CDC. (2021, July 22). *Sexually Transmitted Infections Treatment Guidelines,2021.* Retrieved from Adolescents: https://www.cdc.gov/std/treatment-guidelines/adolescents.htm#:~:text=All%2050%20states%20and%20the,the%20allowable%20deductible%20is%20reached

CDC. (2023). *National Overview of STIs in 2023.* Retrieved from STI Statistics: https://www.cdc.gov/sti-statistics/annual/summary.html

CDC. (2024, December 10). *Disability Impacts All of Us Infographic.* Disability and Health. https://www.cdc.gov/disability-and-health/articles-documents/disability-impacts-all-of-us-infographic.html?CDC_AAref_Val=https://www.cdc.gov/ncbddd/disabilityandhealth/infographic-disability-impacts-all.html

CDC. (n.d.). *Centers for Disease Control and Prevention User guide to the 2016 Period Linked Birth/Infant Death Public Use File.* https://ftp.cdc.gov/pub/Health_Statistics/NCHS/Dataset_Documentation/DVS/periodlinked/LinkPE16Guide.pdf

Charter, R., Ussher, J., Perz, J., & Robinson, K. (2021). Negotiating mental health amongst transgender parents in Australia. *International Journal of Transgender Health, 23*(3), 308–320. DOI: 10.1080/26895269.2021.1875951 PMID: 35799955

Chin, M. G., LaGuardia, J. S., Morgan, K. B. J., Ngo, H., Moghadam, S., Huang, K. X., & Lee, J. C. (2023). *United States health policies on gender-affirming care in 2022. Plastic &Amp.* Reconstructive Surgery. DOI: 10.1097/PRS.0000000000010594

Chiper, S. (2013). Teaching intercultural communication: ICT resources and best practices. *Procedia Social and Behavioral Sciences, 93*(2012), 1641–1645.

Chrisler, J. C., Barney, A., & Palatino, B. (2016). Ageism can be hazardous to women's health: Ageism, sexism, and stereotypes of older women in the healthcare system. *The Journal of Social Issues, 72*(1), 86–104. DOI: 10.1111/josi.12157

Clayton, J. A., & Tannenbaum, C. (2016). Sex and gender reporting in health research: Why it matters. *Journal of the American Medical Association, 316*(18), 1863–1864. PMID: 27802482

Cole, E. (2009). Intersectionality and research in psychology. *The American Psychologist, 64*(3), 170–180. DOI: 10.1037/a0014564 PMID: 19348518

Collins, F. S., Morgan, M., & Patrinos, A. (2003). The Human Genome Project: Lessons from Large-Scale Biology. *Science, 300*(5617), 286–290. DOI: 10.1126/science.1084564 PMID: 12690187

Cooper Owens, D. (2017). *Medical Bondage: Race, Gender, and the Origins of American Gynecology.* University of Georgia Press., DOI: 10.2307/j.ctt1pwt69x

Coria, A., McKelvey, T. G., Charlton, P., Woodworth, M., & Lahey, T. (2013). The design of a medical school social justice and curriculum. *Academic Medicine*, *88*(10), 1442–1449. DOI: 10.1097/ACM.0b013e3182a325be PMID: 23969356

Corneau, S. & Stergiopoulos, V. (2012) More than being against it: Anti-racism and anti-oppression in mental health services. Academic Press.

Coutinho, A. J., Nguyen, B., Kelly, C., Lin, K., Gits, A., Crichlow, R., & Moreno, G. (2020). Formal advocacy curricula in family medicine residencies: A CERA survey of program directors. *Family Medicine*, *52*(4), 255–261. PMID: 32267520

Craig, K., Holmes, C., Hudspith, M., Moor, G., Moosa-Mitha, M., Varcoe, C., & Wallace, B. (2019). Pain in persons who are marginalized by social conditions. *Pain*, *161*(2), 261–265. DOI: 10.1097/j.pain.0000000000001719 PMID: 31651578

Creanga, A. A.. (2017). Racial and ethnic disparities in maternal mortality. *American Journal of Obstetrics and Gynecology*, *217*(6), 689–699.

D'Alton, M. E., Friedman, A. M., Bernstein, P. S., Brown, H. L., Callaghan, W. M., Clark, S. L., Grobman, W. A., Kilpatrick, S. J., O'Keeffe, D. F., Montgomery, D. M., Srinivas, S. K., Wendel, G. D., Wenstrom, K. D., & Foley, M. R. (2019). Putting the "M" back in maternal-fetal medicine: A 5-year report card on a collaborative effort to address maternal morbidity and mortality in the United States. *American Journal of Obstetrics and Gynecology*, *221*(4), 311–317.e1. DOI: 10.1016/j.ajog.2019.02.055 PMID: 30849353

Davis Moore, T. (2023). Can Provider Bias Impact Patient Treatment Outcomes: A Qualitative Analysis. https://digitalcommons.memphis.edu/etd/3025/

Delevan, K. (2023, November 4). *Research Guides: FYS 101: Intersectionality*. Researchguides.library.syr.edu. https://researchguides.library.syr.edu/fys101/intersectionality#:~:text=Intersectionality%20(or%20intersectional%20theory)%20is

Denevi, E., & Paston, N. (2006, Winter). Helping Whites Develop Anti-Racist Identities: Overcoming their resistance to fighting racism. *Multicultural Education*, 70–71.

Devereaux, P. J., Choi, P. T., Lacchetti, C., Weaver, B., Schünemann, H. J., Haines, T., Lavis, J. N., Grant, B. J. B., Haslam, D. R. S., Bhandari, M., Sullivan, T., Cook, D. J., Walter, S. D., Meade, M., Khan, H., Bhatnagar, N., & Guyatt, G. H. (2002). A systematic review and meta-analysis of studies comparing mortality rates of private for-profit and private not-for-profit hospitals. *Canadian Medical Association Journal*, *166*(11), 1399–1406. https://www.cmaj.ca/content/166/11/1399.short PMID: 12054406

DeVoss, D., Jasken, J., & Hayden, D. (2002). Teaching Intracultural and Intercultural Communication: A critique suggested method. *Journal of Business and Technical Communication, 16*(1), 69–94.

Dhanani, L. Y., & Totton, R. R. (2023). Have You Heard the News? The Effects of Exposure to News About Recent Transgender Legislation on Transgender Youth and Young Adults. *Sexuality Research & Social Policy, 20*(4), 1345–1359. DOI: 10.1007/s13178-023-00810-6 PMID: 37363351

Dimitrov, N., Dawson, D., Olsen, K., & Meadows, K. N. (2014). Developing the intercultural competence of graduate students. *Canadian Journal of Higher Education, 44*(3), 86–103.

Dobbs, J. (2023). *Navy Federal faces lawsuit, allegations of racial bias in mortgage lending. American Banker, N.* PAG.

Dobie, S. (2007). Reflections on a Well-Traveled Path: Self-awareness, mindful practice, and relationship centered care as foundations for medical education. *Academic Medicine, 82*(4). PMID: 17414201

Drake, P., Tolbert, J., Rudowitz, R., & Damico, A. (2024, February 26). *How Many Uninsured Are in the Coverage Gap and How Many Could be Eligible if All States Adopted the Medicaid Expansion?* Retrieved from KFF: https://www.kff.org/medicaid/issue-brief/how-many-uninsured-are-in-the-coverage-gap-and-how-many-could-be-eligible-if-all-states-adopted-the-medicaid-expansion/

Dutko, P., Ver Ploeg, M., & Farrigan, T. (2012). *Characteristics and Influential Factors of Food Deserts*. United States Department of Agriculture: Economic Research Service.

Dyrbye, L. N., Thomas, M. R., Huschka, M. M., Lawson, K. L., Novotny, P. J., Sloan, J. A., & Shanafellt, T. D. (2006). A multicenter study of burnout, depression, and quality of life in minority and nonminority US medical students. *Mayo Clinic Proceedings, 8*(11), 1435–1442. PMID: 17120398

Ehrenreich, B., & English, D. (1973). *Witches, Midwives, and Nurses: A History of Non-male individuals Healers*. Feminist Press.

Eisenchlas, S., & Trevaskes, S. (2007). Developing intercultural communication skills through intergroup interaction. *Intercultural Education, 18*(5), 413–425. DOI: 10.1080/14675980701685271

Elkadi, J., Chudleigh, C., Maguire, A., Ambler, G., Scher, S., & Kozlowska, K. (2023). Developmental pathway choices of young people presenting to a gender service with gender distress: A prospective follow-up study. *Children (Basel, Switzerland)*, *10*(2), 314. DOI: 10.3390/children10020314 PMID: 36832443

Evans, M. (2019). *Fits and starts: A genealogy of hysteria in modern France*. Cornell University Press.

Fabian, A. (2010). *The Skull Collectors: Race, Science and America's Unburied Dead*. University of Chicago Press. DOI: 10.7208/chicago/9780226233499.001.0001

Falck, F., & Bränström, R. (2023). The significance of structural stigma towards transgender people in health care encounters across Europe: Health care access, gender identity disclosure, and discrimination in health care as a function of national legislation and public attitudes. *BMC Public Health*, *23*(1), 1031. Advance online publication. DOI: 10.1186/s12889-023-15856-9 PMID: 37259082

Faulkner, S., Haas, M., Wang, D., Walker, C., Lee-Parritz, A., Perkins, R., & Chinkam, S. (2021). The effects of removing race from the VBAC calculator: Implications for counseling. *American Journal of Obstetrics and Gynecology*, *224*(2), S467–S468. DOI: 10.1016/j.ajog.2020.12.769

FitzGerald, C., & Hurst, S. (2017). Implicit bias in healthcare professionals: A systematic review. *BMC Medical Ethics*, *18*(1), 1–18. DOI: 10.1186/s12910-017-0179-8 PMID: 28249596

Flexner, A. (1910). Medical education in the United States and Canada. *Science*, *32*(810), 41–50. DOI: 10.1126/science.32.810.41 PMID: 17745880

Flood, S., McMurry, J., Sojourner, A., & Wiswall, M. (2022). Inequality in Early Care Experienced by US Children. *The Journal of Economic Perspectives: a Journal of the American Economic Association*, 199–222.

Foronda, C., Baptiste, D., Reinholdt, M. M., & Ousman, K. (2016). Cultural Humility: A Concept Analysis. *Journal of Transcultural Nursing*, *27*(3), 210–217. PMID: 26122618

Fuertes, J. N., Toporovsky, A., Reyes, M., & Osborne, J. B. (2017). The physician-patient working alliance: Theory, research, and future possibilities. *Patient Education and Counseling*, *100*(4), 610–615. DOI: 10.1016/j.pec.2016.10.018 PMID: 27773600

Funk, C., & Lopez, M. H. (2022). Hispanic Americans' Trust in and Engagement with Science. Pew Research Center. https://www.pewresearch.org/science/2022/06/14/hispanic-americans-trust-in-and-engagement-with-science/

Garcia, C. L., Abreu, L. C., Ramos, J. L. S., Castro, C. F. D., Smiderle, F. R. N., Santos, J. A. D., & Bezerra, I. M. P. (2019). Influence of Burnout on Patient Safety: Systematic Review and Meta-Analysis. *Medicina (Kaunas, Lithuania)*, *55*(9), 553. DOI: 10.3390/medicina55090553 PMID: 31480365

George, S., Duran, N., & Norris, K. (2014). A Systematic Review of Barriers and Facilitators to Minority Research Participation Among African Americans, Latinos, Asian Americans, and Pacific Islanders. *American Journal of Public Health*, *104*(2), e16–e31. DOI: 10.2105/AJPH.2013.301706 PMID: 24328648

Geter, A., Herron, A., & Sutton, M. (2018). Hiv-related stigma by healthcare providers in the united states: A systematic review. *AIDS Patient Care and STDs*, *32*(10), 418–424. DOI: 10.1089/apc.2018.0114 PMID: 30277814

Goetz, T., & Wolk, C. B. (2023). Moving toward targeted eating disorder care for transgender, non-binary, and gender-expansive patients in the United States. *International Journal of Eating Disorders*, *56*(12), 2210–2222. DOI: 10.1002/eat.24055 PMID: 37638738

Goodman, A. (2020, June 25). *Race Is Real, But It's Not Genetic*. Discover Magazine.

Goodwin, M. (2017). How the Criminalization of Pregnancy Robs Women of Reproductive Autonomy. *The Hastings Center Report*, *47*(S3), S19–S27. DOI: 10.1002/hast.791 PMID: 29171895

Greenwood, B. N. (2020). Physician-patient racial concordance and disparities in infant mortality. *Proceedings of the National Academy of Sciences of the United States of America*, *117*(35), 21194–21200. PMID: 32817561

Guzman, G., & Kollar, M. (2023, September 23). *Income in the United States:2022*. Retrieved from United States Census Bureau: https://www.census.gov/library/publications/2023/demo/p60-279.html

Hagihigi, A. S. (2023). Biases in healthcare: An overview. *Medical News Today*. https://www.medicalnewstoday.com/articles/biases-in-healthcare

Haines, M. (n.d.). *Fertility and Mortality in the United States*. Eh.net; Economic History Association. https://eh.net/encyclopedia/fertility-and-mortality-in-the-united-states/

Hareli, S., Karnieli-Miller, O., Hermoni, D., & Eidelman, S. (2007). Factors in the doctor–patient relationship that accentuate physicians' hurt feelings when patients terminate the relationship with them. *Patient Education and Counseling*, *67*(1-2), 169–175. DOI: 10.1016/j.pec.2007.03.010 PMID: 17448620

Hart, T., Sharvendiran, R., Chikermane, V., Kidwai, A., & Grace, D. (2021). At the intersection of homophobia and racism: Sociocultural context and the sexual health of south asian canadian gay and bisexual men. *Stigma and Health*. Advance online publication. DOI: 10.1037/sah0000295

Hassen, N., Lofters, A., Michael, S., Mall, A., Pinto, A. D., & Rackal, J. (2021). Implementing Anti-Racism Interventions in Healthcare Settings: A Scoping Review. *International Journal of Environmental Research and Public Health, 18*(6), 2993. Advance online publication. DOI: 10.3390/ijerph18062993 PMID: 33803942

Hausmann, L., Jones, A., McInnes, S., & Zickmund, S. (2020). Identifying health-care experiences associated with perceptions of racial/ethnic discrimination among veterans with pain: A cross-sectional mixed methods survey. *PLoS One, 15*(9), e0237650. DOI: 10.1371/journal.pone.0237650 PMID: 32881940

Hawkins, B. D. (2023). New Beginnings. *Diverse Issues in Higher Education, 40*(9), 31–33.

HealthCare.gov. (n.d.). *What Marketplace health insurance plans cover*. Retrieved May 2023, from Health benefits & coverage: https://www.healthcare.gov/coverage/what-marketplace-plans-cover/

Hear Her Campaign. (2022, September 8). *Clinical Resources and Tools | CDC*. Www.cdc.gov. https://www.cdc.gov/hearher/healthcare-providers/clinical-resources-tools.html

Heller, J. (2022, July 25). *AP exposes the Tuskegee Syphilis Study: The 50th Anniversary*. Associated Press.

Herbeck, D. M., West, J. C., Ruditis, I., Duffy, F. F., Fitek, D. J., Bell, C. C., & Snowden, L. R. (2004). Variations in use of second-generation antipsychotic medication by race among adult psychiatric patients. *Psychiatric Services (Washington, D.C.), 55*(6), 677–684. DOI: 10.1176/appi.ps.55.6.677 PMID: 15175466

Herrmann, L., Barkmann, C., Bindt, C., Fahrenkrug, S., Breu, F., Grebe, J., & Becker-Hébly, I. (2023). Binary and non-binary gender identities, internalizing problems, and treatment wishes among adolescents referred to a gender identity clinic in Germany. *Archives of Sexual Behavior, 53*(1), 91–106. DOI: 10.1007/s10508-023-02674-8 PMID: 37563319

Hilliard, C. B. (2016). High osteoporosis risk among East Africans linked to lactase persistence genotype. *BoneKEy Reports, 5*. Advance online publication. DOI: 10.1038/bonekey.2016.30 PMID: 27408710

Himmelstein, G., Bates, D., & Zhou, L. (2022). Examination of Stigmatizing Language in the Electronic Health Record. *JAMA Network Open*, *5*(1), e2144967. Advance online publication. DOI: 10.1001/jamanetworkopen.2021.44967 PMID: 35084481

Hines, D., Laury, E., & Habermann, B. (2019). They just do not get me: A qualitative analysis of transgender women's health care experiences and clinician interactions. *The Journal of the Association of Nurses in AIDS Care: JANAC*, *30*(5), e82–e95. DOI: 10.1097/JNC.0000000000000023 PMID: 31461741

Hobson, J., Gilstrap, S., Owens, M., Gloston, G., Ho, M., Gathright, J., Dotson, H. F., White, D. M., Cody, S. L., Justin Thomas, S., & Goodin, B. (2022). Intersectional hiv and chronic pain stigma: Implications for mood, sleep, and pain severity. *Journal of the International Association of Providers of AIDS Care*, *21*, 232595822210779. DOI: 10.1177/23259582221077941 PMID: 35200070

Hoffman, K. M. (2016). Racial bias in pain assessment and treatment recommendations. *Proceedings of the National Academy of Sciences of the United States of America*, *113*(16), 4296–4301. PMID: 27044069

Hoffman, K. M., Trawalter, S., Axt, J. R., & Oliver, M. N. (2016). Racial bias in pain assessment and treatment recommendations, and false beliefs about biological differences between blacks and whites. *Proceedings of the National Academy of Sciences of the United States of America*, *113*(16), 4296–4301. DOI: 10.1073/pnas.1516047113 PMID: 27044069

Holdt Somer, S. J., Sinkey, R. G., & Bryant, A. S. (2017). Epidemiology of racial/ethnic disparities in severe maternal morbidity and mortality. *Seminars in Perinatology*, *41*(5), 258–265. DOI: 10.1053/j.semperi.2017.04.001 PMID: 28888263

Holt, N., Hope, D., Mocarski, R., & Woodruff, N. (2023). The often-circuitous path to affirming mental health care for transgender and gender-diverse adults. *Current Psychiatry Reports*, *25*(3), 105–111. DOI: 10.1007/s11920-023-01410-2 PMID: 36773177

Hopkins, C. S.-B., & Kennedy, E. B.-A.-P. (2024). Caring for survivors of sexual violence in primary care. *Women's Health Care*, *11*(1), 25–30. DOI: 10.51256/WHC022425

Horrigan, B., Lewis, S., Abrams, D., & Pechura, C. (2012). Integrative medicine in america—-how integrative medicine is being practiced in clinical centers across the united states. *Global Advances in Health and Medicine : Improving Healthcare Outcomes Worldwide*, *1*(3), 18–52. DOI: 10.7453/gahmj.2012.1.3.006

Hostetter, C., Call, J., Gerke, D. R., Holloway, B. T., Walls, N. E., & Greenfield, J. C. (2022). "we are doing the absolute most that we can, and no one is listening": Barriers and facilitators to health literacy within transgender and nonbinary communities. *International Journal of Environmental Research and Public Health, 19*(3), 1229. DOI: 10.3390/ijerph19031229 PMID: 35162254

Howe, L. C., Hardebeck, E. J., Eberhardt, J. L., Markus, H. R., & Crum, A. J. (2022). White patients' physical responses to healthcare treatments are influenced by provider race and gender. *Proceedings of the National Academy of Sciences of the United States of America, 119*(27), e2007717119. DOI: 10.1073/pnas.2007717119 PMID: 35749352

Hoyert, D. (2023, March 16). *Maternal Mortality Rates in the United States, 2021.* Www.cdc.govCenters for Disease Control and Prevention. https://www.cdc.gov/nchs/data/hestat/maternal-mortality/2021/maternal-mortality-rates-2021.htm#:~:text=In%202021%2C%20the%20maternal%20mortality

Hughto, J., Rose, A., Pachankis, J., & Reisner, S. (2017). Barriers to gender transition-related healthcare: Identifying underserved transgender adults in Massachusetts. *Transgender Health, 2*(1), 107–118. DOI: 10.1089/trgh.2017.0014 PMID: 29082331

Human Rights Watch. (2017). "I Want to Be Like Nature Made Me": Medically Unnecessary Surgeries on Intersex Children in the U.S. *Journal of the American Medical Association, 316*(22), 2353-2354.

Hunt, B. (2019). *Redlining*. Chicagohistory.org. http://www.encyclopedia.chicagohistory.org/pages/1050.html

Hunter, K., & Thompson, B. (2019). A Scoping review of Social Determinants of Health Curricula in Post-Graduate Medical Education. *Canadian Medical Education Journal, 10*(3), e61–e71. PMID: 31388378

Huynh, L. N. (2020, March). *Employment barriers within low- and moderate-income communities*. Retrieved from U.S. Bureau of Labor Statistics: https://www.bls.gov/opub/mlr/2020/beyond-bls/employment-barriers-within-low-and-moderate-income-communities.htm

Ibrahim, A., Clarke, J., Beischel, W. J., & van Anders, S. M. (2023). Gender/sex markers, bio/logics, and U.S. identity documents. *Feminism & Psychology, 34*(1), 132–150. DOI: 10.1177/09593535231193232

Inoue, A. B. (2020). Teaching antiracist writing. *Journal of College Reading and Learning, 50*(1), 1–23.

Institute of Medicine (US) Committee on Understanding and Eliminating Racial and Ethnic Disparities in Health Care. (2003). *Unequal Treatment: Confronting Racial and Ethnic Disparities in Health Care* (Smedley, B. D., Stith, A. Y., & Nelson, A. R., Eds.). National Academies Press. DOI: 10.17226/12875

Institute of Medicine (US) Roundtable on Health Literacy. (2011). Innovations in Health Literacy Research: Workshop Summary. National Academies Press (US). Available from: https://www.ncbi.nlm.nih.gov/books/NBK209674/

Iversen, J. (2024, February 27). *Medicaid's Look-Back Period Explained: Exceptions & Penalties*. Retrieved from Paying for Senior Care: https://www.payingforseniorcare.com/medicaid/look-back-period

Jang, C., & Lee, H. (2022). A Review of Racial Disparities in Infant Mortality in the US. *Children (Basel, Switzerland)*, *9*(2), 257. DOI: 10.3390/children9020257 PMID: 35204976

Janz H. L. (2019). Ableism: the undiagnosed malady afflicting medicine. CMAJ: Canadian Medical Association journal = journal de l'Association medicale canadienne, 191(17), E478–E479. DOI: 10.1503/cmaj.180903

Javaid, M., & Bellware, K. (2024, January 3). She miscarried in her bathroom. Now she's charged with abuse of a corpse. *Washington Post*. https://www.washingtonpost.com/nation/2023/12/15/ohio-woman-miscarriage-abuse-of-corpse-grand-jury/

Jean, C., & Cyr, E. (2022). Accessible Medical Education & TIC: Increasing Equitable Care for Disabled Patients. *Harvard Public Health Review (Cambridge, Mass.)*, *44*. https://hphr.org/edition-44-su/ and https://pmc.ncbi.nlm.nih.gov/articles/PMC9518008/#R40 PMID: 36176338

Job, C., Adenipekun, B., Cleves, A., & Samuriwo, R. (2022). Health professional's implicit bias of adult patients with low socioeconomic status (SES) and its effects on clinical decision-making: A scoping review protocol. *BMJ Open*, *12*(12), e059837. DOI: 10.1136/bmjopen-2021-059837 PMID: 36523234

Johansson, C., & Chinworth, S. A. (2018). *Mobility in context: Principles of patient care skills*. FA Davis.

Johnson, C. D. (2023). The MONROE Method: A Methodology on Navigating Race, Oppression, and Equity in Medical Education through Physician Cultural Responsibility. https://aura.antioch.edu/etds/979

Johnson, C. (2022). Conquering the health disparities of structural racism. *Journal of Public Health Management and Practice*, *28*(Supplement 1), S15–S17. DOI: 10.1097/PHH.0000000000001431 PMID: 34797256

Johnson, C., Rastetter, M., & Olayiwola, J. N. (2022). Pathways to Equity: Implementing a Health Equity Leadership Curriculum in Residency Education as an Antidote to Systemic Racism. *Journal of the National Medical Association, 114*(2), 141–146. DOI: 10.1016/j.jnma.2021.12.015 PMID: 35078671

Jorgensen, S. C. J. (2023). Transition Regret and Detransition: Meanings and Uncertainties. *Archives of Sexual Behavior, 52*(5), 2173–2184. DOI: 10.1007/s10508-023-02626-2 PMID: 37266795

Jorgensen, S., Hunter, P., Regenstreif, L., Sinai, J., & Malone, W. (2022). Puberty blockers for gender dysphoric youth: A lack of sound science. *Journal of the American College of Clinical Pharmacy: JAACP, 5*(9), 1005–1007. DOI: 10.1002/jac5.1691

Kamran, R., Jackman, L., Chan, C., Suk, Y., Jacklin, C., Deck, E., Wietek, N., Stepney, M., Harrison, C., Jain, A., & Rodrigues, J. (2023). Implementation of Patient-Reported Outcome Measures for Gender-Affirming Care Worldwide: A Systematic Review. *JAMA Network Open, 6*(4), e236425. DOI: 10.1001/jamanetworkopen.2023.6425 PMID: 37010869

Karas, K. (2005). Must Doctors Report Underage Sex as Abuse? *The Virtual Mentor*, •••, 234–238. PMID: 23249492

Kasden, D. (2008, May 15). *Victory in the Regina McKnight Case | News & Commentary*. American Civil Liberties Union. https://www.aclu.org/news/reproductive-freedom/victory-regina-mcknight-case

Katz, J. (2002). *The silent world of doctor and patient*. Jhu Press. https://www.google.co.in/books/edition/The_Silent_World_of_Doctor_and_Patient/x1DNCNNX8AIC?hl=en&gbpv=1&dq=Patients+can+listen+to+physicians+provide+guidance+and+truest+for+the+obligations+it+is+outcome+assessment+in+the+better+health+conditions.&pg=PR9&printsec=frontcover

Katz, J., Rosenbloom, B., & Fashler, S. (2015). Chronic pain, psychopathology, and dsm-5 somatic symptom disorder. *Canadian Journal of Psychiatry, 60*(4), 160–167. DOI: 10.1177/070674371506000402 PMID: 26174215

Katznelson, I. (2005). *When Affirmative Action was White: An Untold History of Racial Inequality in Twentieth-century America*. W.W. Norton.

Katznelson, I., & Mettler, S. (2008). On Race and Policy History: A Dialogue about the G.I. Bill. *Perspectives on Politics, 6*(3), 519–537. https://www.jstor.org/stable/20446759. DOI: 10.1017/S1537592708081267

Kennedy, M., & Kennedy, M. (2014). Bogan bias: Addressing class-based prejudice in physician-patient interactions. *Journal of Social Inclusion, 5*(2), 27–43. DOI: 10.36251/josi74

King, S. H., & Castenell, L. A. (2001). *Racism and racial inequality: Implications for teacher education.* AACTE Publications.

Kleinsinger, F. (2010). Working with the noncompliant patient. *The Permanente Journal, 14*(1), 54–60. DOI: 10.7812/TPP/09-064 PMID: 20740133

Kondrat, M. E. (1999). Who is the "self" in self-aware: Professional self-awareness from a critical theory perspective. *The Social Service Review, 73*(4), 451–477. DOI: 10.1086/514441

Krebs, D., Harris, R., Steinbaum, A., Pilcher, S., Guss, C., Kremen, J., Roberts, S. A., Baskaran, C., Carswell, J., & Millington, K. (2022). Care for transgender young people. *Hormone Research in Paediatrics, 95*(5), 405–414. DOI: 10.1159/000524030 PMID: 35272283

Lagu, T., Haywood, C., Reimold, K., DeJong, C., Walker Sterling, R., & Iezzoni, L. I. (2022). "I Am Not The Doctor For You": Physicians' Attitudes About Caring For People With Disabilities. *Health Affairs, 41*(10), 1387–1395. DOI: 10.1377/hlthaff.2022.00475 PMID: 36190896

Landon, B. E., Onnela, J.-P., Meneades, L., & James O'malley, M. (2021). Assessment of Racial Disparities in Primary Care Physician Specialty Referrals. *JAMA Network Open, 4*(1), 2029238. DOI: 10.1001/jamanetworkopen.2020.29238 PMID: 33492373

LaVeist, T. A., Isaac, L. A., & Williams, K. P. (2009). Mistrust of Health Care Organizations Is Associated with Underutilization of Health Services. *Health Services Research, 44*(6), 2093–2105. DOI: 10.1111/j.1475-6773.2009.01017.x PMID: 19732170

Lawrence, J. (2000). The Indian Health Service and the Sterilization of Native American Women. *American Indian Quarterly, 24*(3), 400–419. DOI: 10.1353/aiq.2000.0008 PMID: 17089462

Laws, T. (2021). How Should We Respond to Racist Legacies in Health Professions Education Originating in the Flexner Report? *AMA Journal of Ethics, 23*(3), 271–275. DOI: 10.1001/amajethics.2021.271 PMID: 33818380

Lee, J. Y., & Rosenthal, S. M. (2023). Gender-Affirming Care of Transgender and Gender-Diverse Youth: Current Concepts. *Annual Review of Medicine, 74*(1), 107–116. DOI: 10.1146/annurev-med-043021-032007 PMID: 36260812

Lee, P., Le Saux, M., Siegel, R., Goyal, M., Chen, C., Ma, Y., & Meltzer, A. C. (2019). Racial and ethnic disparities in the management of acute pain in US emergency departments: Meta-analysis and systematic review. *The American Journal of Emergency Medicine*, *37*(9), 1770–1777. DOI: 10.1016/j.ajem.2019.06.014 PMID: 31186154

Lee, R. J., Madan, R. A., Kim, J., Posadas, E. M., & Yu, E. Y. (2021). Disparities in Cancer Care and the Asian American Population. *The Oncologist*, *26*(6), 453–460. DOI: 10.1002/onco.13748 PMID: 33683795

Lewis, J. A., & Tabacco Mar, R. (2022). Sexism. *Moving Toward Antibigotry*, 175-185.

Lewis, J. R. (1994). Patient views on quality care in general practice: Literature review. *Social Science & Medicine*, *39*(5), 655–670. DOI: 10.1016/0277-9536(94)90022-1 PMID: 7973865

Loza, O., Hernandez, P., Calderon-Mora, J., Laks, S., Leiner, M., Reddy, S., Lara, P., & Granados, H. (2018). Developing trans-affirming health services in an underserved area: An intersectional approach. *Transgender Health*, *3*(1), 127–135. DOI: 10.1089/trgh.2018.0011 PMID: 30023431

Lucey, C. R., & Johnston, S. C. (2020). The Transformational Effects of COVID-19 on Medical Education. *Journal of the American Medical Association*, *324*(11), 1033. Advance online publication. DOI: 10.1001/jama.2020.14136 PMID: 32857137

Lyon, W. (2021). Virtue and medical ethics education. *Philosophy, Ethics, and Humanities in Medicine; PEHM*, *16*(1), 2. DOI: 10.1186/s13010-021-00100-2 PMID: 34039382

Macchia, L. (2023, January 30). Rising Physical Pain Is Linked to More 'Deaths of Despair.' Scientific American. https://www.scientificamerican.com/article/rising physical-pain-is-linked-to-more-deaths-of-despair1/

Macias-Konstantopoulos, W. L., Collins, K. A., Diaz, R., Duber, H. C., Edwards, C. D., Hsu, A. P., Ranney, M. L., Riviello, R. J., Wettstein, Z. S., & Sachs, C. J. (2023). Race, Healthcare, and Health Disparities: A Critical Review and Recommendations for Advancing Health Equity. *The Western Journal of Emergency Medicine*, *24*(5), 906–918. DOI: 10.5811/WESTJEM.58408 PMID: 37788031

MacSorley, R., White, J., Conerly, V., Walker, J., Lofton, S., Ragland, G., Davey, D. B., & Robertson, A. (2014). Pain assessment and management strategies for elderly patients. *Home Healthcare Nurse*, *32*(5), 272–285. DOI: 10.1097/NHH.0000000000000065 PMID: 24802598

Mailhot Amborski, A., Bussières, E.-L., Vaillancourt-Morel, M.-P., & Joyal, C. C. (2021). Sexual Violence Against Persons With Disabilities: A Meta-Analysis. *Trauma, Violence & Abuse*, *23*(4), 152483802199597. DOI: 10.1177/1524838021995975 PMID: 33657931

Malfait, F., Colman, M., Vroman, R., Wandele, I., Rombaut, L., Miller, R., & Syx, D. (2021). Pain in the ehlers–danlos syndromes: Mechanisms, models, and challenges. *American Journal of Medical Genetics. Part C, Seminars in Medical Genetics*, *187*(4), 429–445. DOI: 10.1002/ajmg.c.31950 PMID: 34797601

Manary, M. P., Boulding, W., Staelin, R., & Glickman, S. W. (2013). The patient experience and health outcomes. *The New England Journal of Medicine*, *368*(3), 201–203. DOI: 10.1056/NEJMp1211775 PMID: 23268647

Mannucci, P. M., Schutgens, R. E., Santagostino, E., & Mauser-Bunschoten, E. P. (2009). How I treat age-related morbidities in elderly persons with hemophilia. *Blood*, *114*(26), 5256–5263. DOI: 10.1182/blood-2009-07-215665 PMID: 19837978

Marshall, S. A., Stewart, M. K., Barham, C., Ounpraseuth, S., & Curran, G. M. (2022). Facilitators and barriers to providing affirming care for transgender patients in primary care practices in Arkansas. *The Journal of Rural Health*, *39*(1), 251–261. DOI: 10.1111/jrh.12683 PMID: 35644535

Masters, C., Robinson, D., Faulkner, S., Patterson, E., McIlraith, T., & Ansari, A. (2019). Addressing Biases in Patient Care with The 5Rs of Cultural Humility, a Clinician Coaching Tool. *Journal of General Internal Medicine*, *34*(4), 627–630. DOI: 10.1007/s11606-018-4814-y PMID: 30623383

Masumori, N., Baba, T., Abe, T., & Niwa, K. (2021). What is the most anticipated change induced by treatment using gender-affirming hormones in individuals with gender incongruence? *International Journal of Urology*, *28*(5), 526–529. DOI: 10.1111/iju.14499 PMID: 33465834

Mayne, S. L., Yellayi, D., Pool, L. R., Grobman, W. A., & Kershaw, K. N. (2018). Racial Residential Segregation and Hypertensive Disorder of Pregnancy Among Women in Chicago: Analysis of Electronic Health Record Data. *American Journal of Hypertension*, *31*(11), 1221–1227. DOI: 10.1093/ajh/hpy112 PMID: 30010764

McGurran, B. (9, May 2023). *College Tuition Inflation: Compare The Cost Of College Over Time*. Retrieved from Forbes Advisor: https://www.forbes.com/advisor/student-loans/college-tuition-inflation/

Medicare.gov. (n.d.). *Costs in the coverage gap*. Retrieved from Medicare.gov: https://www.medicare.gov/drug-coverage-part-d/costs-for-medicare-drug-coverage/costs-in-the-coverage-gap

Meghani, S. (2011). Corporatization of pain medicine: Implications for widening pain care disparities. *Pain Medicine*, *12*(4), 634–644. DOI: 10.1111/j.1526-4637.2011.01074.x PMID: 21392249

Mehta, L. S. (2016). Acute myocardial infarction in non-male individuals: A scientific statement from the American Heart Association. *Circulation*, *133*(9), 916–947. PMID: 26811316

Mikovits, J. (2022). "I do not feel like I am a person": Nursing knowledge of transgender care through the lens of transgender people. *Journal of Advanced Nursing*, *78*(9), 3012–3024. DOI: 10.1111/jan.15308 PMID: 35642833

Mills, A. M., Shofer, F. S., Boulis, A. K., Holena, D. N., & Abbuhl, S. B. (2011). Racial disparity in analgesic treatment for ED patients with abdominal or back pain. *The American Journal of Emergency Medicine*, *29*(7), 752–756. DOI: 10.1016/j.ajem.2010.02.023 PMID: 20825892

Mills, A., Astle, K., & Frazier, C. (2022). "affirming" journey: Narrative review and practice considerations on gender-affirming care. *Journal of the American College of Clinical Pharmacy: JAACP*, *5*(7), 697–706. DOI: 10.1002/jac5.1621

Morantz-Sanchez, R. (1985). *Sympathy and Science: Non-male individuals Physicians in American Medicine*. University of North Carolina Press.

Morris, M. A., Hamer, M. K., Eberle, K., Jensen, K. M., & Wong, A. A. (2021). Implementation of Collection of Patients' Disability Status by Centralized Scheduling. *Joint Commission Journal on Quality and Patient Safety*, *47*(10), 627–636. DOI: 10.1016/j.jcjq.2021.05.007 PMID: 34144917

Moustakli, E., & Tsonis, O. (2023). Exploring hormone therapy effects on reproduction and health in transgender individuals. *Medicina*, *59*(12), 2094. DOI: 10.3390/medicina59122094 PMID: 38138197

Muntinga, M., Krajenbrink, V., Peerdeman, S., Croiset, G., & Verdonk, P. (2015). Toward diversity-responsive medical education: Taking an intersectionality-based approach to a curriculum evaluation. *Advances in Health Sciences Education : Theory and Practice*, *21*(3), 541–559. DOI: 10.1007/s10459-015-9650-9 PMID: 26603884

Murray, B., & McCrone, S. (2015). An integrative review of promoting trust in the patient–primary care provider relationship. *Journal of Advanced Nursing*, *71*(1), 3–23. DOI: 10.1111/jan.12502 PMID: 25113235

NACE. (2025). *Principles for Ethical Professional Practice*. Retrieved from NACE: https://naceweb.org/career-development/organizational-structure/principles-for-ethical-professional-practice/

Nall, M. C. (2020, March 4). *What is the Medicare donut hole?* Retrieved from Medical News Today: https://www.medicalnewstoday.com/articles/what-is-the-medicare-donut-hole#donut-hole-in-2020

National Cancer Institute. (n.d.). *Socioeconomic Status*. Retrieved May 2024, from National Cancer Institute: https://www.cancer.gov/publications/dictionaries/cancer-terms/def/socioeconomic-status

National Center for Chronic Disease Prevention and Health Promotion (NCCD-PHP). (n.d.). https://www.cdc.gov/chronicdisease/healthequity/health-equity-communications/nccdphp-health-equity-glossary.html#:~:text=Implicit%20Bias%3A%20A%20form%20of

National Institutes of Health. (2007). *Cultural Awareness Glossary of Key Terms*. https://www.niehs.nih.gov/news/events/pastmtg/hazmat/assets/2007/wtp_2007ntec_wruc_latino_tips_glossary_508.pdf

Nazar, M., Kendall, K., Day, L., & Nazar, H. (2015). Decolonising medical curricula through diversity education: Lessons from students. *Medical Teacher*, *37*(4), 385–393. DOI: 10.3109/0142159X.2014.947938 PMID: 25156358

Nelson, K. M., Skinner, A., & Underhill, K. (2022). Minor Consent Laws for Sexually Transmitted Infection and HIV Services. *Journal of the American Medical Association*, *328*(7), 674–676. DOI: 10.1001/jama.2022.10777 PMID: 35972493

Nie, J. B., Cheng, Y., Zou, X., Gong, N., Tucker, J. D., Wong, B., & Kleinman, A. (2018). The vicious circle of patient–physician mistrust in China: Health professionals' perspectives, institutional conflict of interest, and building trust through medical professionalism. *Developing World Bioethics*, *18*(1), 26–36. DOI: 10.1111/dewb.12170 PMID: 28922547

Njoku, A., Evans, M., Nimo-Sefah, L., & Bailey, J. (2023). Listen to the Whispers before They Become Screams: Addressing Black Maternal Morbidity and Mortality in the United States. *Health Care*, *11*(3), 438. DOI: 10.3390/healthcare11030438 PMID: 36767014

Nolan, I., Blasdel, G., Dubin, S., Goetz, T., Greene, R., & Morrison, S. (2020). The current state of transgender medical education in the United States and Canada: Update to a scoping review. *Journal of Medical Education and Curricular Development*, *7*. Advance online publication. DOI: 10.1177/2382120520934813 PMID: 32637641

Novak, N. L., Lira, N., O'Connor, K. E., Harlow, S. D., Kardia, S. L. R., & Stern, A. M. (2018). Disproportionate Sterilization of Latinos Under California's Eugenic Sterilization Program, 1920–1945. *American Journal of Public Health, 108*(5), 611–613. DOI: 10.2105/AJPH.2018.304369 PMID: 29565671

Nunez-Smith, M. (2010). Institutional culture and minority faculty career success in academic medicine. *Journal of the American Medical Association, 304*(12), 1373–1379.

Odlum, M., Moise, N., Kronish, I. M., Broadwell, P., Alcántara, C., Davis, N. J., Cheung, Y. K. K., Perotte, A., & Yoon, S. (2020). Trends in Poor Health Indicators Among Black and Hispanic Middle-aged and Older Adults in the United States, 1999-2018. *JAMA Network Open, 3*(11), e2025134. DOI: 10.1001/jamanetworkopen.2020.25134 PMID: 33175177

Office of Disease Prevention and Health Promotion. (n.d.). Social Determinants of Health. *Healthy People 2030*. U.S. Department of Health and Human Services. https://odphp.health.gov/healthypeople/priority-areas/social-determinants-health

Olaisen, R. H., Schluchter, M. D., Flocke, S. A., Smyth, K. A., Koroukian, S. M., & Stange, K. C. (2020). Assessing the longitudinal impact of physician-patient relationship on functional health. *Annals of Family Medicine, 18*(5), 422–429. DOI: 10.1370/afm.2554 PMID: 32928758

Pellegrini, C. A. (2017). Trust: The keystone of the patient-physician relationship. *Journal of the American College of Surgeons, 224*(2), 95–102. DOI: 10.1016/j.jamcollsurg.2016.10.032 PMID: 27773776

Perrot, S. (2019). Fibromyalgia: A misconnection in a multiconnected world? *European Journal of Pain (London, England), 23*(5), 866–873. DOI: 10.1002/ejp.1367 PMID: 30663833

Perugino, F., Angelis, V., Pompili, M., & Martelletti, P. (2022). Stigma and chronic pain. *Pain and Therapy, 11*(4), 1085–1094. DOI: 10.1007/s40122-022-00418-5 PMID: 35930220

Peterson-KFF. (2024, January 12). *How does cost affect access to healthcare?* Retrieved from Health System Tracker: https://www.healthsystemtracker.org/chart-collection/cost-affect-access-care/#Percent%20of%20adults%20reporting%20delaying%20or%20going%20without%20medical%20care%20due%20to%20cost,%20by%20selected%20characteristics,%202000-2022

Peterson-KFF. (2024, January 4). *How do health expenditures vary across the population?* Retrieved from Health System Tracker: https://www.healthsystemtracker.org/chart-collection/health-expenditures-vary-across-population/#Average%20total%20health%20spending,%20by%20age%20and%20sex,%202021%C2%A0

Phelan, S. M., Burgess, D. J., Yeazel, M. W., Hellerstedt, W. L., Griffin, J. M., & van Ryn, M. (2015). Impact of weight bias and stigma on quality of care and outcomes for patients with obesity. *Obesity Reviews, 16*(4), 319–326. DOI: 10.1111/obr.12266 PMID: 25752756

Pieterse, A. L., Utsey, S. O., & Miller, M. J. (2016). Development and initial validation of the anti-racism behavioral inventory (ARBI). *Counselling Psychology Quarterly, 29*(4), 356–381. DOI: 10.1080/09515070.2015.1101534

Powell, W., Richmond, J., Mohottige, D., Yen, I., Joslyn, A., & Corbie-Smith, G. (2019). Medical Mistrust, Racism, and Delays in Preventive Health Screening Among African-American Men. *Behavioral Medicine (Washington, D.C.), 45*(2), 102–117. DOI: 10.1080/08964289.2019.1585327 PMID: 31343960

Presser, H. B. (1969). The Role of Sterilization in Controlling Puerto Rican Fertility. *Population Studies, 23*(3), 343–361. DOI: 10.1080/00324728.1969.10405290 PMID: 22073953

Puckett, J., Tornello, S., Mustanski, B., & Newcomb, M. (2022). Gender variations, generational effects, and mental health of transgender people about timing and status of gender identity milestones. *Psychology of Sexual Orientation and Gender Diversity, 9*(2), 165–178. DOI: 10.1037/sgd0000391 PMID: 35983565

Quick facts: United States. US Census Bureau. (2018). AAMC. Quick facts: United States. US Census Bureau.

Ramani, S., Konings, K., Mann, V., & van der Vluten, C. (2017). Uncovering the unknown: A grounded theory study exploring the impact of self-awareness on the culture of feedback in residency education. *Medical Teacher, 39*(10), 1065–1073. DOI: 10.1080/0142159X.2017.1353071 PMID: 28741446

Reisner, S., Bradford, J., Hopwood, R., González, A., Makadon, H., Todisco, D., & Mayer, K. (2015). Comprehensive transgender healthcare: The gender affirming clinical and public health model of Fenway health. *Journal of Urban Health, 92*(3), 584–592. DOI: 10.1007/s11524-015-9947-2 PMID: 25779756

Restar, A., Jin, H., Jarrett, B. A., Adamson, T., Baral, S., Howell, S., & Beckham, S. W. (2021). Characterizing the impact of COVID-19 environment on mental health, gender-affirming services, and socioeconomic loss in a global sample of transgender and non-binary people: A structural equation modeling. *BMJ Global Health*, *6*(3), e004424. DOI: 10.1136/bmjgh-2020-004424 PMID: 33753401

Richards, C., Bouman, W. P., & Seal, L. (2016). Intersex, Variations of Sex Characteristics, and DSD: The Need for Change. *Journal of Pediatric Endocrinology & Metabolism*, *29*(11), 1263–1268.

Rigsby, E. A. (2016, June 23). *Understanding Exclusionary Zoning and Its Impact on Concentrated Poverty*. Retrieved from The Century Foundation: https://tcf.org/content/facts/understanding-exclusionary-zoning-impact-concentrated-poverty/

Roberts-West, L., Gravatt, A., Guest, N., Hunt, A., Siddique, L., & Serbic, D. (2023). A comparison of social exclusion towards people with depression or chronic back pain. *British Journal of Pain*, *17*(3), 267–280. DOI: 10.1177/20494637221148337 PMID: 37342396

Rouse, M.Jr. (2023). Promoting gender-affirming care: Challenging conflation and embracing complexity. *Policy Insights from the Behavioral and Brain Sciences*, *10*(2), 186–192. DOI: 10.1177/23727322231197148

RTI Health Alliance. (2023, June 27). Addressing Healthcare Bias Among People With Disabilities. Retrieved from RTI Health Alliance: https://healthcare.rti.org/insights/health-inequities-of-disabled-persons

Ruddere, L., & Craig, K. (2016). Understanding stigma and chronic pain: A-state-of-the-art review. *Pain*, *157*(8), 1607–1610. DOI: 10.1097/j.pain.0000000000000512 PMID: 26859821

Ryan-Ndegwa, S., Zamani, R., & Akrami, M. (2021). Assessing demographic access to hip replacement surgery in the united kingdom: A systematic review. *International Journal for Equity in Health*, *20*(1), 224. Advance online publication. DOI: 10.1186/s12939-021-01561-9 PMID: 34641862

Salow, A. D., Pool, L. R., Grobman, W. A., & Kershaw, K. N. (2018). Associations of neighborhood-level racial residential segregation with adverse pregnancy outcomes. *American Journal of Obstetrics and Gynecology*, *218*(3), 351.e1–351.e7. DOI: 10.1016/j.ajog.2018.01.022 PMID: 29421603

Saluja, B., & Bryant, Z. (2021). How Implicit Bias Contributes to Racial Disparities in Maternal Morbidity and Mortality in the United States. *Journal of Women's Health*, *30*(2), 270–273. DOI: 10.1089/jwh.2020.8874 PMID: 33237843

Samulowitz, A., Gremyr, I., Eriksson, E., & Hensing, G. (2018). "Brave Men" and "Emotional Non-male individuals ": A theory-guided literature review on gender bias in health care and gendered norms towards patients with chronic pain. *Pain Research & Management, 2018*, 1–14.

Samulowitz, A., Gremyr, I., Eriksson, E., & Hensing, G. (2018). "Brave Men" and "Emotional Women": A theory-guided literature review on gender bias in health care and gendered norms towards patients with chronic pain. *Pain Research & Management, 2018*, 1–14. DOI: 10.1155/2018/6358624 PMID: 29682130

San, L., & Arranz, B. (2023). Effective patient-physician communication in the era of neuropsychopharmacology. *European Neuropsychopharmacology, 71*, 1–2. DOI: 10.1016/j.euroneuro.2023.02.007 PMID: 36867984

Santas, A. (2000). Teaching antiracism. *Studies in Philosophy and Education, 19*(4), 349–361. DOI: 10.1023/A:1005298916161

Santiago-Rodriguez, E., Rivas, C., Maiorana, A., Pérez, A., Erguera, X., Johnson, M., Christopoulos, K. A., Marquez, C., & Sauceda, J. (2021). Unpacking the "backpack of shame": Exploring intersections of stigma among latinx people living with hiv in san francisco, ca. *Cultural Diversity & Ethnic Minority Psychology, 27*(4), 630–637. DOI: 10.1037/cdp0000487 PMID: 34410754

Savitt, T. L. (1978). *Medicine and Slavery: The Diseases and Health Care of Blacks in Antebellum Virginia*. University of Illinois Press.

Savitt, T. L. (1982). The Use of Blacks for Medical Experimentation and Demonstration in the Old South. *The Journal of Southern History, 48*(3), 331–348. DOI: 10.2307/2207450 PMID: 11645888

Scharff, D. P., Mathews, K. J., Jackson, P., Hoffsuemmer, J., Martin, E., & Edwards, D. (2010). More than Tuskegee: Understanding Mistrust about Research Participation. *Journal of Health Care for the Poor and Underserved, 21*(3), 879–897. DOI: 10.1353/hpu.0.0323 PMID: 20693733

Schatman, M. (2011). Pain and corporatization: More special interests, more disparities, more vulnerability. *Pain Medicine, 12*(4), 632–633. DOI: 10.1111/j.1526-4637.2011.01092.x PMID: 21463473

Scheitle, C. P., Frost, J., & Ecklund, E. H. (2023). The Association between Religious Discrimination and Health: Disaggregating by Types of Discrimination Experiences, Spencer, K. L., & Grace, M. (2016). Social foundations of health care inequality and treatment bias. *Annual Review of Sociology, 42*(1), 101–120. DOI: 10.1146/annurev-soc-091715-074226

Schiebinger, L. (1987). *The history of non-male individuals in medicine.* Signs: Journal of Non-male individuals in Culture and Society, 12(3), 515-531.

Schluger, N. W., Dozor, A. J., & Jung, Y. E. G. (2022). Rethinking the Race Adjustment in Pulmonary Function Testing. *Annals of the American Thoracic Society, 19*(3), 353–356. DOI: 10.1513/AnnalsATS.202107-890PS PMID: 34784493

Schonberger, J. (2024, January 28). *The threat that high childcare costs pose to the US economy.* Retrieved from Yahoo Finance: https://finance.yahoo.com/news/the-threat-that-high-childcare-costs-pose-to-the-us-economy-124248273.html

Schulz, M. (2023, August 10). *Student Loan Debt Statistics.* Retrieved from LendingTree: https://www.lendingtree.com/student/student-loan-debt-statistics/

Schwartz, R. C., & Blankenship, D. M. (2014). Racial disparities in psychotic disorder diagnosis: A review of empirical literature. *World Journal of Psychiatry, 4*(4), 133–140. DOI: 10.5498/wjp.v4.i4.133 PMID: 25540728

Scott, D. (2023, October 16). *Why the US is the only country that ties your health insurance to your job.* Retrieved from Vox: https://www.vox.com/23890764/healthcare-insurance-marketplace-open-enrollment-employer-sponsored-united-blue-cross-shield-aetna

Seelman, K., Colón-Diaz, M., LeCroix, R., Xavier-Brier, M., & Kattari, L. (2017). Transgender noninclusive healthcare and delaying care because of fear: Connections to general health and mental health among transgender adults. *Transgender Health, 2*(1), 17–28. DOI: 10.1089/trgh.2016.0024 PMID: 28861545

Segal, S. P., Bola, J. R., & Watson, M. A. (1996). Race, Quality of Care, and Antipsychotic Prescribing Practices in Psychiatric Emergency Services. *Psychiatric Services (Washington, D.C.), 47*(3), 282–286. DOI: 10.1176/ps.47.3.282 PMID: 8820552

Sengupta, T., Soni, T., Bolock, A. M., Heisey, S. A., Kuchinski, E. C., Piper, B. J., Joyce, J. M., & Carbe, C. J. (2023). Knowledge, attitudes, and beliefs of medical students toward transgender healthcare: A community-driven initiative. *Cureus.* Advance online publication. DOI: 10.7759/cureus.49992 PMID: 38058529

Sex. (2025). In *Merriam-Webster.com.* https://www.merriam-webster.com/dictionary/sex

Sharma, M., Pinto, A. D., & Kumagai, A. K. (2018). Teaching the Social Determinants of Health: A path to equity or a road to nowhere? *Academic Medicine, 2018*(93), 25–30. DOI: 10.1097/ACM.0000000000001689 PMID: 28445214

Shin, S. J., Kumar, A., & Safer, J. D. (2022). Gender-Affirming Surgery: Perioperative Medical Care. Endocrine practice. *Endocrine Practice*, *28*(4), 420–424. DOI: 10.1016/j.eprac.2022.02.007 PMID: 35217191

Silva, K., Nauman, C., Tebbe, E., & Parent, M. (2022). Policy attitudes toward adolescents transitioning gender. *Journal of Counseling Psychology*, *69*(4), 403–415. DOI: 10.1037/cou0000601 PMID: 34968097

Sing, S., Peters, R., Syurina, E., Irwanto, I., Naniche, D., & Zweekhorst, M. (2020). Intersectionality and health-related stigma: Insights from experiences of people living with stigmatized health conditions in indonesia. *International Journal for Equity in Health*, *19*(1), 206. Advance online publication. DOI: 10.1186/s12939-020-01318-w PMID: 33176809

Sjoding, M. W., Dickson, R. P., Iwashyna, T. J., Gay, S. E., & Valley, T. S. (2020). Racial Bias in Pulse Oximetry Measurement. *The New England Journal of Medicine*, *383*(25), 2477–2478. DOI: 10.1056/NEJMc2029240 PMID: 33326721

Sloan, S., & Benson, J. J. (2021). Toward a conceptual model for successful transgender aging. *Qualitative Social Work: Research and Practice*, *21*(2), 455–471. DOI: 10.1177/1473325021994666

Snyder, J. E., Upton, R. D., Hassett, T. C., Lee, H., Nouri, Z., & Dill, M. (2023). Black Representation in the Primary Care Physician Workforce and Its Association With Population Life Expectancy and Mortality Rates in the US. *JAMA Network Open*, *6*(4), e236687. DOI: 10.1001/jamanetworkopen.2023.6687 PMID: 37058307

Solomon, J. (2021, July 26). *Closing the coverage gap would improve Black maternal health.* Center on Budget and Policy Priorities. https://www.cbpp.org/research/health/closing-the-coverage-gap-would-improve-black-maternal-health

Srinivasan, S. (2023). Elderly TB patients in India: Situation Analysis, Tuijin Jishu/Journal of Propulsion Technology, Vol. 44 No. 6 (2023), 364-367. DOI: 10.52783/tjjpt.v44.i6.3140

Srinivasan, S. (2025). Patient-Centric Care in Tuberculosis Management: Addressing Challenges and Improving Health Outcomes. In *Convergence of Population Health Management, Pharmacogenomics, and Patient-Centered Care* (pp. 265-282). IGI Global. DOI: 10.4018/979-8-3693-3260-3.ch012

Staats EB. (1976). *Letter report (HRD-77-3) investigation of allegations concerning Indian Health Service. Comptroller General of the United States*. Author.

Staats, C., Capatosto, K., Wright, R. A., & Contractor, D. (2015). State of the Science: Implicit Bias Review 2015. Academic Press.

Stahnisch, F. W., & Verhoef, M. (2012). The Flexner Report of 1910 and Its Impact on Complementary and Alternative Medicine and Psychiatry in North America in the 20th Century. *Evidence-Based Complementary and Alternative Medicine : eCAM*, *2012*, 1–10. DOI: 10.1155/2012/647896 PMID: 23346209

Stangl, A. L., Earnshaw, V. A., & Logie, C. H. (2019). The Health Stigma and Discrimination Framework: A global, crosscutting framework to inform research, intervention development, and policy on health-related stigmas. *BMC Medicine*, *17*, 31. DOI: 10.1186/s12916-019-1271-3 PMID: 30764826

Stangl, A., Atkins, K., Leddy, A., Sievwright, K., Sevelius, J., Lippman, S., Veras, M. A., Zamudio-Haas, S., Smith, M. K., Pachankis, J. E., Logie, C. H., Rao, D., Weiser, S., & Nyblade, L. (2023). What do we know about interventions to reduce intersectional stigma and discrimination in the context of hiv? a systematic review. *Stigma and Health*, *8*(3), 393–408. DOI: 10.1037/sah0000414

Stone, A. A. (1976). *Mental Health and Law: A System in Transition*. Jason Aronson.

Strasser, J., & Spelocha, H. (2005). How can university professors help their students to understand issues of diversity through interpersonal and intrapersonal intelligences. *Multicultural Education*, *12*(4), 20.

Stringer, K., Turan, B., McCormick, L., Durojaiye, M., Nyblade, L., Kempf, M., Lichtenstein, B., & Turan, J. (2015). Hiv-related stigma among healthcare providers in the deep south. *AIDS and Behavior*, *20*(1), 115–125. DOI: 10.1007/s10461-015-1256-y PMID: 26650383

Stroumsa, D., Shires, D., Richardson, C., Jaffee, K., & Woodford, M. (2019). Transphobia rather than education predicts provider knowledge of transgender health care. *Medical Education*, *53*(4), 398–407. DOI: 10.1111/medu.13796 PMID: 30666699

Syed, M., & McLean, K. (2015). Understanding identity integration: Theoretical, methodological, and applied issues. *Journal of Adolescence*, *47*(1), 109–118. DOI: 10.1016/j.adolescence.2015.09.005 PMID: 26522883

Telusca, N., Gaisey, J., Woods, C., Khan, J., & Mackey, S. (2022). Strategies to promote racial healthcare equity in pain medicine: A call to action. *Pain Medicine*, *23*(7), 1225–1230. DOI: 10.1093/pm/pnac057 PMID: 35412639

Teutsch, C. (2003). Patient–doctor communication. *Medical Clinics*, *87*(5), 1115–1145. https://www.medical.theclinics.com/article/S0025-7125(03)00066-X/abstract PMID: 14621334

The Lancet Series on racism, xenophobia, discrimination, and health. (2022). The Lancet. www.thelancet.com/series/racism-xenophobia-discrimination-health

Thomas, K., & Silver-Greenberg, J. (2022, September 24). How a Hospital Chain Used a Poor Neighborhood to Turn Huge Profits. *The New York Times*. https://www.nytimes.com/2022/09/24/health/bon-secours-mercy-health-profit-poor-neighborhood.html

Tordoff, D. M., Wanta, J. W., Collin, A., Stepney, C., Inwards-Breland, D. J., & Ahrens, K. (2022). Mental Health Outcomes in Transgender and Nonbinary Youths Receiving Gender-Affirming Care. *JAMA Network Open*, *5*(2), e220978. DOI: 10.1001/jamanetworkopen.2022.0978 PMID: 35212746

Trauma Informed Care. (2018, March 20). *What Is Trauma?* Trauma-Informed Care Implementation Resource Center. https://www.traumainformedcare.chcs.org/what-is-trauma/

Tsugawa, Y. (2017). Comparison of hospital mortality and readmission rates for Medicare patients treated by male vs. female physicians. *JAMA Internal Medicine*, *177*(2), 206–213. PMID: 27992617

Tucker, J. D., Wong, B., Nie, J. B., & Kleinman, A. (2016). Rebuilding patient–physician trust in China. *Lancet*, *388*(10046), 755. DOI: 10.1016/S0140-6736(16)31362-9 PMID: 27560268

U.S. Department of Justice Civil Rights Division. (2024). *Introduction to the Americans with Disabilities Act*. ADA.gov. https://www.ada.gov/topics/intro-to-ada/

United Nations. (2025). *What Is The UN Ethics Office?* Retrieved from UN Ethics Office: Listen - Advise - Respect: https://www.un.org/en/ethics/#:~:text=The%20UN%20Ethics%20Office%20promotes,and%20respect%20for%20human%20rights

Uppal, P., Golden, B. L., Panicker, A., Khan, O. A., & Burday, M. J. (2022). The Case Against Race-Based GFR. *Delaware Journal of Public Health*, *8*(3), 86–89. DOI: 10.32481/djph.2022.014 PMID: 36177174

Vaccaro, C., Karageuzian, S. A., & McFadden, E. (2023). The importance of safely prescribing hormones in the transgender community. *Cureus*. Advance online publication. DOI: 10.7759/cureus.44639 PMID: 37799231

Valentine, S. E., Shipherd, J. C., Smith, A. M., & Kauth, M. R. (2021). Improving affirming care for sexual and gender minority veterans. *Psychological Services*, *18*(2), 205–215. DOI: 10.1037/ser0000378 PMID: 31343189

Van Ryn, M., & Burke, J. (2000). The effect of patient race and socio-economic status on physicians' perceptions of patients. *Social Science & Medicine*, *50*(6), 813–828. DOI: 10.1016/S0277-9536(99)00338-X PMID: 10695979

Varkey, B. (2020). Principles of Clinical Ethics and Their Application to Practice. *Medical Principles and Practice : International Journal of the Kuwait University, Health Science Centre*, •••, 17–28. https://pmc.ncbi.nlm.nih.gov/articles/PMC7923912/ PMID: 32498071

Veatch, R. M. (1972). Models for ethical medicine in a revolutionary age. *The Hastings Center Report*, *2*(3), 5–7. DOI: 10.2307/3560825 PMID: 4679693

Vedam, S., Stoll, K., Taiwo, T. K., Rubashkin, N., Cheyney, M., Strauss, N., McLemore, M., Cadena, M., Nethery, E., Rushton, E., Schummers, L., & Declercq, E. (2019). The Giving Voice to Mothers Study: Inequity and mistreatment during pregnancy and childbirth in the United States. *Reproductive Health*, *16*(1), 77. Advance online publication. DOI: 10.1186/s12978-019-0729-2 PMID: 31182118

Vela, M. B., Erondu, A. I., Smith, N. A., Peek, M. E., Woodruff, J. N., & Chin, M. H. (2022). Eliminating Explicit and Implicit Biases in Health Care: Evidence and Research Needs. *Annual Review of Public Health*, *43*(1), 477–501. DOI: 10.1146/annurev-publhealth-052620-103528 PMID: 35020445

Vogel, M., Choi, F., Westenberg, J., Cabanis, M., Nikoo, N., Nikoo, M., Hwang, S. W., Somers, J., Schütz, C. G., & Krausz, M. (2021). Chronic pain among individuals experiencing homelessness and its interdependence with opioid and other substance use and mental illness. *International Journal of Environmental Research and Public Health*, *19*(1), 5. DOI: 10.3390/ijerph19010005 PMID: 35010263

Vyas, D. A., Eisenstein, L. G., & Jones, D. S. (2020). Hidden in Plain Sight — Reconsidering the Use of Race Correction in Clinical Algorithms. *The New England Journal of Medicine*, *383*(9), 874–882. DOI: 10.1056/NEJMms2004740 PMID: 32853499

Walkowska, A., Przymuszała, P., Marciniak-Stępak, P., Nowosadko, M., & Baum, E. (2023). Enhancing cross-cultural competence of medical and healthcare students with the use of simulated patients—A systematic review. *International Journal of Environmental Research and Public Health*, *20*(3), 2505. DOI: 10.3390/ijerph20032505 PMID: 36767872

Wang, K. (2022). Housing Instability and Socioeconomic Disparities in Health: Evidence from the U.S. Economic Recession. *Journal of Racial and Ethnic Health Disparities*, *9*(6), 2451–2467. DOI: 10.1007/s40615-021-01181-7 PMID: 34837164

Ward, P. (2018). Trust and communication in a doctor-patient relationship: A literature review. *Journal of Healthcare Communications*, *3*(3), 36. DOI: 10.4172/2472-1654.100146

Washington, H. A. (2006). *Medical Apartheid.* Doubleday.

Weingartner, L., Noonan, E. J., Bohnert, C., Potter, J., Shaw, M. A., & Holthouser, A. (2022). Gender-Affirming Care With Transgender and Genderqueer Patients: A Standardized Patient Case. *MedEdPORTAL: the Journal of Teaching and Learning Resources, 18*, 11249. DOI: 10.15766/mep_2374-8265.11249 PMID: 35664552

Weisleder, P. (2023). Moral distress, moral injury, and burnout: Clinicians' resilience and adaptability are not the solution. *Annals of the Child Neurology Society, 1*(4), 262–266. DOI: 10.1002/cns3.20048

Wermiel, S. J. (2023, January 6). *Inequitable and Inadequate School Funding*. Retrieved from American Bar Association: Human Rights: https://www.americanbar.org/groups/crsj/publications/human_rights_magazine_home/wealth-disparities-in-civil-rights/inequitable-and-inadequate-school-funding/

Wiederhold, S., Lergetporer, P., Peter, F., & Hermes, H. (2021, December 7). https://cepr.org/voxeu/columns/socioeconomic-gap-childcare-enrolment-role-behavioural-barriers. Retrieved from CEPR: https://cepr.org/voxeu/columns/socioeconomic-gap-childcare-enrolment-role-behavioural-barriers

World Population Review. (2024). *Age of Consent by State 2024*. Retrieved from World Population Review: https://worldpopulationreview.com/state-rankings/age-of-consent-by-state

WPATH (World Professional Association for Transgender Health). (2022). Standards of Care for the Health of Transgender and Gender Diverse People, Version 8. https://www.wpath.org/soc8

Wyman, M. F., Shiovitz-Ezra, S., & Bengel, J. (2018). Ageism in the health care system: Providers, patients, and systems. *Contemporary perspectives on ageism*, 193-212. DOI: 10.1007/978-3-319-73820-8

Yedidia, M. J. (2007). Transforming doctor-patient relationships to promote patient-centered care: Lessons from palliative care. *Journal of Pain and Symptom Management, 33*(1), 40–57. DOI: 10.1016/j.jpainsymman.2006.06.007 PMID: 17196906

York, M., Davidson, L. M., Hemingway, C., Russell, R., Neeley, M., & Fleming, A. (2021). Becoming Active Bystanders and Advocated: Teaching medical students to respond to bias in the clinical setting. *Academic Medicine, 2021*(17).

Zellars, R. (2018, May 31). *Black Subjectivity and the Origins of American Gynecology–AAIHS.* Aaihs.org. https://www.aaihs.org/black-subjectivity-and-the-origins-of-american-gynecology/

Zhang, L., Losin, E. A. R., Ashar, Y. K., Koban, L., & Wager, T. D. (2021). Gender biases in estimation of others' pain. *The Journal of Pain*, *22*(9), 1048–1059. DOI: 10.1016/j.jpain.2021.03.001 PMID: 33684539

Zwick, J., Appleseth, H., & Arndt, S. (2020). Stigma: How it affects the substance use disorder patient. *Substance Abuse Treatment, Prevention, and Policy*, *15*(1), 50. DOI: 10.1186/s13011-020-00288-0 PMID: 32718328

Related References

To continue our tradition of advancing information science and technology research, we have compiled a list of recommended IGI Global readings. These references will provide additional information and guidance to further enrich your knowledge and assist you with your own research and future publications.

Abu Seman, S. A., & Ramayah, T. (2017). Are We Ready to App?: A Study on mHealth Apps, Its Future, and Trends in Malaysia Context. In Pelet, J. (Ed.), *Mobile Platforms, Design, and Apps for Social Commerce* (pp. 69–83). Hershey, PA: IGI Global. DOI: 10.4018/978-1-5225-2469-4.ch005

Adeleke, I. T., & Abdul, Q. B. (2020). Opinions on Cyber Security, Electronic Health Records, and Medical Confidentiality: Emerging Issues on Internet of Medical Things From Nigeria. In Pankajavalli, P., & Karthick, G. (Eds.), *Incorporating the Internet of Things in Healthcare Applications and Wearable Devices* (pp. 199–211). IGI Global. https://doi.org/10.4018/978-1-7998-1090-2.ch012

Aggarwal, S., & Azad, V. (2017). A Hybrid System Based on FMM and MLP to Diagnose Heart Disease. In Bhattacharyya, S., De, S., Pan, I., & Dutta, P. (Eds.), *Intelligent Multidimensional Data Clustering and Analysis* (pp. 293–325). Hershey, PA: IGI Global. DOI: 10.4018/978-1-5225-1776-4.ch011

Al-Busaidi, S. S. (2018). Interdisciplinary Relationships Between Medicine and Social Sciences. In Al-Suqri, M., Al-Kindi, A., AlKindi, S., & Saleem, N. (Eds.), *Promoting Interdisciplinarity in Knowledge Generation and Problem Solving* (pp. 124–137). Hershey, PA: IGI Global. DOI: 10.4018/978-1-5225-3878-3.ch009

Al Kareh, T., & Thoumy, M. (2018). The Impact of Health Information Digitization on the Physiotherapist-Patient Relationship: A Pilot Study of the Lebanese Community. *International Journal of Healthcare Information Systems and Informatics, 13*(2), 29–53. DOI: 10.4018/IJHISI.2018040103

Alenzuela, R. (2017). Research, Leadership, and Resource-Sharing Initiatives: The Role of Local Library Consortia in Access to Medical Information. In Ram, S. (Ed.), *Library and Information Services for Bioinformatics Education and Research* (pp. 199–211). Hershey, PA: IGI Global. DOI: 10.4018/978-1-5225-1871-6.ch012

Ali, S., Samie, A. U., Ali, A., Bhat, A. H., Mir, T., & Prasad, B. V. (2020). Mental Health: A Global Issue Affecting the Pattern of Life in Kashmir. In Taukeni, S. (Ed.), *Biopsychosocial Perspectives and Practices for Addressing Communicable and Non-Communicable Diseases* (pp. 18–29). IGI Global. https://doi.org/10.4018/978-1-7998-2139-7.ch002

Almpani, S., Stefaneas, P., Boley, H., Mitsikas, T., & Frangos, P. (2019). A Rule-Based Model for Compliance of Medical Devices Applied to the European Market. *International Journal of Extreme Automation and Connectivity in Healthcare*, *1*(2), 56–78. https://doi.org/10.4018/IJEACH.2019070104

Alnakhi, W. K. (2021). Medical Travel and Public Health: Definitions, Frameworks, and Future Research. In Singh, M., & Kumaran, S. (Eds.), *Growth of the Medical Tourism Industry and Its Impact on Society: Emerging Research and Opportunities* (pp. 74–94). IGI Global. https://doi.org/10.4018/978-1-7998-3427-4.ch004

Ameri, H., Alizadeh, S., & Noughabi, E. A. (2017). Application of Data Mining Techniques in Clinical Decision Making: A Literature Review and Classification. In Noughabi, E., Raahemi, B., Albadvi, A., & Far, B. (Eds.), *Handbook of Research on Data Science for Effective Healthcare Practice and Administration* (pp. 257–295). Hershey, PA: IGI Global. DOI: 10.4018/978-1-5225-2515-8.ch012

Anand, S. (2017). Medical Image Enhancement Using Edge Information-Based Methods. In Singh, B. (Ed.), *Computational Tools and Techniques for Biomedical Signal Processing* (pp. 123–148). Hershey, PA: IGI Global. DOI: 10.4018/978-1-5225-0660-7.ch006

Anton, J. L., Soriano, J. V., Martinez, M. I., & Garcia, F. B. (2018). Comprehensive E-Learning Appraisal System. In M. Khosrow-Pour, D.B.A. (Ed.), *Encyclopedia of Information Science and Technology, Fourth Edition* (pp. 5787-5799). Hershey, PA: IGI Global. https://doi.org/DOI: 10.4018/978-1-5225-2255-3.ch503

Aslan, F. (2021). Could There Be an Alternative Method of Media Literacy in Promoting Health in Children and Adolescents? Media Literacy and Health Promotion. In G. Sarı (Eds.), *Handbook of Research on Representing Health and Medicine in Modern Media* (pp. 191-199). IGI Global. https://doi.org/10.4018/978-1-7998-6825-5.ch013

Atzori, B., Hoffman, H. G., Vagnoli, L., Messeri, A., & Grotto, R. L. (2018). Virtual Reality as Distraction Technique for Pain Management in Children and Adolescents. In M. Khosrow-Pour, D.B.A. (Ed.), *Encyclopedia of Information Science and Technology, Fourth Edition* (pp. 5955-5965). Hershey, PA: IGI Global. DOI: 10.4018/978-1-5225-2255-3.ch518

Audibert, M., Mathonnat, J., Pélissier, A., & Huang, X. X. (2018). The Impact of the New Rural Cooperative Medical Scheme on Township Hospitals' Utilization and Income Structure in Weifang Prefecture, China. In I. Management Association (Ed.), *Health Economics and Healthcare Reform: Breakthroughs in Research and Practice* (pp. 109-121). Hershey, PA: IGI Global. https://doi.org/DOI: 10.4018/978-1-5225-3168-5.ch007

Aulia, A., & Pratiti, B. (2022). Cyberchondria and Medical Student Syndrome: An Anxious Path to Be an Anxiety Healer? In Aker, H., & Aiken, M. (Eds.), *Handbook of Research on Cyberchondria, Health Literacy, and the Role of Media in Society's Perception of Medical Information* (pp. 98–113). IGI Global. https://doi.org/10.4018/978-1-7998-8630-3.ch006

Babu, A., & Ayyappan, S. (2017). A Methodological Evaluation of Crypto-Watermarking System for Medical Images. In Bhatt, C., & Peddoju, S. (Eds.), *Cloud Computing Systems and Applications in Healthcare* (pp. 189–217). Hershey, PA: IGI Global. DOI: 10.4018/978-1-5225-1002-4.ch010

Bakke, A. (2017). Ethos in E-Health: From Informational to Interactive Websites. In Folk, M., & Apostel, S. (Eds.), *Establishing and Evaluating Digital Ethos and Online Credibility* (pp. 85–103). Hershey, PA: IGI Global. DOI: 10.4018/978-1-5225-1072-7.ch005

Bali, S. (2018). Enhancing the Reach of Health Care Through Telemedicine: Status and New Possibilities in Developing Countries. In Pandey, U., & Indrakanti, V. (Eds.), *Open and Distance Learning Initiatives for Sustainable Development* (pp. 339–354). Hershey, PA: IGI Global. DOI: 10.4018/978-1-5225-2621-6.ch019

Balls-Berry, J. E., & Albold, C. (2019). Asynchronous Education for Graduate Medical Trainees to Reduce Health Disparities and Address Social Determinants of Health: Online Education for Graduate Medical Trainees. In Demiroz, E., & Waldman, S. (Eds.), *Optimizing Medical Education With Instructional Technology* (pp. 1–20). IGI Global. https://doi.org/10.4018/978-1-5225-6289-4.ch001

Barrett, T. E. (2018). Essentials for Education and Training for Tomorrow's Physicians. In Smith, C. (Ed.), *Exploring the Pressures of Medical Education From a Mental Health and Wellness Perspective* (pp. 230–252). Hershey, PA: IGI Global. DOI: 10.4018/978-1-5225-2811-1.ch010

Bazan, V., Jax, M. D., & Zwischenberger, J. B. (2020). Alice in Simulation-Land: Surgical Simulation in Medical Education. In Gotian, R., Kang, Y., & Safdieh, J. (Eds.), *Handbook of Research on the Efficacy of Training Programs and Systems in Medical Education* (pp. 449–458). IGI Global. https://doi.org/10.4018/978-1-7998-1468-9.ch023

Beaudoin, S. (2019). The Hidden Face of Medical Intervention. In C. Albuquerque (Eds.), *Emerging Trends and Innovations in Privacy and Health Information Management* (pp. 188-211). IGI Global. https://doi.org/10.4018/978-1-5225-8470-4.ch008

Bernardes, O., Amorim, V., & Usman, B. (2021). The Good, the Bad, and the Ugly: Don't Blame COVID-19 for Health System Inefficiencies. In J. Santos, & I. Pereira (Ed.), *Management and Marketing for Improved Competitiveness and Performance in the Healthcare Sector* (pp. 115-139). IGI Global. https://doi.org/10.4018/978-1-7998-7263-4.ch006

Berrahal, S., & Boudriga, N. (2017). The Risks of Wearable Technologies to Individuals and Organizations. In Marrington, A., Kerr, D., & Gammack, J. (Eds.), *Managing Security Issues and the Hidden Dangers of Wearable Technologies* (pp. 18–46). Hershey, PA: IGI Global. DOI: 10.4018/978-1-5225-1016-1.ch002

Bhargava, P. (2018). Blended Learning: An Effective Application to Clinical Teaching. In Tang, S., & Lim, C. (Eds.), *Preparing the Next Generation of Teachers for 21st Century Education* (pp. 302–320). Hershey, PA: IGI Global. DOI: 10.4018/978-1-5225-4080-9.ch018

Bird, J. L. (2017). Writing Healing Narratives. In Bryan, V., & Bird, J. (Eds.), *Healthcare Community Synergism between Patients, Practitioners, and Researchers* (pp. 1–28). Hershey, PA: IGI Global. DOI: 10.4018/978-1-5225-0640-9.ch001

Bougoulias, K., Kouris, I., Prasinos, M., Giokas, K., & Koutsouris, D. (2017). Ob/Gyn EMR Software: A Solution for Obstetricians and Gynecologists. In Moumtzoglou, A. (Ed.), *Design, Development, and Integration of Reliable Electronic Healthcare Platforms* (pp. 101–111). Hershey, PA: IGI Global. DOI: 10.4018/978-1-5225-1724-5.ch006

Bouslimi, R., Ayadi, M. G., & Akaichi, J. (2018). Medical Image Retrieval in Healthcare Social Networks. *International Journal of Healthcare Information Systems and Informatics, 13*(2), 13–28. DOI: 10.4018/IJHISI.2018040102

Bouzaabia, O., Bouzaabia, R., & Mejri, K. (2017). Role of Internet in the Development of Medical Tourism Service in Tunisia. In Capatina, A., & Rancati, E. (Eds.), *Key Challenges and Opportunities in Web Entrepreneurship* (pp. 211–241). Hershey, PA: IGI Global. DOI: 10.4018/978-1-5225-2466-3.ch009

Brown-Jackson, K. L. (2018). Telemedicine and Telehealth: Academics Engaging the Community in a Call to Action. In Burton, S. (Ed.), *Engaged Scholarship and Civic Responsibility in Higher Education* (pp. 166–193). Hershey, PA: IGI Global. DOI: 10.4018/978-1-5225-3649-9.ch008

Bwalya, K. J. (2017). Next Wave of Tele-Medicine: Virtual Presence of Medical Personnel. In Moahi, K., Bwalya, K., & Sebina, P. (Eds.), *Health Information Systems and the Advancement of Medical Practice in Developing Countries* (pp. 168–180). Hershey, PA: IGI Global. DOI: 10.4018/978-1-5225-2262-1.ch010

Celik, G. (2018). Determining Headache Diseases With Genetic Algorithm. In Kose, U., Guraksin, G., & Deperlioglu, O. (Eds.), *Nature-Inspired Intelligent Techniques for Solving Biomedical Engineering Problems* (pp. 249–262). Hershey, PA: IGI Global. DOI: 10.4018/978-1-5225-4769-3.ch012

Chakraborty, S., Chatterjee, S., Ashour, A. S., Mali, K., & Dey, N. (2018). Intelligent Computing in Medical Imaging: A Study. In Dey, N. (Ed.), *Advancements in Applied Metaheuristic Computing* (pp. 143–163). Hershey, PA: IGI Global. DOI: 10.4018/978-1-5225-4151-6.ch006

Chandra, L., Downey, C. L., Svavarsdottir, H. S., Skinner, H., & Young, A. L. (2020). Gender Equity in Medical Leadership. In Bellini, M., & Papalois, V. (Eds.), *Gender Equity in the Medical Profession* (pp. 94–109). IGI Global. https://doi.org/10.4018/978-1-5225-9599-1.ch007

Chandran, S. (2019). Medical Data Storage and Compression. In Swarnambiga, A. (Ed.), *Medical Image Processing for Improved Clinical Diagnosis* (pp. 140–154). IGI Global. https://doi.org/10.4018/978-1-5225-5876-7.ch007

Chavez, A., & Kovarik, C. (2017). Open Source Technology for Medical Practice in Developing Countries. In Moahi, K., Bwalya, K., & Sebina, P. (Eds.), *Health Information Systems and the Advancement of Medical Practice in Developing Countries* (pp. 33–59). Hershey, PA: IGI Global. DOI: 10.4018/978-1-5225-2262-1.ch003

Chen, S., Traba, C., Lamba, S., & Soto-Greene, M. (2020). Professional and Career Development of Medical Students. In Gotian, R., Kang, Y., & Safdieh, J. (Eds.), *Handbook of Research on the Efficacy of Training Programs and Systems in Medical Education* (pp. 305–326). IGI Global. https://doi.org/10.4018/978-1-7998-1468-9.ch016

Chien, G. C., Haroutunian, A., England, B., & Candido, K. D. (2019). Optimizing Medical Education With Instructional Technology: Technology to Optimize Teaching Human Anatomy. In Demiroz, E., & Waldman, S. (Eds.), *Optimizing Medical Education With Instructional Technology* (pp. 71–78). IGI Global. https://doi.org/10.4018/978-1-5225-6289-4.ch005

Choudhari, R. H. (2021). Multidimensional Impact of Climate Change on Human Reproduction and Fertility: A Medical Perspective on Changing Dynamics. In K. Wani, & N. Naha (Eds.), *Climate Change and Its Impact on Fertility* (pp. 278-315). IGI Global. https://doi.org/10.4018/978-1-7998-4480-8.ch014

Ciufudean, C. (2018). Innovative Formalism for Biological Data Analysis. In M. Khosrow-Pour, D.B.A. (Ed.), *Encyclopedia of Information Science and Technology, Fourth Edition* (pp. 1814-1824). Hershey, PA: IGI Global. DOI: 10.4018/978-1-5225-2255-3.ch158

Colaguori, R., & Danesi, M. (2017). Medical Semiotics: A Revisitation and an Exhortation. *International Journal of Semiotics and Visual Rhetoric*, *1*(1), 11–18. DOI: 10.4018/IJSVR.2017010102

Cole, A. W., & Salek, T. A. (2017). Adopting a Parasocial Connection to Overcome Professional Kakoethos in Online Health Information. In Folk, M., & Apostel, S. (Eds.), *Establishing and Evaluating Digital Ethos and Online Credibility* (pp. 104–120). Hershey, PA: IGI Global. DOI: 10.4018/978-1-5225-1072-7.ch006

Deperlioglu, O. (2018). Intelligent Techniques Inspired by Nature and Used in Biomedical Engineering. In Kose, U., Guraksin, G., & Deperlioglu, O. (Eds.), *Nature-Inspired Intelligent Techniques for Solving Biomedical Engineering Problems* (pp. 51–77). Hershey, PA: IGI Global. DOI: 10.4018/978-1-5225-4769-3.ch003

Desai, K. P., Shah, M. A., Lapasia, M. C., Patil, S. A., & Pathak, S. P. (2022). Applied Intelligence for Mental Health Detection: ManoVaidya – A Mental Health Therapist. In Thakare, A., Wagh, S., Bhende, M., Anter, A., & Gao, X. (Eds.), *Handbook of Research on Applied Intelligence for Health and Clinical Informatics* (pp. 80–91). IGI Global. https://doi.org/10.4018/978-1-7998-7709-7.ch005

Dey, N., & Ashour, A. S. (2018). Meta-Heuristic Algorithms in Medical Image Segmentation: A Review. In Dey, N. (Ed.), *Advancements in Applied Metaheuristic Computing* (pp. 185–203). Hershey, PA: IGI Global. DOI: 10.4018/978-1-5225-4151-6.ch008

Dey, N., Ashour, A. S., & Althoupety, A. S. (2017). Thermal Imaging in Medical Science. In Santhi, V. (Ed.), *Recent Advances in Applied Thermal Imaging for Industrial Applications* (pp. 87–117). Hershey, PA: IGI Global. DOI: 10.4018/978-1-5225-2423-6.ch004

Di Virgilio, F., Camillo, A. A., & Camillo, I. C. (2017). The Impact of Social Network on Italian Users' Behavioural Intention for the Choice of a Medical Tourist Destination. *International Journal of Tourism and Hospitality Management in the Digital Age*, *1*(1), 36–49. DOI: 10.4018/IJTHMDA.2017010103

Dobani, F., Pennington, M. L., Coe, E., Morrison, P., & Gulliver, S. B. (2020). Bridging the Gaps: Toward Effective Collaboration Between Peer Supporters and Behavioral Health Professionals. In Bowers, C., Beidel, D., & Marks, M. (Eds.), *Mental Health Intervention and Treatment of First Responders and Emergency Workers* (pp. 190–204). IGI Global. https://doi.org/10.4018/978-1-5225-9803-9.ch011

Dogra, A. K., & Dogra, P. (2017). The Medical Tourism Industry in the BRIC Nations: An Indian Analysis. In Dhiman, M. (Ed.), *Opportunities and Challenges for Tourism and Hospitality in the BRIC Nations* (pp. 320–336). Hershey, PA: IGI Global. DOI: 10.4018/978-1-5225-0708-6.ch020

Doublestein, B. A., Lee, W. T., & Pfohl, R. M. (2020). Overview of Professionalism Competence: Bringing Balance to the Medical Education Continuum. In Selladurai, R., Hobson, C., Selladurai, R., & Greer, A. (Eds.), *Evaluating Challenges and Opportunities for Healthcare Reform* (pp. 215–231). IGI Global. https://doi.org/10.4018/978-1-7998-2949-2.ch010

Drowos, J. L., & Wood, S. K. (2017). Preparing Future Physicians to Adapt to the Changing Health Care System: Promoting Humanism through Curricular Design. In Bryan, V., & Bird, J. (Eds.), *Healthcare Community Synergism between Patients, Practitioners, and Researchers* (pp. 106–125). Hershey, PA: IGI Global. DOI: 10.4018/978-1-5225-0640-9.ch006

Dulam, K. (2017). Medical Patents and Impact on Availability and Affordability of Essential Medicines in India. In Aggarwal, R., & Kaur, R. (Eds.), *Patent Law and Intellectual Property in the Medical Field* (pp. 41–57). Hershey, PA: IGI Global. DOI: 10.4018/978-1-5225-2414-4.ch003

Dutta, P. (2017). Decision Making in Medical Diagnosis via Distance Measures on Interval Valued Fuzzy Sets. *International Journal of System Dynamics Applications*, *6*(4), 63–83. DOI: 10.4018/IJSDA.2017100104

Dutta, P. (2021). Medical Pre-Screening of Common Diseases: An Interval-Valued Fuzzy Set Approach. In Azar, A., & Kamal, N. (Eds.), *Handbook of Research on Modeling, Analysis, and Control of Complex Systems* (pp. 267–292). IGI Global. https://doi.org/10.4018/978-1-7998-5788-4.ch011

Dwivedi, M. K., Pandey, S. K., & Singh, P. K. (2021). Public Health Surveillance System: Infectious Diseases. In Yadav, D., Bansal, A., Bhatia, M., Hooda, M., & Morato, J. (Eds.), *Diagnostic Applications of Health Intelligence and Surveillance Systems* (pp. 201–220). IGI Global. https://doi.org/10.4018/978-1-7998-6527-8.ch010

El Guemhioui, K., & Demurjian, S. A. (2017). Semantic Reconciliation of Electronic Health Records Using Semantic Web Technologies. *International Journal of Information Technology and Web Engineering*, *12*(2), 26–48. DOI: 10.4018/IJITWE.2017040102

Etim, A., Etim, D. N., & Scott, J. (2020). Mobile Health and Telemedicine: Awareness, Adoption and Importance of Health Study. *International Journal of Healthcare Information Systems and Informatics*, *15*(1), 81–96. https://doi.org/10.4018/IJHISI.2020010105

Fino, E., & Hanna-Khalil, B. (2020). Psychometric Post-Examination Analysis in Medical Education Training Programs. In Gotian, R., Kang, Y., & Safdieh, J. (Eds.), *Handbook of Research on the Efficacy of Training Programs and Systems in Medical Education* (pp. 221–242). IGI Global. https://doi.org/10.4018/978-1-7998-1468-9.ch012

Fishback, J. L., & Klein, R. M. (2019). Collaborative Learning for Histopathology Education. In Demiroz, E., & Waldman, S. (Eds.), *Optimizing Medical Education With Instructional Technology* (pp. 177–193). IGI Global. https://doi.org/10.4018/978-1-5225-6289-4.ch010

Fisher, J. (2018). Sociological Perspectives on Improving Medical Diagnosis Emphasizing CAD. In M. Khosrow-Pour, D.B.A. (Ed.), *Encyclopedia of Information Science and Technology, Fourth Edition* (pp. 1017-1024). Hershey, PA: IGI Global. DOI: 10.4018/978-1-5225-2255-3.ch088

Franco Santos, D., Branco Silva, A. R., Novo, M. D., & Vaz de Almeida, C. (2022). Medical Burnout: Is Mindfulness an Effective Coping Strategy? In Gupta, S. (Ed.), *Handbook of Research on Clinical Applications of Meditation and Mindfulness-Based Interventions in Mental Health* (pp. 184–194). IGI Global. https://doi.org/10.4018/978-1-7998-8682-2.ch012

Frank, E. M. (2018). Healthcare Education: Integrating Simulation Technologies. In Bryan, V., Musgrove, A., & Powers, J. (Eds.), *Handbook of Research on Human Development in the Digital Age* (pp. 163–182). Hershey, PA: IGI Global. DOI: 10.4018/978-1-5225-2838-8.ch008

Gambhir, P. (2021). Enhancing Mental Health: A Role for Technology. In Hooke, A. (Ed.), *Technological Breakthroughs and Future Business Opportunities in Education, Health, and Outer Space* (pp. 264–269). IGI Global. https://doi.org/10.4018/978-1-7998-6772-2.ch017

Garcia-Santa, N., San Miguel, B., & Ugai, T. (2019). Converging Semantic Knowledge and Deep Learning for Medical Coding. *International Journal of Privacy and Health Information Management, 7*(2), 33–52. https://doi.org/10.4018/IJPHIM.2019070103

Garner, G. (2018). Foundations for Yoga Practice in Rehabilitation. In Telles, S., & Singh, N. (Eds.), *Research-Based Perspectives on the Psychophysiology of Yoga* (pp. 263–307). Hershey, PA: IGI Global. DOI: 10.4018/978-1-5225-2788-6.ch015

Garrote Andújar, S. A., Araújo Vila, N., Brea, J. A., & de Araújo, A. F. (2021). Medical Tourism: Analysis and Expectations Worldwide. In Borges, A., & Rodrigues, P. (Eds.), *New Techniques for Brand Management in the Healthcare Sector* (pp. 84–102). IGI Global. https://doi.org/10.4018/978-1-7998-3034-4.ch006

Gavurová, B., Kováč, V., & Šoltés, M. (2018). Medical Equipment and Economic Determinants of Its Structure and Regulation in the Slovak Republic. In M. Khosrow-Pour, D.B.A. (Ed.), *Encyclopedia of Information Science and Technology, Fourth Edition* (pp. 5841-5852). Hershey, PA: IGI Global. DOI: 10.4018/978-1-5225-2255-3.ch508

Ge, X., Wang, Q., Huang, K., Law, V., & Thomas, D. C. (2017). Designing Simulated Learning Environments and Facilitating Authentic Learning Experiences in Medical Education. In Stefaniak, J. (Ed.), *Advancing Medical Education Through Strategic Instructional Design* (pp. 77–100). Hershey, PA: IGI Global. DOI: 10.4018/978-1-5225-2098-6.ch004

Gewald, H., & Gewald, C. (2018). Inhibitors of Physicians' Use of Mandatory Hospital Information Systems (HIS). *International Journal of Healthcare Information Systems and Informatics, 13*(1), 29–44. DOI: 10.4018/IJHISI.2018010103

Ghosh, D., & Dinda, S. (2017). Health Infrastructure and Economic Development in India. In Das, R. (Ed.), *Social, Health, and Environmental Infrastructures for Economic Growth* (pp. 99–119). Hershey, PA: IGI Global. DOI: 10.4018/978-1-5225-2364-2.ch006

Ghosh, K., & Sen, K. C. (2017). The Potential of Crowdsourcing in the Health Care Industry. In Wickramasinghe, N. (Ed.), *Handbook of Research on Healthcare Administration and Management* (pp. 418–427). Hershey, PA: IGI Global. DOI: 10.4018/978-1-5225-0920-2.ch024

Gonzalez-Urquijo, M., Macias-Rodriguez, Y., & Davila-Rivas, J. A. (2022). The Role of Telemedicine and Globalization in Medical Education. In Lopez, M. (Ed.), *Advancing Health Education With Telemedicine* (pp. 288–295). IGI Global. https://doi.org/10.4018/978-1-7998-8783-6.ch015

Gopalan, V., Chan, E., & Ho, D. T. (2018). Deliberate Self-Harm and Suicide Ideology in Medical Students. In Smith, C. (Ed.), *Exploring the Pressures of Medical Education From a Mental Health and Wellness Perspective* (pp. 122–143). Hershey, PA: IGI Global. DOI: 10.4018/978-1-5225-2811-1.ch005

Goswami, N. (2021). Effects of Spaceflight, Aging, and Bedrest on Falls: Aging Meets Spaceflight! In Eklund, P. (Ed.), *Integrated Care and Fall Prevention in Active and Healthy Aging* (pp. 91–106). IGI Global. https://doi.org/10.4018/978-1-7998-4411-2.ch005

Goswami, S., Dey, U., Roy, P., Ashour, A., & Dey, N. (2017). Medical Video Processing: Concept and Applications. In Dey, N., Ashour, A., & Patra, P. (Eds.), *Feature Detectors and Motion Detection in Video Processing* (pp. 1–17). Hershey, PA: IGI Global. DOI: 10.4018/978-1-5225-1025-3.ch001

Goswami, S., Mahanta, K., Goswami, S., Jigdung, T., & Devi, T. P. (2018). Ageing and Cancer: The Epigenetic Basis, Alternative Treatment, and Care. In Prasad, B., & Akbar, S. (Eds.), *Handbook of Research on Geriatric Health, Treatment, and Care* (pp. 206–235). Hershey, PA: IGI Global. DOI: 10.4018/978-1-5225-3480-8.ch012

Gouva, M. I. (2017). The Psychological Impact of Medical Error on Patients, Family Members, and Health Professionals. In Riga, M. (Ed.), *Impact of Medical Errors and Malpractice on Health Economics, Quality, and Patient Safety* (pp. 171–196). Hershey, PA: IGI Global. DOI: 10.4018/978-1-5225-2337-6.ch007

Gündüz, U., & Pembecioğlu, N. (2021). Case Study of Gender and Career Choices: Being and Becoming Medical People. In G. Sarı (Ed.), *Handbook of Research on Representing Health and Medicine in Modern Media* (pp. 269-307). IGI Global. https://doi.org/10.4018/978-1-7998-6825-5.ch018

Gupta, A. (2021). Artificial Intelligence Approaches to Detect Neurodegenerative Disease From Medical Records: A Perspective. In Rani, G., & Tiwari, P. (Eds.), *Handbook of Research on Disease Prediction Through Data Analytics and Machine Learning* (pp. 254–267). IGI Global. https://doi.org/10.4018/978-1-7998-2742-9.ch013

Gürcü, M., & Tengilimoğlu, D. (2017). Health Tourism-Based Destination Marketing. In Bayraktar, A., & Uslay, C. (Eds.), *Strategic Place Branding Methodologies and Theory for Tourist Attraction* (pp. 308–331). Hershey, PA: IGI Global. DOI: 10.4018/978-1-5225-0579-2.ch015

Gürsel, G. (2017). For Better Healthcare Mining Health Data. In Bhattacharyya, S., De, S., Pan, I., & Dutta, P. (Eds.), *Intelligent Multidimensional Data Clustering and Analysis* (pp. 135–158). Hershey, PA: IGI Global. DOI: 10.4018/978-1-5225-1776-4.ch006

Gyaase, P. O., Darko-Lartey, R., William, H., & Borkloe, F. (2017). Towards an Integrated Electronic Medical Records System for Quality Healthcare in Ghana: An Exploratory Factor Analysis. *International Journal of Computers in Clinical Practice*, *2*(2), 38–55. DOI: 10.4018/IJCCP.2017070103

Hagle, H. N., Liu, Y., Murphy, D. M., & Krom, L. (2022). Innovative Adaptation of Training and Technical Assistance: Education for the Behavioral Health Workforce. In Ford, C., & Garza, K. (Eds.), *Handbook of Research on Updating and Innovating Health Professions Education: Post-Pandemic Perspectives* (pp. 239–264). IGI Global. https://doi.org/10.4018/978-1-7998-7623-6.ch011

Halis, M., & Halis, M. (2021). The Relationship Between Organizational Culture and Organizational Commitment: A Research in Private Health Institutions. In G. Sarı (Ed.), *Handbook of Research on Representing Health and Medicine in Modern Media* (pp. 308-329). IGI Global. https://doi.org/10.4018/978-1-7998-6825-5.ch019

Halis, M., Tepret, S., Çamlibel, Z., & Halis, M. (2021). Competitiveness in Medical Tourism: An Evaluation on Kocaeli Medical Tourism Market. In G. Sarı (Ed.), *Handbook of Research on Representing Health and Medicine in Modern Media* (pp. 239-268). IGI Global. https://doi.org/10.4018/978-1-7998-6825-5.ch017

Hanel, P. (2017). Is China Catching Up?: Health-Related Applications of Biotechnology. In Bas, T., & Zhao, J. (Eds.), *Comparative Approaches to Biotechnology Development and Use in Developed and Emerging Nations* (pp. 465–520). Hershey, PA: IGI Global. DOI: 10.4018/978-1-5225-1040-6.ch016

Hartman, A., & Brown, S. (2017). Synergism through Therapeutic Visual Arts. In Bryan, V., & Bird, J. (Eds.), *Healthcare Community Synergism between Patients, Practitioners, and Researchers* (pp. 29–48). Hershey, PA: IGI Global. DOI: 10.4018/978-1-5225-0640-9.ch002

Heck, A. J., Cross, C. E., & Tatum, V. Y. (2020). Early Medical Education Readiness Interventions: Enhancing Undergraduate Preparedness. In Gotian, R., Kang, Y., & Safdieh, J. (Eds.), *Handbook of Research on the Efficacy of Training Programs and Systems in Medical Education* (pp. 283–304). IGI Global. https://doi.org/10.4018/978-1-7998-1468-9.ch015

Hemant, B., Arasappa, R. G. I., Udupa, K., & Varambally, S. (2021). Yoga for Mental Health Disorders: Research and Practice. In Telles, S., & Gupta, R. (Eds.), *Handbook of Research on Evidence-Based Perspectives on the Psychophysiology of Yoga and Its Applications* (pp. 179–198). IGI Global. https://doi.org/10.4018/978-1-7998-3254-6.ch011

Herdeiro, M. T., Gouveia, N., & Roque, F. (2021). Clinical Research and Regulatory Affairs: Skills and Tools in Pharmacy Education. In Figueiredo, I., & Cavaco, A. (Eds.), *Pedagogies for Pharmacy Curricula* (pp. 160–184). IGI Global. https://doi.org/10.4018/978-1-7998-4486-0.ch008

Hosoda, M., & Hosoda, M. (2019). Supporting Patient-led Initiatives to Improve Healthcare: An Investigation of Cancer and ME/CFS Support Groups and Prefectural Medical Councils in Japan. *International Journal of Patient-Centered Healthcare, 9*(2), 44–56. https://doi.org/10.4018/IJPCH.20190701.oa2

Iqbal, S., Ahmad, S., & Willis, I. (2017). Influencing Factors for Adopting Technology Enhanced Learning in the Medical Schools of Punjab, Pakistan. *International Journal of Information and Communication Technology Education, 13*(3), 27–39. DOI: 10.4018/IJICTE.2017070103

Jagiello, K., Sosnowska, A., Mikolajczyk, A., & Puzyn, T. (2017). Nanomaterials in Medical Devices: Regulations' Review and Future Perspectives. *Journal of Nanotoxicology and Nanomedicine, 2*(2), 1–11. DOI: 10.4018/JNN.2017070101

Jagtap, R., Phulare, K., Kurhade, M., & Gawande, K. S. (2021). Healthcare Conversational Chatbot for Medical Diagnosis. In Patil, B., & Vohra, M. (Eds.), *Handbook of Research on Engineering, Business, and Healthcare Applications of Data Science and Analytics* (pp. 401–415). IGI Global. https://doi.org/10.4018/978-1-7998-3053-5.ch020

Janosek, D. M. (2022). What Is the "Public Good" in a Pandemic? Who Decides?: Policy Makers and the Need for Leadership in Society's Perception of Medical Information. In Aker, H., & Aiken, M. (Eds.), *Handbook of Research on Cyberchondria, Health Literacy, and the Role of Media in Society's Perception of Medical Information* (pp. 1–15). IGI Global. https://doi.org/10.4018/978-1-7998-8630-3.ch001

Jena, T. K. (2018). Skill Training Process in Medicine Through Distance Mode. In Pandey, U., & Indrakanti, V. (Eds.), *Optimizing Open and Distance Learning in Higher Education Institutions* (pp. 228–243). Hershey, PA: IGI Global. DOI: 10.4018/978-1-5225-2624-7.ch010

Joseph, V., & Miller, J. M. (2018). Medical Students' Perceived Stigma in Seeking Care: A Cultural Perspective. In Smith, C. (Ed.), *Exploring the Pressures of Medical Education From a Mental Health and Wellness Perspective* (pp. 44–67). Hershey, PA: IGI Global. DOI: 10.4018/978-1-5225-2811-1.ch002

Joyce, B. L., & Swanberg, S. M. (2017). Using Backward Design for Competency-Based Undergraduate Medical Education. In Stefaniak, J. (Ed.), *Advancing Medical Education Through Strategic Instructional Design* (pp. 53–76). Hershey, PA: IGI Global. DOI: 10.4018/978-1-5225-2098-6.ch003

Kalder, M., & Kostev, K. (2021). Epidemiology of Gynaecological and Breast Cancers: Incidence, Survival, and Mental Health. In Dinas, K., Petousis, S., Kalder, M., & Mavromatidis, G. (Eds.), *Handbook of Research on Oncological and Endoscopical Dilemmas in Modern Gynecological Clinical Practice* (pp. 1–21). IGI Global. https://doi.org/10.4018/978-1-7998-4213-2.ch001

Kaljo, K., & Jacques, L. (2018). Flipping the Medical School Classroom. In M. Khosrow-Pour, D.B.A. (Ed.), *Encyclopedia of Information Science and Technology, Fourth Edition* (pp. 5800-5809). Hershey, PA: IGI Global. DOI: 10.4018/978-1-5225-2255-3.ch504

Karanfiloglu, M. (2021). The Role of Social Media Use in Health Communication: Digitized Health Communication During COVID-19 Pandemic. In G. Sarı (Eds.), *Handbook of Research on Representing Health and Medicine in Modern Media* (pp. 84-104). IGI Global. https://doi.org/10.4018/978-1-7998-6825-5.ch006

Karthikeyan, P., Vasuki, S., & Karthik, K. (2019). Non-Subsampled Contourlet Transform-Based Effective Denoising of Medical Images: Denoising of Medical Images Using Contourlet. In Swarnambiga, A. (Ed.), *Medical Image Processing for Improved Clinical Diagnosis* (pp. 155–183). IGI Global. https://doi.org/10.4018/978-1-5225-5876-7.ch008

Kashyap, R., & Rahamatkar, S. (2019). Medical Image Segmentation: An Advanced Approach. In Paul, S., Bhattacharya, P., & Bit, A. (Eds.), *Early Detection of Neurological Disorders Using Machine Learning Systems* (pp. 292–321). IGI Global. https://doi.org/10.4018/978-1-5225-8567-1.ch015

Kasina, H., Bahubalendruni, M. V., & Botcha, R. (2017). Robots in Medicine: Past, Present and Future. *International Journal of Manufacturing, Materials, and Mechanical Engineering*, *7*(4), 44–64. DOI: 10.4018/IJMMME.2017100104

Katehakis, D. G. (2018). Electronic Medical Record Implementation Challenges for the National Health System in Greece. *International Journal of Reliable and Quality E-Healthcare*, *7*(1), 16–30. DOI: 10.4018/IJRQEH.2018010102

Katehakis, D. G., & Kouroubali, A. (2022). Digital Transformation Challenges for the Development of Quality Electronic Medical Records in Greece. In Moumtzoglou, A. (Ed.), *Quality of Healthcare in the Aftermath of the COVID-19 Pandemic* (pp. 112–134). IGI Global. https://doi.org/10.4018/978-1-7998-9198-7.ch007

Kaur, P. D., & Sharma, P. (2017). Success Dimensions of ICTs in Healthcare. In Singh, B. (Ed.), *Computational Tools and Techniques for Biomedical Signal Processing* (pp. 149–173). Hershey, PA: IGI Global. DOI: 10.4018/978-1-5225-0660-7.ch007

Kaushik, P. (2018). Comorbidity of Medical and Psychiatric Disorders in Geriatric Population: Treatment and Care. In Prasad, B., & Akbar, S. (Eds.), *Handbook of Research on Geriatric Health, Treatment, and Care* (pp. 448–474). Hershey, PA: IGI Global. DOI: 10.4018/978-1-5225-3480-8.ch025

Khachane, M. Y. (2017). Organ-Based Medical Image Classification Using Support Vector Machine. *International Journal of Synthetic Emotions*, *8*(1), 18–30. DOI: 10.4018/IJSE.2017010102

Kharbanda, V., Madaan, R., & Bhatia, K. K. (2021). Incautious Usage of Social Media: Impact on Emotional Intelligence and Health Concerns. In Yadav, D., Bansal, A., Bhatia, M., Hooda, M., & Morato, J. (Eds.), *Diagnostic Applications of Health Intelligence and Surveillance Systems* (pp. 172–186). IGI Global. https://doi.org/10.4018/978-1-7998-6527-8.ch008

Kirci, P. (2018). Intelligent Techniques for Analysis of Big Data About Healthcare and Medical Records. In Shah, N., & Mittal, M. (Eds.), *Handbook of Research on Promoting Business Process Improvement Through Inventory Control Techniques* (pp. 559–582). Hershey, PA: IGI Global. DOI: 10.4018/978-1-5225-3232-3.ch029

Kldiashvili, E. (2018). Cloud Approach for the Medical Information System: MIS on Cloud. In Khosrow-Pour, M. (Ed.), *Incorporating Nature-Inspired Paradigms in Computational Applications* (pp. 238–261). Hershey, PA: IGI Global. DOI: 10.4018/978-1-5225-5020-4.ch008

Ko, H., Mesicek, L., Choi, J., Choi, J., & Hwang, S. (2018). A Study on Secure Contents Strategies for Applications With DRM on Cloud Computing. *International Journal of Cloud Applications and Computing*, *8*(1), 143–153. DOI: 10.4018/IJCAC.2018010107

Komendziński, T., Mikołajewska, E., & Mikołajewski, D. (2018). Cross-Cultural Decision-Making in Healthcare: Theory and Practical Application in Real Clinical Conditions. In Rosiek-Kryszewska, A., & Leksowski, K. (Eds.), *Healthcare Administration for Patient Safety and Engagement* (pp. 276–298). Hershey, PA: IGI Global. DOI: 10.4018/978-1-5225-3946-9.ch015

Konecny, L. T. (2018). Medical School Wellness Initiatives. In Smith, C. (Ed.), *Exploring the Pressures of Medical Education From a Mental Health and Wellness Perspective* (pp. 209–228). Hershey, PA: IGI Global. DOI: 10.4018/978-1-5225-2811-1.ch009

Kromrei, H., Solomonson, W. L., & Juzych, M. S. (2017). Teaching Residents How to Teach. In Stefaniak, J. (Ed.), *Advancing Medical Education Through Strategic Instructional Design* (pp. 164–185). Hershey, PA: IGI Global. DOI: 10.4018/978-1-5225-2098-6.ch008

Kulkarni, S., Savyanavar, A., Kulkarni, P., Stranieri, A., & Ghorpade, V. (2018). Framework for Integration of Medical Image and Text-Based Report Retrieval to Support Radiological Diagnosis. In Kolekar, M., & Kumar, V. (Eds.), *Biomedical Signal and Image Processing in Patient Care* (pp. 86–122). Hershey, PA: IGI Global. DOI: 10.4018/978-1-5225-2829-6.ch006

Kumar, A., & Sarkar, B. K. (2018). Performance Analysis of Nature-Inspired Algorithms-Based Bayesian Prediction Models for Medical Data Sets. In Singh, U., Tiwari, A., & Singh, R. (Eds.), *Soft-Computing-Based Nonlinear Control Systems Design* (pp. 134–155). Hershey, PA: IGI Global. DOI: 10.4018/978-1-5225-3531-7.ch007

Labbadi, W., & Akaichi, J. (2017). Efficient Algorithm for Answering Fuzzy Medical Requests in Pervasive Healthcare Information Systems. *International Journal of Healthcare Information Systems and Informatics*, *12*(2), 46–64. DOI: 10.4018/IJHISI.2017040103

Lagumdzija, A., & Swing, V. K. (2017). Health, Digitalization, and Individual Empowerment. In Topor, F. (Ed.), *Handbook of Research on Individualism and Identity in the Globalized Digital Age* (pp. 380–402). Hershey, PA: IGI Global. DOI: 10.4018/978-1-5225-0522-8.ch017

Lamey, T. W., & Davidson-Shivers, G. V. (2017). Instructional Strategies and Sequencing. In Stefaniak, J. (Ed.), *Advancing Medical Education Through Strategic Instructional Design* (pp. 30–52). Hershey, PA: IGI Global. DOI: 10.4018/978-1-5225-2098-6.ch002

Lee, D. C., & Gefen, D. (2020). Promises and Challenges of Medical Patient Healthcare Portals in Underserved Communities: The Case of Einstein Medical Center Philadelphia (EMCP). In McHaney, R., Reychev, I., Azuri, J., McHaney, M., & Moshonov, R. (Eds.), *Impacts of Information Technology on Patient Care and Empowerment* (pp. 219–251). IGI Global. https://doi.org/10.4018/978-1-7998-0047-7.ch012

Leon, G. (2017). The Role of Forensic Medicine in Medical Errors. In Riga, M. (Ed.), *Impact of Medical Errors and Malpractice on Health Economics, Quality, and Patient Safety* (pp. 144–170). Hershey, PA: IGI Global. DOI: 10.4018/978-1-5225-2337-6.ch006

Leung, L. Y. (2020). Representation of Gender Equality From the Perspective of the Medical Trainee and its Ripple Effect: Highlighting Gender Inequality in Medical Student Experiences. In Bellini, M., & Papalois, V. (Eds.), *Gender Equity in the Medical Profession* (pp. 29–50). IGI Global. https://doi.org/10.4018/978-1-5225-9599-1.ch003

Lopes, M. J., Fonseca, C., & Barbosa, P. (2020). The Individual Care Plan as Electronic Health Record: A Tool for Management, Integration of Care, and Better Health Results. In Mendes, D., Fonseca, C., Lopes, M., García-Alonso, J., & Murillo, J. (Eds.), *Exploring the Role of ICTs in Healthy Aging* (pp. 1–12). IGI Global. https://doi.org/10.4018/978-1-7998-1937-0.ch001

Love, L., & McDowelle, D. (2018). Developing a Comprehensive Wellness Program for Medical Students. In Smith, C. (Ed.), *Exploring the Pressures of Medical Education From a Mental Health and Wellness Perspective* (pp. 190–208). Hershey, PA: IGI Global. DOI: 10.4018/978-1-5225-2811-1.ch008

Lovell, K. L. (2017). Development and Evaluation of Neuroscience Computer-Based Modules for Medical Students: Instructional Design Principles and Effectiveness. In Stefaniak, J. (Ed.), *Advancing Medical Education Through Strategic Instructional Design* (pp. 262–276). Hershey, PA: IGI Global. DOI: 10.4018/978-1-5225-2098-6.ch013

Lubin, R., & Hamlin, M. D. (2018). Medical Student Burnout: A Social Cognitive Learning Perspective on Medical Student Mental Health and Wellness. In Smith, C. (Ed.), *Exploring the Pressures of Medical Education From a Mental Health and Wellness Perspective* (pp. 92–121). Hershey, PA: IGI Global. DOI: 10.4018/978-1-5225-2811-1.ch004

Luk, C. Y. (2018). Moving Towards Universal Health Coverage: Challenges for the Present and Future in China. In Fong, B., Ng, A., & Yuen, P. (Eds.), *Sustainable Health and Long-Term Care Solutions for an Aging Population* (pp. 19–45). Hershey, PA: IGI Global. DOI: 10.4018/978-1-5225-2633-9.ch002

Mackintosh, S. E., & Katsaros, E. (2020). Building Interprofessional Competencies Into Medical Education and Assessment. In Waldman, S., & Bowlin, S. (Eds.), *Building a Patient-Centered Interprofessional Education Program* (pp. 84–112). IGI Global. https://doi.org/10.4018/978-1-7998-3066-5.ch005

Magalhães, J. L., Quoniam, L., Hartz, Z., Silveira, H., & Rito, P. D. (2022). Knowledge Management in Big Data Times for Global Health: Challenges for Quality in One Health. In Lima de Magalhães, J., Hartz, Z., Jamil, G., Silveira, H., & Jamil, L. (Eds.), *Handbook of Research on Essential Information Approaches to Aiding Global Health in the One Health Context* (pp. 149–163). IGI Global. https://doi.org/10.4018/978-1-7998-8011-0.ch008

Mahat, M., & Pettigrew, A. (2017). The Regulatory Environment of Non-Profit Higher Education and Research Institutions and Its Implications for Managerial Strategy: The Case of Medical Education and Research. In West, L., & Worthington, A. (Eds.), *Handbook of Research on Emerging Business Models and Managerial Strategies in the Nonprofit Sector* (pp. 336–351). Hershey, PA: IGI Global. DOI: 10.4018/978-1-5225-2537-0.ch017

Maitra, I. K., & Bandhyopadhyaay, S. K. (2017). Adaptive Edge Detection Method towards Features Extraction from Diverse Medical Imaging Technologies. In Bhattacharyya, S., De, S., Pan, I., & Dutta, P. (Eds.), *Intelligent Multidimensional Data Clustering and Analysis* (pp. 159–192). Hershey, PA: IGI Global. DOI: 10.4018/978-1-5225-1776-4.ch007

Mane, V. M., Patki, S., Dhumma, A. V., & Apte, K. J. (2022). Telehealth System for Effective Treatment in COVID-19 Pandemics. In Thakare, A., Wagh, S., Bhende, M., Anter, A., & Gao, X. (Eds.), *Handbook of Research on Applied Intelligence for Health and Clinical Informatics* (pp. 328–339). IGI Global. https://doi.org/10.4018/978-1-7998-7709-7.ch019

Mangu, V. P. (2017). Mobile Health Care: A Technology View. In Bhatt, C., & Peddoju, S. (Eds.), *Cloud Computing Systems and Applications in Healthcare* (pp. 1–18). Hershey, PA: IGI Global. DOI: 10.4018/978-1-5225-1002-4.ch001

Manirabona, A., Fourati, L. C., & Boudjit, S. (2017). Investigation on Healthcare Monitoring Systems: Innovative Services and Applications. *International Journal of E-Health and Medical Communications*, *8*(1), 1–18. DOI: 10.4018/IJEHMC.2017010101

Martins, C. L., Martinho, D., Marreiros, G., Conceição, L., Faria, L., & Simões de Almeida, R. (2022). Artificial Intelligence in Digital Mental Health. In Marques, A., & Queirós, R. (Eds.), *Digital Therapies in Psychosocial Rehabilitation and Mental Health* (pp. 201–225). IGI Global. https://doi.org/10.4018/978-1-7998-8634-1.ch010

Marwan, M., Kartit, A., & Ouahmane, H. (2018). A Framework to Secure Medical Image Storage in Cloud Computing Environment. *Journal of Electronic Commerce in Organizations*, *16*(1), 1–16. DOI: 10.4018/JECO.2018010101

Mason, A., Bhati, S., Jiang, R., & Spencer, E. A. (2020). Medical Tourism Patient Mortality: Considerations From a 10-Year Review of Global News Media Representations. In Merviö, M. (Ed.), *Global Issues and Innovative Solutions in Healthcare, Culture, and the Environment* (pp. 206–225). IGI Global. https://doi.org/10.4018/978-1-7998-3576-9.ch011

Masoud, M. P., Nejad, M. K., Darebaghi, H., Chavoshi, M., & Farahani, M. (2018). The Decision Support System and Conventional Method of Telephone Triage by Nurses in Emergency Medical Services: A Comparative Investigation. *International Journal of E-Business Research*, *14*(1), 77–88. DOI: 10.4018/IJEBR.2018010105

Mathew, N. E., Walter, A., & Eapen, V. (2020). Mental Health Challenges in Children With Intellectual Disabilities. In Gopalan, R. (Ed.), *Developmental Challenges and Societal Issues for Individuals With Intellectual Disabilities* (pp. 13–39). IGI Global. https://doi.org/10.4018/978-1-7998-1223-4.ch002

Mazzola, A. (2020). The Social Mandate to Deal With Mental Health: A Comparison Between Interventions in a Mental Health Center, a School, and a Psychoanalytic Office. In Padmanaban, S., & Subudhi, C. (Eds.), *Psycho-Social Perspectives on Mental Health and Well-Being* (pp. 234–254). IGI Global. https://doi.org/10.4018/978-1-7998-1185-5.ch012

McDonald, W. G., Martin, M., & Salzberg, L. D. (2018). From Medical Student to Medical Resident: Graduate Medical Education and Mental Health in the United States. In Smith, C. (Ed.), *Exploring the Pressures of Medical Education From a Mental Health and Wellness Perspective* (pp. 145–169). Hershey, PA: IGI Global. DOI: 10.4018/978-1-5225-2811-1.ch006

McGrowder, D. A., Miller, F. G., Nwokocha, C., Wilson-Clarke, C. F., Anderson, M., Anderson-Jackson, L., Williams, L., & Alexander-Lindo, R. (2021). Medical Herbs and the Treatment of Diabetes Mellitus: Mechanisms of Action. In Hussain, A., & Behl, S. (Eds.), *Treating Endocrine and Metabolic Disorders With Herbal Medicines* (pp. 48–73). IGI Global. https://doi.org/10.4018/978-1-7998-4808-0.ch003

Medhekar, A. (2017). The Role of Social Media for Knowledge Dissemination in Medical Tourism: A Case of India. In Chugh, R. (Ed.), *Harnessing Social Media as a Knowledge Management Tool* (pp. 25–54). Hershey, PA: IGI Global. DOI: 10.4018/978-1-5225-0495-5.ch002

Medhekar, A. (2020). Digital Health Innovation Enhancing Patient Experience in Medical Travel. In Sandhu, K. (Ed.), *Opportunities and Challenges in Digital Healthcare Innovation* (pp. 13–35). IGI Global. https://doi.org/10.4018/978-1-7998-3274-4.ch002

Medhekar, A., & Haq, F. (2018). Urbanization and New Jobs Creation in Healthcare Services in India: Challenges and Opportunities. In Benna, U., & Benna, I. (Eds.), *Urbanization and Its Impact on Socio-Economic Growth in Developing Regions* (pp. 198–218). Hershey, PA: IGI Global. DOI: 10.4018/978-1-5225-2659-9.ch010

Mehta, P. (2017). Framework of Indian Healthcare System and its Challenges: An Insight. In Bryan, V., & Bird, J. (Eds.), *Healthcare Community Synergism between Patients, Practitioners, and Researchers* (pp. 247–271). Hershey, PA: IGI Global. DOI: 10.4018/978-1-5225-0640-9.ch011

Mendes, E., Sousa, B. B., & Gonçalves, M. (2021). The Role of Technologies in Relationship Management and Internal Marketing: An Approach in the Health Sector. In J. Santos, & I. Pereira (Ed.), *Management and Marketing for Improved Competitiveness and Performance in the Healthcare Sector* (pp. 213-237). IGI Global. https://doi.org/10.4018/978-1-7998-7263-4.ch010

Meyer, T. M., & Simen, J. H. (2020). Geriatric Interprofessional Education: A Practical Guide for Health Professions Educators. In Waldman, S., & Bowlin, S. (Eds.), *Building a Patient-Centered Interprofessional Education Program* (pp. 120–136). IGI Global. https://doi.org/10.4018/978-1-7998-3066-5.ch007

Mi, M. (2017). Informal Learning in Medical Education. In Stefaniak, J. (Ed.), *Advancing Medical Education Through Strategic Instructional Design* (pp. 225–244). Hershey, PA: IGI Global. DOI: 10.4018/978-1-5225-2098-6.ch011

Mishra, K., & Thomas, R. (2022). Low Cost, User-Controlled Peroneal Stimulator for Foot Drop in Patients With Stroke: An Experiment in Indian Rehabilitation Set-Up. In Stasolla, F. (Ed.), *Assistive Technologies for Assessment and Recovery of Neurological Impairments* (pp. 279–303). IGI Global. https://doi.org/10.4018/978-1-7998-7430-0.ch014

Mishra, S., & Panda, M. (2019). Artificial Intelligence in Medical Science. In Bouchemal, N. (Ed.), *Intelligent Systems for Healthcare Management and Delivery* (pp. 306–330). IGI Global. https://doi.org/10.4018/978-1-5225-7071-4.ch014

Mosadeghrad, A. M., & Woldemichael, A. (2017). Application of Quality Management in Promoting Patient Safety and Preventing Medical Errors. In Riga, M. (Ed.), *Impact of Medical Errors and Malpractice on Health Economics, Quality, and Patient Safety* (pp. 91–112). Hershey, PA: IGI Global. DOI: 10.4018/978-1-5225-2337-6.ch004

Moumtzoglou, A. (2017). Digital Medicine: The Quality Standpoint. In Moumtzoglou, A. (Ed.), *Design, Development, and Integration of Reliable Electronic Healthcare Platforms* (pp. 179–195). Hershey, PA: IGI Global. DOI: 10.4018/978-1-5225-1724-5.ch011

Moumtzoglou, A., & Pouliakis, A. (2018). Population Health Management and the Science of Individuality. *International Journal of Reliable and Quality E-Healthcare*, *7*(2), 1–26. DOI: 10.4018/IJRQEH.2018040101

Mukhtar, W. F., & Abuelyaman, E. S. (2017). Opportunities and Challenges of Big Data in Healthcare. In Wickramasinghe, N. (Ed.), *Handbook of Research on Healthcare Administration and Management* (pp. 47–58). Hershey, PA: IGI Global. DOI: 10.4018/978-1-5225-0920-2.ch004

Munugala, S., Brar, G. K., Syed, A., Mohammad, A., & Halgamuge, M. N. (2018). The Much Needed Security and Data Reforms of Cloud Computing in Medical Data Storage. In Lytras, M., & Papadopoulou, P. (Eds.), *Applying Big Data Analytics in Bioinformatics and Medicine* (pp. 99–113). Hershey, PA: IGI Global. DOI: 10.4018/978-1-5225-2607-0.ch005

Naha, N., & Manickavachagam, G. (2021). Textile Industry and Health Hazards: Impact of Climate Change Issues and Fertility Potential. In K. Wani, & N. Naha (Ed.), *Climate Change and Its Impact on Fertility* (pp. 42-69). IGI Global. https://doi.org/10.4018/978-1-7998-4480-8.ch003

Nair, L. D. (2019). Childhood Neurodegenerative Disorders. In Uddin, M., & Amran, M. (Eds.), *Handbook of Research on Critical Examinations of Neurodegenerative Disorders* (pp. 385–412). IGI Global. https://doi.org/10.4018/978-1-5225-5282-6.ch018

Nayak, S. R., & Mishra, J. (2019). Analysis of Medical Images Using Fractal Geometry. In Dey, N., Ashour, A., Kalia, H., Goswami, R., & Das, H. (Eds.), *Histopathological Image Analysis in Medical Decision Making* (pp. 181–201). IGI Global. https://doi.org/10.4018/978-1-5225-6316-7.ch008

Netto, J. T., Hartz, Z., & de Magalhães, J. L. (2022). One Health and Information Management Using Big Data in Health: A Brazilian Case Study for COVID-19. In Lima de Magalhães, J., Hartz, Z., Jamil, G., Silveira, H., & Jamil, L. (Eds.), *Handbook of Research on Essential Information Approaches to Aiding Global Health in the One Health Context* (pp. 36–51). IGI Global. https://doi.org/10.4018/978-1-7998-8011-0.ch003

Ngara, R. (2017). Multiple Voices, Multiple Paths: Towards Dialogue between Western and Indigenous Medical Knowledge Systems. In Ngulube, P. (Ed.), *Handbook of Research on Theoretical Perspectives on Indigenous Knowledge Systems in Developing Countries* (pp. 332–358). Hershey, PA: IGI Global. DOI: 10.4018/978-1-5225-0833-5.ch015

Nikumbh, D. D., Sayyad, S., Joshi, R. R., Dubey, K. S., Mehta, D. V., & Matta, D. K. (2022). Applied Intelligence for Medical Diagnosing. In Thakare, A., Wagh, S., Bhende, M., Anter, A., & Gao, X. (Eds.), *Handbook of Research on Applied Intelligence for Health and Clinical Informatics* (pp. 44–79). IGI Global. https://doi.org/10.4018/978-1-7998-7709-7.ch004

O'Connor, Y., & Heavin, C. (2018). Defining and Characterising the Landscape of eHealth. In M. Khosrow-Pour, D.B.A. (Ed.), *Encyclopedia of Information Science and Technology, Fourth Edition* (pp. 5864-5875). Hershey, PA: IGI Global. DOI: 10.4018/978-1-5225-2255-3.ch510

Ochonogor, W. C., & Okite-Amughoro, F. A. (2018). Building an Effective Digital Library in a University Teaching Hospital (UTH) in Nigeria. In Tella, A., & Kwanya, T. (Eds.), *Handbook of Research on Managing Intellectual Property in Digital Libraries* (pp. 184–204). Hershey, PA: IGI Global. DOI: 10.4018/978-1-5225-3093-0.ch010

Olivares, S. L., Cruz, A. G., Cabrera, M. V., Regalado, A. I., & García, J. E. (2017). An Assessment Study of Quality Model for Medical Schools in Mexico. In Mukerji, S., & Tripathi, P. (Eds.), *Handbook of Research on Administration, Policy, and Leadership in Higher Education* (pp. 404–439). Hershey, PA: IGI Global. DOI: 10.4018/978-1-5225-0672-0.ch016

Omoruyi, E. A., & Omidele, F. (2018). Resident Physician and Medical Academic Faculty Burnout: A Review of Current Literature. In Smith, C. (Ed.), *Exploring the Pressures of Medical Education From a Mental Health and Wellness Perspective* (pp. 171–189). Hershey, PA: IGI Global. DOI: 10.4018/978-1-5225-2811-1.ch007

Pandey, A., Singh, B., Saini, B. S., & Sood, N. (2019). Medical Data Security Tools and Techniques in E-Health Applications. In Singh, B., Saini, B., Singh, D., & Pandey, A. (Eds.), *Medical Data Security for Bioengineers* (pp. 124–131). IGI Global. https://doi.org/10.4018/978-1-5225-7952-6.ch006

Papadopoulou, P., Lytras, M., & Marouli, C. (2018). Bioinformatics as Applied to Medicine: Challenges Faced Moving from Big Data to Smart Data to Wise Data. In Lytras, M., & Papadopoulou, P. (Eds.), *Applying Big Data Analytics in Bioinformatics and Medicine* (pp. 1–25). Hershey, PA: IGI Global. DOI: 10.4018/978-1-5225-2607-0.ch001

Paraskou, A., & George, B. P. (2018). An Overview of Reproductive Tourism. In *Legal and Economic Considerations Surrounding Reproductive Tourism: Emerging Research and Opportunities* (pp. 1–17). Hershey, PA: IGI Global. DOI: 10.4018/978-1-5225-2694-0.ch001

Pereira, S., Silva, L., Machado, J., & Cabral, A. (2020). The Clinical Informatization in Portugal: An Approach to the National Health Service Certification. *International Journal of Reliable and Quality E-Healthcare*, *9*(2), 34–47. https://doi.org/10.4018/IJRQEH.2020040103

Phuritsabam, B., & Devi, A. B. (2017). Information Seeking Behavior of Medical Scientists at Jawaharlal Nehru Institute of Medical Science: A Study. In Ram, S. (Ed.), *Library and Information Services for Bioinformatics Education and Research* (pp. 177–187). Hershey, PA: IGI Global. DOI: 10.4018/978-1-5225-1871-6.ch010

Pieczka, B. (2018). Management of Risk and Adverse Events in Medical Entities. In Rosiek-Kryszewska, A., & Leksowski, K. (Eds.), *Healthcare Administration for Patient Safety and Engagement* (pp. 31–46). Hershey, PA: IGI Global. DOI: 10.4018/978-1-5225-3946-9.ch003

Poduval, J. (2017). Medical Errors: Impact on Health Care Quality. In Riga, M. (Ed.), *Impact of Medical Errors and Malpractice on Health Economics, Quality, and Patient Safety* (pp. 33–60). Hershey, PA: IGI Global. DOI: 10.4018/978-1-5225-2337-6.ch002

Politis, D., Stagiopoulos, P., Aidona, S., Kyriafinis, G., & Constantinidis, I. (2018). Autonomous Learning and Skill Accreditation: A Paradigm for Medical Studies. In Kumar, A. (Ed.), *Optimizing Student Engagement in Online Learning Environments* (pp. 266–296). Hershey, PA: IGI Global. DOI: 10.4018/978-1-5225-3634-5.ch012

Pomares-Quimbaya, A., González, R. A., Sierra, A., Daza, J. C., Muñoz, O., García, A., & Bohórquez, W. R. (2017). ICT for Enabling the Quality Evaluation of Health Care Services: A Case Study in a General Hospital. In Moumtzoglou, A. (Ed.), *Design, Development, and Integration of Reliable Electronic Healthcare Platforms* (pp. 196–210). Hershey, PA: IGI Global. DOI: 10.4018/978-1-5225-1724-5.ch012

Ponnuswamy, P., Paul, A. S., & Jose, A. B. (2021). Pre-, Peri-, and Post-Natal Risk Factors in ADHD. In Gopalan, R. (Ed.), *New Developments in Diagnosing, Assessing, and Treating ADHD* (pp. 43–54). IGI Global. https://doi.org/10.4018/978-1-7998-5495-1.ch003

Pouliakis, A., Margari, N., Karakitsou, E., Archondakis, S., & Karakitsos, P. (2018). Emerging Technologies Serving Cytopathology: Big Data, the Cloud, and Mobile Computing. In El Naqa, I. (Ed.), *Emerging Developments and Practices in Oncology* (pp. 114–152). Hershey, PA: IGI Global. DOI: 10.4018/978-1-5225-3085-5.ch005

Praveenkumar, P., Santhiyadevi, R., & Amirtharajan, R. (2019). Medical Data Are Safe: An Encrypted Quantum Approach. In Singh, B., Saini, B., Singh, D., & Pandey, A. (Eds.), *Medical Data Security for Bioengineers* (pp. 142–165). IGI Global. https://doi.org/10.4018/978-1-5225-7952-6.ch008

Punhani, R., Saini, S., Varun, N., & Rustagi, R. (2021). mHealth: A Resolution in Improving Global Health. In D. Yadav, A. Bansal, M. Bhatia, M. Hooda, & J. Morato (Ed.), *Diagnostic Applications of Health Intelligence and Surveillance Systems* (pp. 86-105). IGI Global. https://doi.org/10.4018/978-1-7998-6527-8.ch004

Quintela, A., & Veiga, A. (2022). An Integrated Approach (Social and Health) in the Elderly With Diabetes: An Increase in Health Literacy. In Vaz de Almeida, C., & Ramos, S. (Eds.), *Handbook of Research on Assertiveness, Clarity, and Positivity in Health Literacy* (pp. 134–142). IGI Global. https://doi.org/10.4018/978-1-7998-8824-6.ch008

Rai, A., Kothari, R., & Singh, D. P. (2017). Assessment of Available Technologies for Hospital Waste Management: A Need for Society. In Singh, R., Singh, A., & Srivastava, V. (Eds.), *Environmental Issues Surrounding Human Overpopulation* (pp. 172–188). Hershey, PA: IGI Global. DOI: 10.4018/978-1-5225-1683-5.ch010

Rajagopalan, S., Janakiraman, S., & Rengarajan, A. (2019). Medical Image Encryption: Microcontroller and FPGA Perspective. In Singh, B., Saini, B., Singh, D., & Pandey, A. (Eds.), *Medical Data Security for Bioengineers* (pp. 278–304). IGI Global. https://doi.org/10.4018/978-1-5225-7952-6.ch014

Ramamoorthy, S., & Sivasubramaniam, R. (2018). Image Processing Including Medical Liver Imaging: Medical Image Processing from Big Data Perspective, Ultrasound Liver Images, Challenges. In Lytras, M., & Papadopoulou, P. (Eds.), *Applying Big Data Analytics in Bioinformatics and Medicine* (pp. 380–392). Hershey, PA: IGI Global. DOI: 10.4018/978-1-5225-2607-0.ch016

Rathor, G. P., & Gupta, S. K. (2017). Improving Multimodality Image Fusion through Integrate AFL and Wavelet Transform. In Tiwari, V., Tiwari, B., Thakur, R., & Gupta, S. (Eds.), *Pattern and Data Analysis in Healthcare Settings* (pp. 143–157). Hershey, PA: IGI Global. DOI: 10.4018/978-1-5225-0536-5.ch008

Rexhepi, H., & Persson, A. (2017). Challenges to Implementing IT Support for Evidence Based Practice Among Nurses and Assistant Nurses: A Qualitative Study. *Journal of Electronic Commerce in Organizations*, *15*(2), 61–76. DOI: 10.4018/JECO.2017040105

Ribeiro, A. D., Ribeiro, L. P., Silva, C. A., & Magalhães-Ribeiro, L. P. (2021). Patient Safety: The Patient's Perspective From Public Sector Health Institutions in the Algarve Region, Portugal. In Eklund, P. (Ed.), *Integrated Care and Fall Prevention in Active and Healthy Aging* (pp. 200–222). IGI Global. https://doi.org/10.4018/978-1-7998-4411-2.ch011

Rodrigues, H., & Brochado, A. (2021). Going for Silver-Senior Consumers' Reviews of Medical Tourism. In Borges, A., & Rodrigues, P. (Eds.), *New Techniques for Brand Management in the Healthcare Sector* (pp. 64–83). IGI Global. https://doi.org/10.4018/978-1-7998-3034-4.ch005

Rodrigues, J. M., Oliveira, F., Ribeiro, C. P., & Santos, R. C. (2022). Mobile Mental Health for Depression Assistance: Research Directions, Obstacles, Advantages, and Disadvantages of Implementing mHealth. In Marques, A., & Queirós, R. (Eds.), *Digital Therapies in Psychosocial Rehabilitation and Mental Health* (pp. 21–40). IGI Global. https://doi.org/10.4018/978-1-7998-8634-1.ch002

Ros, M., Weaver, L., & Neuwirth, L. S. (2020). Virtual Reality Stereoscopic 180-Degree Video-Based Immersive Environments: Applications for Training Surgeons and Other Medical Professionals. In Stefaniak, J. (Ed.), *Cases on Instructional Design and Performance Outcomes in Medical Education* (pp. 92–119). IGI Global. https://doi.org/10.4018/978-1-7998-5092-2.ch005

Rosiek, A. (2018). The Assessment of Actions of the Environment and the Impact of Preventive Medicine for Public Health in Poland. In Rosiek-Kryszewska, A., & Leksowski, K. (Eds.), *Healthcare Administration for Patient Safety and Engagement* (pp. 106–119). Hershey, PA: IGI Global. DOI: 10.4018/978-1-5225-3946-9.ch006

Rosiek, A., & Rosiek-Kryszewska, A. (2018). Managed Healthcare: Doctor Life Satisfaction and Its Impact on the Process of Communicating With the Patient. In Rosiek-Kryszewska, A., & Leksowski, K. (Eds.), *Healthcare Administration for Patient Safety and Engagement* (pp. 244–261). Hershey, PA: IGI Global. DOI: 10.4018/978-1-5225-3946-9.ch013

Rosiek-Kryszewska, A., & Rosiek, A. (2018). The Involvement of the Patient and his Perspective Evaluation of the Quality of Healthcare. In Rosiek-Kryszewska, A., & Leksowski, K. (Eds.), *Healthcare Administration for Patient Safety and Engagement* (pp. 121–144). Hershey, PA: IGI Global. DOI: 10.4018/978-1-5225-3946-9.ch007

Rosiek-Kryszewska, A., & Rosiek, A. (2018). The Impact of Management and Leadership Roles in Building Competitive Healthcare Units. In Rosiek-Kryszewska, A., & Leksowski, K. (Eds.), *Healthcare Administration for Patient Safety and Engagement* (pp. 13–30). Hershey, PA: IGI Global. DOI: 10.4018/978-1-5225-3946-9.ch002

Rouzbehani, K. (2017). Health Policy Implementation: Moving Beyond Its Barriers in United States. In Wickramasinghe, N. (Ed.), *Handbook of Research on Healthcare Administration and Management* (pp. 541–552). Hershey, PA: IGI Global. DOI: 10.4018/978-1-5225-0920-2.ch032

Sajjad, N., Hassan, S., Qadir, J., Ali, R., & Shah, D. (2020). Analyses of the Recycling Potential of Medical Plastic Wastes. In Wani, K., Ariana, L., & Zuber, S. (Eds.), *Handbook of Research on Environmental and Human Health Impacts of Plastic Pollution* (pp. 178–199). IGI Global. https://doi.org/10.4018/978-1-5225-9452-9.ch010

Sam, S. (2017). Mobile Phones and Expanding Human Capabilities in Plural Health Systems. In Moahi, K., Bwalya, K., & Sebina, P. (Eds.), *Health Information Systems and the Advancement of Medical Practice in Developing Countries* (pp. 93–114). Hershey, PA: IGI Global. DOI: 10.4018/978-1-5225-2262-1.ch006

Santos-Trigo, M., Suaste, E., & Figuerola, P. (2018). Technology Design and Routes for Tool Appropriation in Medical Practices. In M. Khosrow-Pour, D.B.A. (Ed.), *Encyclopedia of Information Science and Technology, Fourth Edition* (pp. 3794-3804). Hershey, PA: IGI Global. DOI: 10.4018/978-1-5225-2255-3.ch329

Sarivougioukas, J., Vagelatos, A., Parsopoulos, K. E., & Lagaris, I. E. (2018). Home UbiHealth. In M. Khosrow-Pour, D.B.A. (Ed.), *Encyclopedia of Information Science and Technology, Fourth Edition* (pp. 7765-7774). Hershey, PA: IGI Global. DOI: 10.4018/978-1-5225-2255-3.ch675

Sarkar, B. K. (2017). Big Data and Healthcare Data: A Survey. *International Journal of Knowledge-Based Organizations, 7*(4), 50–77. DOI: 10.4018/IJKBO.2017100104

Sarkar, K., & Li, B. (2021). Deep Learning for Medical Image Segmentation. In Saxena, S., & Paul, S. (Eds.), *Deep Learning Applications in Medical Imaging* (pp. 40–77). IGI Global. https://doi.org/10.4018/978-1-7998-5071-7.ch002

Savani, M. M. (2021). Commitment Devices for Health: Theory and Evidence on Weight Loss. In Mihaila, V. (Ed.), *Behavioral-Based Interventions for Improving Public Policies* (pp. 35–54). IGI Global. https://doi.org/10.4018/978-1-7998-2731-3.ch003

Saxena, K., & Banodha, U. (2017). An Essence of the SOA on Healthcare. In Bhadoria, R., Chaudhari, N., Tomar, G., & Singh, S. (Eds.), *Exploring Enterprise Service Bus in the Service-Oriented Architecture Paradigm* (pp. 283–304). Hershey, PA: IGI Global. DOI: 10.4018/978-1-5225-2157-0.ch018

Saxena, N. (2020). Considerations for Stakeholders of Medical Tourism: A Comprehensive Examination. In Paul, S., & Kulshreshtha, S. (Eds.), *Global Developments in Healthcare and Medical Tourism* (pp. 23–37). IGI Global. https://doi.org/10.4018/978-1-5225-9787-2.ch002

Segura-Azuara, N. D., Guzman-Segura, J. G., Guzmán-Segura, N. M., & Guzmán-Segura, J. P. (2022). Disease Awareness Campaigns: Education for Citizenship in Medical Schools. In Lopez, M. (Ed.), *Advancing Health Education With Telemedicine* (pp. 113–122). IGI Global. https://doi.org/10.4018/978-1-7998-8783-6.ch006

Sekaran, P. A. (2022). Smart Medical Kit in Chronic Kidney Disease Management. In Jeya Mala, D. (Ed.), *Integrating AI in IoT Analytics on the Cloud for Healthcare Applications* (pp. 24–40). IGI Global. https://doi.org/10.4018/978-1-7998-9132-1.ch002

Sen, K., & Ghosh, K. (2018). Incorporating Global Medical Knowledge to Solve Healthcare Problems: A Framework for a Crowdsourcing System. *International Journal of Healthcare Information Systems and Informatics*, *13*(1), 1–14. DOI: 10.4018/IJHISI.2018010101

Senanayake, B., Tyagi, N., Zhou, X., & Edirippulige, S. (2020). Workforce Readiness and Digital Health Integration. In Sandhu, K. (Ed.), *Opportunities and Challenges in Digital Healthcare Innovation* (pp. 170–185). IGI Global. https://doi.org/10.4018/978-1-7998-3274-4.ch010

Shakdher, A., & Pandey, K. (2017). REDAlert+: Medical/Fire Emergency and Warning System using Android Devices. *International Journal of E-Health and Medical Communications*, *8*(1), 37–51. DOI: 10.4018/IJEHMC.2017010103

Shekarian, E., Abdul-Rashid, S. H., & Olugu, E. U. (2017). An Integrated Fuzzy VIKOR Method for Performance Management in Healthcare. In Tavana, M., Szabat, K., & Puranam, K. (Eds.), *Organizational Productivity and Performance Measurements Using Predictive Modeling and Analytics* (pp. 40–61). Hershey, PA: IGI Global. DOI: 10.4018/978-1-5225-0654-6.ch003

Shijina, V., & John, S. J. (2017). Multiple Relations and its Application in Medical Diagnosis. *International Journal of Fuzzy System Applications*, *6*(4), 47–62. DOI: 10.4018/IJFSA.2017100104

Shipley, N., & Chakraborty, J. (2018). Big Data and mHealth: Increasing the Usability of Healthcare Through the Customization of Pinterest – Literary Perspective. In Machado, J., Abelha, A., Santos, M., & Portela, F. (Eds.), *Next-Generation Mobile and Pervasive Healthcare Solutions* (pp. 46–66). Hershey, PA: IGI Global. DOI: 10.4018/978-1-5225-2851-7.ch004

Shridevi, S., & Saleena, B. (2019). Semantic Technologies for Medical Knowledge Representation. In Puratchikody, A., Prabu, S., & Umamaheswari, A. (Eds.), *Computer Applications in Drug Discovery and Development* (Vol. 5, pp. 260–275). IGI Global. https://doi.org/10.4018/978-1-5225-7326-5.ch012

Simões de Almeida, R. (2022). Mobile Mental Health: Opportunities and Challenges. In Marques, A., & Queirós, R. (Eds.), *Digital Therapies in Psychosocial Rehabilitation and Mental Health* (pp. 1–20). IGI Global. https://doi.org/10.4018/978-1-7998-8634-1.ch001

Simões de Almeida, R., & da Silva, T. P. (2022). AI Chatbots in Mental Health: Are We There Yet? In Marques, A., & Queirós, R. (Eds.), *Digital Therapies in Psychosocial Rehabilitation and Mental Health* (pp. 226–243). IGI Global. https://doi.org/10.4018/978-1-7998-8634-1.ch011

Singh, A., & Dutta, M. K. (2017). A Reversible Data Hiding Scheme for Efficient Management of Tele-Ophthalmological Data. *International Journal of E-Health and Medical Communications*, *8*(3), 38–54. DOI: 10.4018/IJEHMC.2017070103

Skourti, P. K., & Pavlakis, A. (2017). The Second Victim Phenomenon: The Way Out. In Riga, M. (Ed.), *Impact of Medical Errors and Malpractice on Health Economics, Quality, and Patient Safety* (pp. 197–222). Hershey, PA: IGI Global. DOI: 10.4018/978-1-5225-2337-6.ch008

Smith, C. R. (2018). Medical Students' Quest Towards the Long White Coat: Impact on Mental Health and Well-Being. In Smith, C. (Ed.), *Exploring the Pressures of Medical Education From a Mental Health and Wellness Perspective* (pp. 1–42). Hershey, PA: IGI Global. DOI: 10.4018/978-1-5225-2811-1.ch001

Smith, S. I., & Dandignac, M. (2018). Perfectionism: Addressing Lofty Expectations in Medical School. In Smith, C. (Ed.), *Exploring the Pressures of Medical Education From a Mental Health and Wellness Perspective* (pp. 68–91). Hershey, PA: IGI Global. DOI: 10.4018/978-1-5225-2811-1.ch003

Soczywko, J., & Rutkowska, D. (2018). The Patient/Provider Relationship in Emergency Medicine: Organization, Communication, and Understanding. In Rosiek-Kryszewska, A., & Leksowski, K. (Eds.), *Healthcare Administration for Patient Safety and Engagement* (pp. 74–105). Hershey, PA: IGI Global. DOI: 10.4018/978-1-5225-3946-9.ch005

Soni, P. (2018). Implications of HIPAA and Subsequent Regulations on Information Technology. In Gupta, M., Sharman, R., Walp, J., & Mulgund, P. (Eds.), *Information Technology Risk Management and Compliance in Modern Organizations* (pp. 71–98). Hershey, PA: IGI Global. DOI: 10.4018/978-1-5225-2604-9.ch004

Souza, T. de V. I. E. (2020). Certifications for Medical Interpreters: A Comparative Analysis. In I. Souza, & E. Fragkou (Eds.), *Handbook of Research on Medical Interpreting* (pp. 26-53). IGI Global. https://doi.org/10.4018/978-1-5225-9308-9.ch002

Srivastava, A., & Aggarwal, A. K. (2018). Medical Image Fusion in Spatial and Transform Domain: A Comparative Analysis. In Anwar, M., Khosla, A., & Kapoor, R. (Eds.), *Handbook of Research on Advanced Concepts in Real-Time Image and Video Processing* (pp. 281–300). Hershey, PA: IGI Global. DOI: 10.4018/978-1-5225-2848-7.ch011

Srivastava, S. K., & Roy, S. N. (2018). Recommendation System: A Potential Tool for Achieving Pervasive Health Care. In Machado, J., Abelha, A., Santos, M., & Portela, F. (Eds.), *Next-Generation Mobile and Pervasive Healthcare Solutions* (pp. 111–127). Hershey, PA: IGI Global. DOI: 10.4018/978-1-5225-2851-7.ch008

Stanimirovic, D. (2017). Digitalization of Death Certification Model: Transformation Issues and Implementation Concerns. In Saeed, S., Bamarouf, Y., Ramayah, T., & Iqbal, S. (Eds.), *Design Solutions for User-Centric Information Systems* (pp. 22–43). Hershey, PA: IGI Global. DOI: 10.4018/978-1-5225-1944-7.ch002

Subbaraman, K., Singh, M., & Johar, I. P. (2021). Medical Tourism: History, Global Scenario, and Indian Perspectives. In Singh, M., & Kumaran, S. (Eds.), *Growth of the Medical Tourism Industry and Its Impact on Society: Emerging Research and Opportunities* (pp. 1–18). IGI Global. https://doi.org/10.4018/978-1-7998-3427-4.ch001

Sukkird, V., & Shirahada, K. (2018). E-Health Service Model for Asian Developing Countries: A Case of Emergency Medical Service for Elderly People in Thailand. In Khosrow-Pour, M. (Ed.), *Optimizing Current Practices in E-Services and Mobile Applications* (pp. 214–232). Hershey, PA: IGI Global. DOI: 10.4018/978-1-5225-5026-6.ch011

Talbot, T. B. (2017). Making Lifelike Medical Games in the Age of Virtual Reality: An Update on "Playing Games with Biology" from 2013. In Dubbels, B. (Ed.), *Transforming Gaming and Computer Simulation Technologies across Industries* (pp. 103–119). Hershey, PA: IGI Global. DOI: 10.4018/978-1-5225-1817-4.ch006

Tarver, E. (2022). Virtual Simulation: A Flipped Classroom Teaching Tool for Healthcare Education. In Coelho, L., Queirós, R., & Reis, S. (Eds.), *Emerging Advancements for Virtual and Augmented Reality in Healthcare* (pp. 65–81). IGI Global. https://doi.org/10.4018/978-1-7998-8371-5.ch005

Tripathi, S., & Musiolik, T. H. (2022). Fairness and Ethics in Artificial Intelligence-Based Medical Imaging. In Musiolik, T., & Dingli, A. (Eds.), *Ethical Implications of Reshaping Healthcare With Emerging Technologies* (pp. 71–85). IGI Global. https://doi.org/10.4018/978-1-7998-7888-9.ch004

Turcu, C. E., & Turcu, C. O. (2017). Social Internet of Things in Healthcare: From Things to Social Things in Internet of Things. In Reis, C., & Maximiano, M. (Eds.), *Internet of Things and Advanced Application in Healthcare* (pp. 266–295). Hershey, PA: IGI Global. DOI: 10.4018/978-1-5225-1820-4.ch010

Tutgun Ünal, A., Ekinci, Y., & Tarhan, N. (2022). Health Literacy and Cyberchondria. In Aker, H., & Aiken, M. (Eds.), *Handbook of Research on Cyberchondria, Health Literacy, and the Role of Media in Society's Perception of Medical Information* (pp. 276–297). IGI Global. https://doi.org/10.4018/978-1-7998-8630-3.ch015

Unwin, D. W., Sanzogni, L., & Sandhu, K. (2017). Developing and Measuring the Business Case for Health Information Technology. In Moahi, K., Bwalya, K., & Sebina, P. (Eds.), *Health Information Systems and the Advancement of Medical Practice in Developing Countries* (pp. 262–290). Hershey, PA: IGI Global. DOI: 10.4018/978-1-5225-2262-1.ch015

Ustun, A. B., Yilmaz, R., & Yilmaz, F. G. (2020). Virtual Reality in Medical Education. In Umair, S. (Ed.), *Mobile Devices and Smart Gadgets in Medical Sciences* (pp. 56–73). IGI Global. https://doi.org/10.4018/978-1-7998-2521-0.ch004

Vamsi, D., & Reddy, P. (2020). Electronic Health Record Security in Cloud: Medical Data Protection Using Homomorphic Encryption Schemes. In Chakraborty, C. (Ed.), *Smart Medical Data Sensing and IoT Systems Design in Healthcare* (pp. 22–47). IGI Global. https://doi.org/10.4018/978-1-7998-0261-7.ch002

Vartholomaios, P., Ramdani, N., Christophorou, C., Georgiadis, D., Guilcher, T., Blouin, M., Rebiai, M., Panayides, A. S., Pattichis, C. S., Sarafidis, M., Costarides, V., Vellidou, E., & Koutsouris, D. (2019). ENDORSE Concept: An Integrated Indoor Mobile Robotic System for Medical Diagnostic Support. *International Journal of Reliable and Quality E-Healthcare*, *8*(3), 47–59. https://doi.org/10.4018/IJRQEH.2019070104

Vasant, P. (2018). A General Medical Diagnosis System Formed by Artificial Neural Networks and Swarm Intelligence Techniques. In Kose, U., Guraksin, G., & Deperlioglu, O. (Eds.), *Nature-Inspired Intelligent Techniques for Solving Biomedical Engineering Problems* (pp. 130–145). Hershey, PA: IGI Global. DOI: 10.4018/978-1-5225-4769-3.ch006

Vaz de Almeida, C. (2022). ACP Model-Assertiveness, Clarity, and Positivity: A Communication and Health Literacy Model for Health Professionals. In Vaz de Almeida, C., & Ramos, S. (Eds.), *Handbook of Research on Assertiveness, Clarity, and Positivity in Health Literacy* (pp. 1–22). IGI Global. https://doi.org/10.4018/978-1-7998-8824-6.ch001

Verma, K. (2022). Modeling Digital Healthcare Services Using NLP and IoT in Smart Cities. In Thomas, J., Geropanta, V., Karagianni, A., Panchenko, V., & Vasant, P. (Eds.), *Smart Cities and Machine Learning in Urban Health* (pp. 138–155). IGI Global. https://doi.org/10.4018/978-1-7998-7176-7.ch007

Viswanathan, J., Saranya, N., & Inbamani, A. (2021). Deep Learning Applications in Medical Imaging: Introduction to Deep Learning-Based Intelligent Systems for Medical Applications. In Saxena, S., & Paul, S. (Eds.), *Deep Learning Applications in Medical Imaging* (pp. 156–177). IGI Global. https://doi.org/10.4018/978-1-7998-5071-7.ch007

Wang, X., Su, K., & Su, L. (2019). Research on Improved Apriori Algorithm Based on Data Mining in Electronic Cases. *International Journal of Healthcare Information Systems and Informatics*, *14*(3), 16–28. https://doi.org/10.4018/IJHISI.2019070102

Wickramasinghe, N. (2020). Minority Health and Wellness: A Digital Health Opportunity. In Wickramasinghe, N. (Ed.), *Handbook of Research on Optimizing Healthcare Management Techniques* (pp. 116–126). IGI Global. https://doi.org/10.4018/978-1-7998-1371-2.ch008

Wickramasinghe, N., Geholt, V., Sloane, E., Smart, P. J., & Schaffer, J. L. (2021). Using Health 4.0 to Enable Post-Operative Wellness Monitoring: The Case of Colorectal Surgery. In Wickramasinghe, N. (Ed.), *Optimizing Health Monitoring Systems With Wireless Technology* (pp. 233–247). IGI Global. https://doi.org/10.4018/978-1-5225-6067-8.ch016

Wilcox, S., Huzo, O., Minhas, A., Walters, N., Adada, J. E., Pennington, M., Roseme, L., Mohammed, D., Dusic, A., & Zeine, R. (2022). The Impact of Medical or Health-Related Internet Searches on Patient Compliance: The Dr. Net Study. In Aker, H., & Aiken, M. (Eds.), *Handbook of Research on Cyberchondria, Health Literacy, and the Role of Media in Society's Perception of Medical Information* (pp. 72–97). IGI Global. https://doi.org/10.4018/978-1-7998-8630-3.ch005

Witzke, K., & Specht, O. (2017). M-Health Telemedicine and Telepresence in Oral and Maxillofacial Surgery: An Innovative Prehospital Healthcare Concept in Structurally Weak Areas. *International Journal of Reliable and Quality E-Healthcare*, *6*(4), 37–48. DOI: 10.4018/IJRQEH.2017100105

Wong, A. K., & Lo, M. F. (2018). Using Pervasive Computing for Sustainable Healthcare in an Aging Population. In Fong, B., Ng, A., & Yuen, P. (Eds.), *Sustainable Health and Long-Term Care Solutions for an Aging Population* (pp. 187–202). Hershey, PA: IGI Global. DOI: 10.4018/978-1-5225-2633-9.ch010

Wu, W., Martin, B. C., & Ni, C. (2017). A Systematic Review of Competency-Based Education Effort in the Health Professions: Seeking Order Out of Chaos. In Rasmussen, K., Northrup, P., & Colson, R. (Eds.), *Handbook of Research on Competency-Based Education in University Settings* (pp. 352–378). Hershey, PA: IGI Global. DOI: 10.4018/978-1-5225-0932-5.ch018

Yadav, S., Ekbal, A., Saha, S., Pathak, P. S., & Bhattacharyya, P. (2017). Patient Data De-Identification: A Conditional Random-Field-Based Supervised Approach. In S. Saha, A. Mandal, A. Narasimhamurthy, S. V, & S. Sangam (Eds.), *Handbook of Research on Applied Cybernetics and Systems Science* (pp. 234-253). Hershey, PA: IGI Global. DOI: 10.4018/978-1-5225-2498-4.ch011

Yu, B., Wijesekera, D., & Costa, P. C. (2017). Informed Consent in Healthcare: A Study Case of Genetic Services. In Moumtzoglou, A. (Ed.), *Design, Development, and Integration of Reliable Electronic Healthcare Platforms* (pp. 211–242). Hershey, PA: IGI Global. DOI: 10.4018/978-1-5225-1724-5.ch013

Yu, B., Wijesekera, D., & Costa, P. C. (2017). Informed Consent in Electronic Medical Record Systems. In I. Management Association (Ed.), *Healthcare Ethics and Training: Concepts, Methodologies, Tools, and Applications* (pp. 1029-1049). Hershey, PA: IGI Global. DOI: 10.4018/978-1-5225-2237-9.ch049

Yu, M., Li, J., & Wang, W. (2017). Creative Life Experience among Students in Medical Education. In Zhou, C. (Ed.), *Handbook of Research on Creative Problem-Solving Skill Development in Higher Education* (pp. 158–184). Hershey, PA: IGI Global. DOI: 10.4018/978-1-5225-0643-0.ch008

Zanetti, C. A., George, A., Stiegmann, R. A., & Phelan, D. (2020). Digital Health. In Gotian, R., Kang, Y., & Safdieh, J. (Eds.), *Handbook of Research on the Efficacy of Training Programs and Systems in Medical Education* (pp. 404–426). IGI Global. https://doi.org/10.4018/978-1-7998-1468-9.ch021

Zangão, M. O. (2020). Self-Perceived Health Status. In Fonseca, C., Lopes, M., Mendes, D., Mendes, F., & García-Alonso, J. (Eds.), *Handbook of Research on Health Systems and Organizations for an Aging Society* (pp. 1–11). IGI Global. DOI: 10.4018/978-1-5225-9818-3.ch001

Zarour, K. (2017). Towards a Telehomecare in Algeria: Case of Diabetes Measurement and Remote Monitoring. *International Journal of E-Health and Medical Communications*, *8*(4), 61–80. DOI: 10.4018/IJEHMC.2017100104

Zavyalova, Y. V., Korzun, D. G., Meigal, A. Y., & Borodin, A. V. (2017). Towards the Development of Smart Spaces-Based Socio-Cyber-Medicine Systems. *International Journal of Embedded and Real-Time Communication Systems*, *8*(1), 45–63. DOI: 10.4018/IJERTCS.2017010104

Zeinali, A. A. (2018). Word Formation Study in Developing Naming Guidelines in the Translation of English Medical Terms Into Persian. In M. Khosrow-Pour, D.B.A. (Ed.), *Encyclopedia of Information Science and Technology, Fourth Edition* (pp. 5136-5147). Hershey, PA: IGI Global. DOI: 10.4018/978-1-5225-2255-3.ch446

Zineldin, M., & Vasicheva, V. (2018). Reducing Medical Errors and Increasing Patient Safety: TRM and 5 Q's Approaches for Better Quality of Life. In *Technological Tools for Value-Based Sustainable Relationships in Health: Emerging Research and Opportunities* (pp. 87–115). Hershey, PA: IGI Global. DOI: 10.4018/978-1-5225-4091-5.ch005

About the Contributors

Christen D. Johnson, MD, EdD, MPH, FAAFP, DipABLM, is a champion for health equity and double board-certified family and lifestyle medicine physician. She specializes in inclusive practice and serving the underserved in Columbus, Ohio. Dr. Johnson lives the phrase "To whom much is given, much is required" through her career path in medicine and medical education, research pursuits, leadership activities, and dedication to serving the most vulnerable communities. She has been honored as a Gates Millennium Scholar, National Health Service Corps Scholar, in the 2017 NBC Black 28 under 28, and in the 2020 National Minority Quality Forum 40 Under 40 Leaders in Health among others. Her research interests include health disparities, medical education, and inclusive medical practice which have facilitated numerous local, regional, and national research presentations, and publications in peer-reviewed journals, textbooks, and grants.

***

Katherine Art, MD(c), is graduating from Wright State University Boonshoft School of Medicine in Dayton, Ohio and will be completing a residency in Internal Medicine. She is from Columbus, Ohio.

Jasmine Bauknight, MD, ABOSD, FAAOS, is a board-certified Orthopaedic Surgeon from New Jersey who specializes in hand and upper extremity surgery. She attended Brown for undergraduate and medical school, completed her Orthopedic Surgery residency at Howard, and completed a hand and upper extremity fellowship at Allegheny General Hospital. She is also a mosaic artist and enjoys spending time with her dog.

Brittany Iris Hugue, MD(c), is a native of Richmond, VA and is passionate about serving diverse communities. She has a background in Chemistry and pharmaceutical development. In addition to her involvement in STEM, she served as a community doula advocate to expectant mothers with challenging circumstances. She is a 2025 graduate of Wright State University Boonshoft School of Medicine where she served as the leader of the AAFP Primary Care Leadership Collaborative and a United Health/NMF Diverse Medical Scholar for her research in improving breastfeeding rates for Black women in Dayton, OH. Dr. Hugue also interned at American Academy of Family Physicians in their inaugural Health Equity Internship Program where she co-created an action guide which addressed anti-racism in medicine. She is a Certified Lactation Counselor (CLC) and a family medicine physician. In her free time, she enjoys spending time with her husband and son, reading, HIIT workouts and eating different cultural cuisines.

Antoinette Leonard-Jean Charles is a dedicated scholar, researcher, and advocate with a passion for advancing health equity and education. She holds an EdD in Educational and Professional Practice with a focus on anti-racism and multiculturalism, alongside two master's degrees in Microbiology (Immunology concentration) and Exercise Science and Nutrition. With over six years of experience, Antoinette has contributed to health education through roles in clinical research, patient advocacy, and academic teaching. Her publications explore critical topics such as health disparities, microaggressions in medical education, and the intersection of technology and medicine. Her publications explore critical topics such as health disparities, microaggressions in medical education, and the intersection of technology and medicine.

Nassim Louail is a resident physician at Mercy St. Rita's Medical Center, specializing in Internal Medicine. He is Algerian and was raised in Columbus, Ohio, He has been a long-standing Buckeye fan, along with attending The Ohio State University for undergraduate studies. He strives to be able to give back to his community and be able to provide students and physicians the necessary resources to successfully manage their symptoms. He has been involved in genetic research with The Ehlers-Danlos Society and has developed a special interest in connective tissue diseases. He hopes to continue to be an advocate and resource for individuals with EDS throughout his career.

Tamika M. Reese, EdD, MBA, is the CEO and Principal Consultant for ShiftView Consulting, LLC. Her company works collaboratively with educational, non-profits and financial organizations to develop transformative solutions to promote diversity, equity, inclusion, cultural humility, and anti-racism policies and practices into their institutions. Dr. Reese brings over 25 years of DEI work into this practice, primarily from her experience in the education sector, where she held positions such as Director, Assistant Superintendent of Curriculum and Instruction,

Assistant Superintendent of Personnel and Operations, and Acting Superintendent. Additionally, she has experience in finance, having been employed as an international banker for Citibank, a financial troubleshooter, and a member of the Chief Financial Officer's inner team for the Port Authority of New York and New Jersey. Throughout her career, Dr. Reese has been called upon to navigate challenging and complex situations for organizations and has achieved success due to her collaborative nature and "out-of-the-box" thinking. This competency has been a hallmark of her work with organizations. Her understanding of the intricacies and nuances of implementing change across a system has enabled her to leverage this knowledge to meet transformative organizational goals sustainably. Dr. Reese received her doctorate in Professional and Educational Practice at Antioch University, specializing in Multicultural and Antiracist Education, and was featured in an article entitled, "EdD Student Shifting Views in Education and Centering Black Girls." Although she officially retired as a New Jersey school administrator, she is highly sought after for starting up, restructuring, or reorganizing human resource departments in school districts due to her extensive knowledge of human resource policies, practices, and procedures, particularly those related to diversity and equity inclusion.

R. Vallipriya has been working in the Department of Physical Sciences at the Institute of Education (Affiliated to Tamilnadu Teacher Education University) as an Assistant Professor. With a wealth of experience, Mrs. R.Vallipriya has accumulated 12 years of extensive teaching. Her scholarly contributions include publishing 7 papers, with 1 peer review in various UGC-CARE, SCOPUS, and peer-reviewed journals.

Srinivasan Vasan has been working in the Department of Humanities and Social Sciences at Graphic Era (Deemed to be University) as an Assistant Professor. With a wealth of experience, Mr. Srinivasan has accumulated 14 years of extensive teaching and field-level expertise. Prior to his current role, he served in the Ministry of Health and Family Welfare, Government of India, and gained valuable experience. He also contributed as a Guest Faculty at the university level and served for nearly 2 years in the State Government Public Works Department as a Mobilization Training Specialist. In the past year, Mr. S. Srinivasan has enriched his experience by actively participating in a tuberculosis project funded by GFATM and USAID, providing a platform for further exploration of his research and practical field-based knowledge. His scholarly contributions include publishing 25 papers, with 18 more under peer review in various UGC-CARE, SCOPUS, and peer-reviewed journals.

Index

I

L

M

N

O

P

R

S

T

www.ingramcontent.com/pod-product-compliance
Lightning Source LLC
LaVergne TN
LVHW080641011026
849160LV00014B/1286
* 9 7 9 8 3 3 7 3 0 0 9 1 7 *